Cancer Drug Discovery and Development

Cancer Drug Discovery and Development

Edited by Lindsay Evans

hayle
medical

New York

Hayle Medical,
750 Third Avenue, 9th Floor,
New York, NY 10017, USA

Visit us on the World Wide Web at:
www.haylemedical.com

ISBN: 978-1-63241-877-7

Cataloging-in-Publication Data

Cancer drug discovery and development / edited by Lindsay Evans.
  p. cm.
Includes bibliographical references and index.
ISBN 978-1-63241-877-7
1. Antineoplastic agents--Development. 2. Antineoplastic agents--Design. 3. Cancer--Chemotherapy.
4. Drugs--Design. 5. Cancer--Treatment. I. Evans, Lindsay.
RS431.A64 C36 2020
616.994 061--dc23

Table of Contents

Preface

Cancer can be treated by a number of different therapeutic modalities that comprise of surgery, radiation therapy, chemotherapy, hormonal therapy, targeted therapy and synthetic lethality. A particular cancer therapy is chosen as per the grade, location and stage of the tumor as well as the performance status of the patient. The complete removal of the cancer without causing any damage to the rest of the body is the ideal goal of cancer treatment. Besides curative intent, treatment also seeks to suppress the cancer to a subclinical state and thereby maintain a quality of life for patients with the chronic condition, and provide palliative care in advanced-stage metastatic cancers. To achieve clinical progress against cancer, it is vital to continue research in cancer drug discovery and development. Since each tumor exhibits a unique set of genomic alterations irrespective of the tissue of origin, it can lead to a wide variability in terms of drug responses. As a result, new human cancer models need to be developed and investigated to achieve better drug discovery and development. This book covers in detail some existing theories and innovative concepts revolving around cancer drug discovery and development. It explores all the important aspects of cancer drugs in the present day scenario. This book is meant for students who are looking for an elaborate reference text on cancer medicine.

This book is the end result of constructive efforts and intensive research done by experts in this field. The aim of this book is to enlighten the readers with recent information in this area of research. The information provided in this profound book would serve as a valuable reference to students and researchers in this field.

At the end, I would like to thank all the authors for devoting their precious time and providing their valuable contribution to this book. I would also like to express my gratitude to my fellow colleagues who encouraged me throughout the process.

Editor

Towards Metabolic Engineering of Podophyllotoxin Production

Christel L. C. Seegers, Rita Setroikromo and

Wim J. Quax

Abstract

The pharmaceutically important anticancer drugs etoposide and teniposide are derived from podophyllotoxin, a natural product isolated from roots of *Podophyllum hexandrum* growing in the wild. The overexploitation of this endangered plant has led to the search for alternative sources. Metabolic engineering aimed at constructing the pathway in another host cell is very appealing, but for that approach, an in-depth knowledge of the pathway toward podophyllotoxin is necessary. In this chapter, we give an overview of the lignan pathway leading to podophyllotoxin. Subsequently, we will discuss the engineering possibilities to produce podophyllotoxin in a heterologous host. This will require detailed knowledge on the cellular localization of the enzymes of the lignan biosynthesis pathway. Due to the high number of enzymes involved and the scarce information on compartmentalization, the heterologous production of podophyllotoxin still remains a tremendous challenge. At the moment, research is focusing on the last step(s) in the conversion of deoxypodophyllotoxin to (epi)podophyllotoxin and 4′-demethyldesoxypodophyllotoxin by plant cytochromes.

Keywords: etoposide, podophyllotoxin, *Podophyllum hexandrum*, *Anthriscus sylvestris*, metabolic engineering

1. Introduction

The high demand of podophyllotoxin derivatives for chemotherapy gives a severe pressure on the natural sources, such as *Podophyllum hexandrum* and *Podophyllum peltatum* [1]. The highest concentration of podophyllotoxin is found in *P. hexandrum* roots, with reported yields up to 6.6% dry weight (d.w.) [2]. The excessive harvesting has resulted in inclusion of *P. hexandrum* in the Convention on International Trade in Endangered Species (CITES) [3]. Chemical synthesis of podophyllotoxin is difficult due to the presence of four contiguous chiral centers and the presence of a base sensitive *trans*-lactone moiety [4]. The shortest synthesis described contains five steps from the commercially available 6-bromopiperonal into (epi) podophyllotoxin [5]. As an alternative, cell suspension cultures have been explored, but these produce only low amounts (max. 0.65% d.w.) of podophyllotoxin [6, 7]. As neither chemical synthesis nor *in vitro* production of podophyllotoxin is economically competitive with the extraction of podophyllotoxin from *P. hexandrum* roots, other alternatives are being searched for. Metabolic engineering aimed at constructing the pathway in a heterologous host is very appealing, but for that approach, an in-depth knowledge of the biosynthetic pathway toward podophyllotoxin is necessary.

2. Lignans and their biological activities

In 1936, Haworth was the first to describe a group of phenylpropanoid dimers (C_6C_3) linked by the central carbon (C8) as lignans [8]. The Haworth's definition of lignan has been adopted by the IUPAC nomenclature recommendations in 2000 [9]. According to this nomenclature, lignans can be divided into eight subgroups based on the oxygen incorporation into the skeleton and the cyclization pattern [10]. In the lignan pathway toward podophyllotoxin, six subgroups of lignans can be defined in the order of occurrence: furofuran, furan, dibenzylbutane, dibenzylbutyrolactol, dibenzylbutyrolactone, and aryltetralin (**Figure 1**). The other two subgroups are arylnaphthalene and dibenzocyclooctadiene. Dibenzylbutanes are only linked by the 8,8' bond. An additional oxygen bridge is found in furofurans, furans, dibenzylbutyrolactols, and dibenzylbutyrolactones. A second carbon-carbon link is found in aryltetralins, arylnaphthalenes, and dibenzocyclooctadienes [10, 11]. The majority of the lignans has oxygen at the C9 (C9') carbon; however, some lignans in the dibenzylbutanes, furans, and dibenzocyclooctadiene subgroups are missing this oxygen [10]. Humans metabolize the furofurans pinoresinol and sesamin, the furan lariciresinol, the dibenzylbutane secoisolariciresinol, and the dibenzylbutyrolactone matairesinol. These lignans are phytoestrogens, which can be converted into enterolactone or enterodiol by intestinal bacteria [12, 13]. Enterolactone and enterodiol have antioxidant, estrogenic, and anti-estrogenic activities in humans; furthermore, they may protect against certain chronic diseases [14]. Several lignans have been described to have antiviral properties; however, therapeutic applications are limited due to the toxicity [15]. The extract, podophyllin, of *Podophyllum* roots and rhizome was included in the U.S. Pharmacopeia in 1820. In 1942, it was removed, because of its severe gastrointestinal toxicity [16]. However, Kaplan described in 1944, the successful treatment of venereal warts (*Condylomata acuminata*) in 200 members of the military by topically applied podophyllin [17]. The aryltetralin podophyllotoxin is the active ingredient in podophyllin, which has been commercialized as a treatment for warts caused by the human papilloma virus [18]. Semisynthetic derivatives of podophyllotoxin were designed as chemotherapy compounds for oral administration or for intravenous treatment [19, 20].

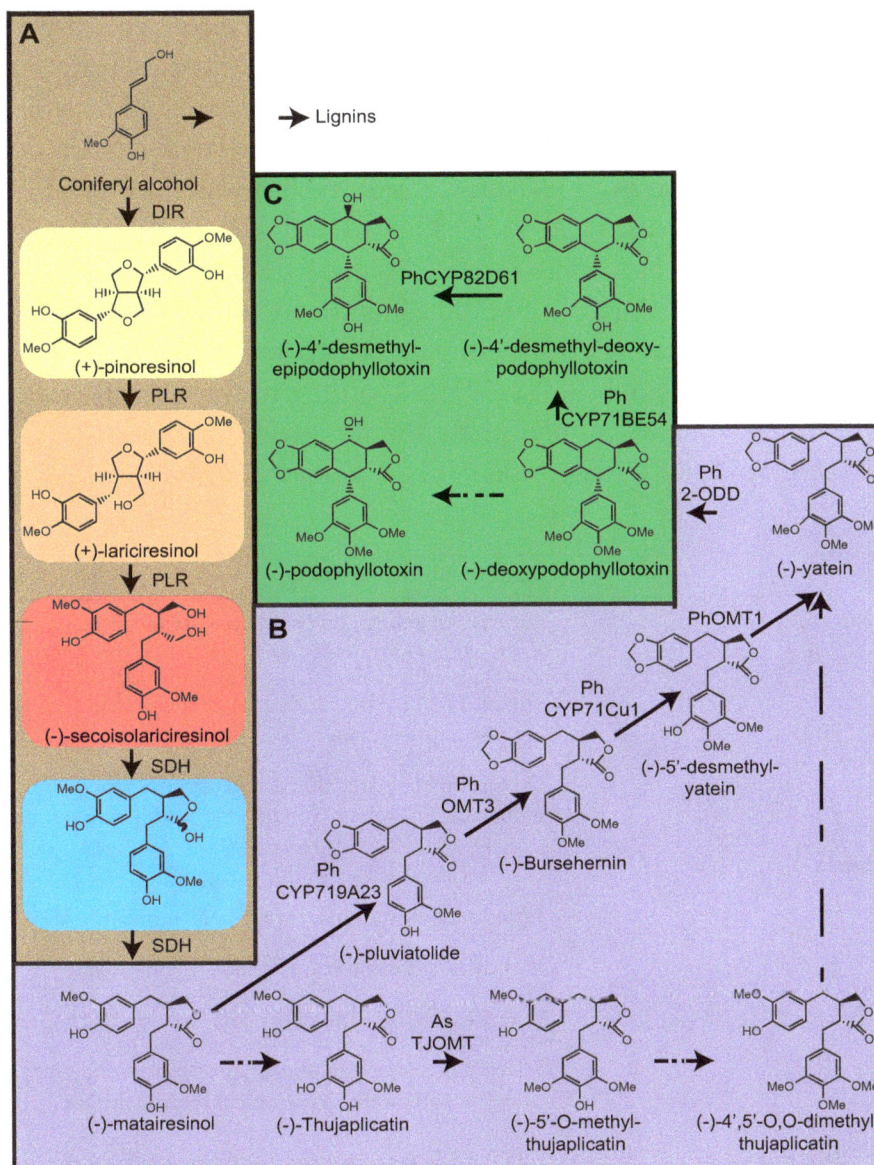

Figure 1. Lignan pathway in *Podophyllum hexandrum* and *Anthriscus sylvestris*. (A) Coniferyl alcohol toward matairesinol (brown box), (B) matairesinol toward deoxypodophyllotoxin (purple box), and (C) deoxypodophyllotoxin toward podophyllotoxin and demethyldesoxypodophyllotoxin (green box). Lignan subgroups are shown by various colors: yellow = furofuran, orange = furan, red = dibenzylbutane, blue = dibenzylbutyrolactol, purple = dibenzylbutyrolactone, and green = aryltetralin.

3. Importance of podophyllotoxin and derivatives for chemotherapy

Podophyllotoxin is a tubulin-interacting agent that inhibits mitotic spindle formation [21]. As podophyllotoxin is severely toxic if applied systemic, a number of less toxic derivatives have been generated and these are now widely used in cancer chemotherapy. Interestingly, the derivatives currently used in the clinic, etoposide, and teniposide, have a different mode of action than podophyllotoxin. They inhibit topoisomerase II by stabilizing its binding to DNA, which results in double-stranded breaks in the DNA and arrest of the cell cycle in the G2 phase [21]. Etoposide (VP-16, VePesid®) was synthesized in 1966 by Sandoz and was further developed by Bristol-Meyers from 1978 onwards. In 1983, it was approved by the FDA for the treatment of testicular cancer [22]. As etoposide is poorly soluble in water, the etoposide prodrug etoposide phosphate (Etopophos®) was designed by Bristol-Meyers Squibb, which was approved by the FDA in 1996 [23]. The prodrug is converted to etoposide within 30 min presumably by alkaline phosphatases. Furthermore, the pharmacokinetics and toxicity of etoposide phosphate are equal to etoposide [24, 25]. According to the National Cancer Institute and the Dutch government etoposide, phosphate should be used in combination therapy for various cancers (**Table 1**) [26–28]. Teniposide (VM-26, Vumon®) was synthesized in 1967 by

Cancer	Combination of drugs
Hodgkin lymphoma in children	Vincristine sulfate, etoposide phosphate, prednisone, doxorubicin hydrochloride
	Doxorubicin hydrochloride, bleomycin, vincristine sulfate, etoposide phosphate
	Doxorubicin hydrochloride, bleomycin, vincristine sulfate, etoposide phosphate, prednisone, cyclophosphamide
Non-hodgkin lymphoma	
- All	Rituximab, ifosfamide, carboplatin, etoposide phosphate
	Etoposide phosphate, ifosfamide, methotrexate
	Lomustine, etoposide phosphate, chlorambucil, prednisolone
- B-cell	Rituximab, etoposide phosphate, prednisone, vincristine sulfate, cyclophosphamide, doxorubicin hydrochloride
Malignant germ cell tumors	
- Nonbrain	Cisplatin, etoposide phosphate, bleomycin
- Ovarian/testicular	Bleomycin, etoposide phosphate, cisplatin
- Advanced testicular	Etoposide phosphate, ifosfamide, cisplatin
Acute myeloid leukemia	
- Children	Cytarabine, daunorubicin hydrochloride, etoposide phosphate
- Phase II	Cytarabine and amsacrine, etoposide or mitoxantrone
High-risk retinoblastoma in children	Carboplatin, etoposide phosphate, vincristine sulfate
Small cell lung cancer	Etoposide with cisplatin or carboplatin
	Cisplatin, cyclophosphamide, doxorubicin, vincristine, methotrexate
Relapsed Wilms tumor	Ifosfamide, carboplatin, and etoposide

Table 1. Cancer chemotherapy combination treatments with etoposide.

Sandoz and was further developed by Bristol-Meyers from 1978 onwards [22]. It is used in the treatment of acute myeloid leukemia and myelodysplastic syndromes in children and in acute lymphocytic leukemia [29, 30]. Toxicity problems are still an issue with etoposide; therefore, novel derivatives were designed and evaluated in preclinical and clinical studies [31]. The derivatives NK611, Gl-311, and TOP-53 were discontinued after phase I or II studies [22, 32, 33]. NK611, which is more water soluble than etoposide, shows similar toxic effects in humans as etoposide. However, only few patients showed efficacy in phase I studies [34–36]. No data of the phase I or II studies were found for GL-311 and TOP-53. Four newer derivatives are tafluposide, F14512, Adva-27a, and QS-ZYX-1-61 [31, 32]. Tafluposide (F-11782), a pentafluorinated epipodophylloid, inhibits topoisomerase I and II activity [37, 38]. In phase I study, stable disease was observed in 7 out of 21 patients with advanced solid tumors, such as choroid and skin melanoma [39]. Increasing the selectivity of anticancer agents is of great interest. As the polyamine transport system is upregulated in cancer cells, F14512 was designed to target the transport system by linking the epipodophyllotoxin core to a spermine chain [40]. Phase I study in adult patients with acute meloid leukemia showed clinical activity in relapsed patients, but limited activity in refractory patients [41]. F14512 will be tested in combination with cytarabine in a phase II study [41]. The minimal therapeutic effect of etoposide on dogs with relapsing lymphomas has resulted in a phase I study of F14512, which showed a strong therapeutic efficacy [42]. The derivative adva-27a, a GEM-difluorinated C-glycoside derivate of podophyllotoxin, is effective against multidrug resistant cancer cells [43]. Preparations are being made for a phase I study in pancreatic and breast cancer patients in Canada [44]. The derivative QS-ZYX-1-61 induces apoptosis by inhibition of topoisomerase II in human non–small-cell lung cancer [45]. Further investigations are necessary for this compound.

4. Overview of the lignan biosynthetic pathway

Podophyllotoxin is produced in the lignan pathway, which we will discuss in more detail in this section (**Figure 1**). Lignins and lignans are the major metabolic products of the phenylpropanoid pathway in vascular plants. Lignins are derived from coumaryl, coniferyl, and sinapyl alcohol, whereas lignans are derived from coniferyl alcohol [46].

4.1. Coniferyl alcohol toward matairesinol

The pathway toward podophyllotoxin starts with pinoresinol, lariciresinol, secoisolariciresinol, and matairesinol. Pinoresinol and lariciresinol are found in most vascular plants, such as *Arabidopsis thaliana*. Some species follow the lignan pathway toward podophyllotoxin until the branch point matairesinol, such as the *Forsythia* species. Lignans further downstream toward podophyllotoxin are found in more specialized plants. An interesting question is whether the capability of podophyllotoxin production is restricted to a limited number of plants, or that other closely related plants have cryptic pathways as shown in bacteria [47]. To answer this question, an in-depth discussion of the lignan pathway is necessary as we do below. Coniferyl alcohol is converted into matairesinol in five steps by three enzymes: dirigent protein, pinoresinol-lariciresinol reductase, and secoisolariciresinol dehydrogenase (**Figure 1A**).

4.1.1. Dirigent protein

In 1997, Davin and coworker showed that the dirigent protein (DIR) from *Forsythia suspensa* can couple two coniferyl alcohols stereospecific to (+)-pinoresinol after their oxidation by a nonspecific oxidase or nonenzymatic single-electron oxidant [48]. Davin and coworkers showed that the DIR protein lacks a detectable catalytic active (oxidative) center and that the rate of dimeric lignan formation is similar in the presence or absence of DIR protein; however, the DIR protein is necessary for enantioselectivity [48]. Both (+)- and (−)-pinoresinol-forming proteins were found in plants. The (+)-forming DIR protein is important for the lignan pathway in the direction of podophyllotoxin synthesis. (+)-Forming DIRs are the ScDIR protein from *Schisandra chinensis*, the *psd-Fi1* from *Frullania intermedia*, and PsDRR206 from *Pisum sativum* [49–51]. In *A. thaliana*, 16 DIR homologs were found of which four were characterized as follows: two formed (−)-pinoresinol (AtDIR5 and AtDIR6); the other two showed nonstereoselective coupling of coniferyl alcohols [49, 52]. On the other hand, *Linum usitatissimum* has (+)-forming and (−)-forming DIR proteins [53]. Kim and coworkers solved the crystal structure of the (+)-pinoresinol forming PSDRR206 of *P. sativum* to 1.95A [54]. Homology modeling of the (−)-pinoresinol forming AtDIR6 in the PSDRR206 crystal structure showed six additional residues in the longest loop of the (+)-forming DIR, which are present in all (+)-forming DIRs. Site-directed mutagenesis could be used to confirm whether one or more of these residues are responsible for the enantioselectivity of the DIR [54].

4.1.2. Pinoresinol-lariciresinol reductase

In 1996, Dinkova-Kostova and coworkers found the pinoresinol-lariciresinol reductase (PLR) in *F. intermedia*, which could reduce (+)-pinoresinol to (+)-lariciresinol and sequentially to (−)-secoisolariciresinol [55]. The (−)-secoisolariciresinol-forming PLRs are important for podophyllotoxin synthesis. These PLRs were found in *F. intermedia* (PLR-Fi1), *Linum album* (PLR-La1), *L. usitatissimum* (PLR-Lu2) and *Linum corymbulosum* (PLR-Lc1) [56–59]. A PLR with opposite enantioselectivity was found in *L. usitatissimum* (PLR-Lu1) [57, 58]. PLR can have selectivity or preference toward one of the enantiomers. The *Thuja plicata* PLRs accept both enantiomers of pinoresinol; however, they were selective for the lariciresinol substrate, as PLR-TP1 accepts only (−)-lariciresinol and PLR-TP2 only (+)-lariciresinol [60]. In *Linum perenne*, it was found that PLR_Lp1 can convert (±)-pinoresinol to (±)-lariciresinol and (±)-secoisolariciresinol, with a preference for (+)-pinoresinol and (−)-lariciresinol [61]. The *F. intermedia* (PLR-Fi1) and *L. usitatissimum* (PLR-Lu1) PLRs were found to convert (+)-lariciresinol to (−)-secoisolariciresinol before depletion of (−)-pinoresinol [56, 57]. On the other hand, *L. album* (PLR-La1) and *L. perenne* (PLR-LP1) PLRs first seem to convert all (+)-pinoresinol to (+)-lariciresinol before converting (+)-lariciresinol further to (−)-secoisolariciresinol [57, 61]. For *A. thaliana* proteins with strict substrate, specificity toward pinoresinol was found as weak or no activity toward lariciresinol was observed [62]. Therefore, these proteins are annotated as pinoresinol reductases (AtPrRs). AtPrR1 reduces both enantiomers, and AtPrR2 only reduces (−)-pinoresinol [62]. The crystal structures of PLR-Tp1 of *T. plicata* were resolved to 2.5 A, and a homology model of PLR-Tp2 with opposite enantioselectivity was deduced from the PLR-Tp1 structure [63]. Three residues in the substrate binding site were different, which could explain the enantioselectivity [63].

4.1.3. Secoisolariciresinol dehydrogenase

Secoisolariciresinol dehydrogenase (SDH) from *F. intermedia* and *P. peltatum* convert (–)-secoiso-lariciresinol into (–)-matairesinol, through the intermediary (–)-lactol. Neither of them was able to convert the opposite enantiomer [64]. Crystallization of *P. peltatum* SDH (1.6 A) showed that it is a tetramer. The ternary complex was obtained by the addition of cofactors and (–)-matairesinol. Based on the position of (–)-matairesinol, also (–)-secoisolariciresinol could be modeled into the crystal structure. Using the same constrains, (+)-secoisolariciresinol could not be modeled into the crystal structure, which could explain the enantioselectivity [64, 65].

4.2. Matairesinol toward deoxypodophyllotoxin

Plant feeding experiments performed by various groups have revealed the metabolites intermediate between matairesinol and podophyllotoxin, such as yatein and deoxypodo-phyllotoxin in *P. hexandrum* [66, 67]. This was followed by the identification of the enzymes in *P. hexandrum* (**Figure 1B**). Marques and coworkers found that pluviatolide synthases in *P. hexandrum* (CYP719A23) and *P. peltatum* (CYP719A24) can convert (–)-matairesinol into (–)-pluviatolide by formation of the methylenedioxy bridge [68]. Lau and Sattely used tran-scriptome mining in *P. hex``vandrum* to identify four additional biosynthetic enzymes in the lignan pathway, which convert (–)-pluviatolide into deoxypodophyllotoxin [69]. Pluviatolide 4-O-methyltransferase (PhOMT3) converts (–)-pluviatolide into bursehernin by methylation at C4'OH. Bursehernin 5'-hydroxylase (CYP71CU1) incorporates a molecular oxygen at C5' in bursehernin, which results in (–)-5'-desmethyl-yatein. In the following step, 5'-demethyl-yatein O-transferase (OMT1) converts (–)-demethyl-yatein to (–)-yatein by methylation at C5'OH. In the last step, deoxypodophyllotoxin synthase (2-ODD) converts (–)-yatein to (–)-deoxypodophyllotoxin by ring closure between C2 and C7' [69]. Sakakibara and coworkers suggest a different route toward deoxypodophyllotoxin for *Anthriscus sylvestris* (**Figure 1B**) [70]. Feeding experiments showed incorporation of matairesinol, thujaplicatin, 5-methylthujaplicatin, and 4,5-dimethylthujaplicatin into yatein [70]. This was followed by the discovery of the enzyme thujaplicatin O-methyltransferase (AsTJOMT), which methyl-ates thujaplicatin to form 5-O-methylthujaplicatin [71]. Furthermore, they found incorpora-tion of matairesinol and pluviatolide in bursehernin, but no further incorporation into yatein. No literature has been reported in the presence of 5-demethylyatein in *A. sylvestris*. However, feeding of 5-demethylyatein to *A. sylvestris* results in yatein formation [70]. In the transcrip-tome of *L. album*, genes related to OMT3 and CYP71CU1 were found; however, no gene related to CYP719A24 was found (**Figure 1B**) [72, 73]. The differences in the lignan pathways in *P. hexandrum*, *A. sylvestris*, and *L. album* indicate the possibility that the later part of the lignan pathway might have convergently evolved in the various species, which decreases the probability of the presence of a cryptic pathway in other species.

4.3. Conversion of deoxypodophyllotoxin into demethyldesoxypodophyllotoxin

The *P. hexandrum* enzyme that converts deoxypodophyllotoxin into podophyllotoxin has not been identified yet. Lau and Sattely, attempted to find this enzyme, presumably a cytochrome, by mining the publicly available RNA-sequencing data set from the Medicinal Plants Consortium.

Furthermore, they analyzed transcriptome data from *P. hexandrum* after upregulating the podophyllotoxin biosynthesis genes by wounding the leaves. Both methods were successful in identifying podophyllotoxin biosynthesis genes as described in the previous session; however, the enzyme converting deoxypodophyllotoxin into podophyllotoxin was not found (**Figure 1C**). They found two P450 cytochromes that can convert deoxypodophyllotoxin into 4'-desmethylepipodophyllotoxin [69]. In the first step, CYP71BE54 converts (−)-deoxypodophyllotoxin to (−)-4'-demethyldesoxypodophyllotoxin. In the second step (-)-4'-demethyldesoxypodophylltoxin is converted to (−)-4'-desmethylepipodophyllotoxin by CYP82D61.

5. Engineering approaches

In this part, we will focus on genetic engineering approach`es to produce podophyllotoxin in a heterologous system. In order to produce podophyllotoxin in *Escherichia coli* or *Saccharomyces cerevisiae*, the pathway from the easily available glucose toward coniferyl alcohol has to be implemented into these organisms.

5.1. Production of coniferyl alcohol in *E. coli* and *S. cerevisiae*

Coniferyl alcohol can be produced in *E. coli* by a co-culture system. Coumaryl alcohol is produced upon insertion of four phenylpropanoid pathway genes [74]. The production can be increased by addition of four key shikimate pathway genes to overproduce tyrosine [75]. Addition of the genes for methyltransferase and HpaBC in another strain resulted in the accumulation of 125 mg/L coniferyl alcohol after 24 h. Co-culturing was necessary as HpaBC converts tyrosine to an unwanted side product [74]. The full biosynthetic pathway toward coniferyl alcohol has not been tested for expression in *S. cerevisiae* yet. However, production of ±100 mg/L coumaric acid has been shown [76]. To convert coumaric acid to coniferyl alcohol in *S. cerevisiae*, four or five additional genes have to be expressed; therefore, in order to produce coniferyl alcohol levels similar to *E. coli*, further optimization of coumaric acid production is necessary.

5.2. Cellular localization of enzymes from the lignan pathway

In order to engineer the lignan pathway for podophyllotoxin production in a heterologous cell, knowledge about the localization of lignans and their corresponding enzymes is necessary. Localization to the wrong organelle might abolish or lower production, as was shown for penicillin production [77]. The monolignol coniferyl alcohol is synthesized in the cytosol and transported over the plasma membrane for incorporation into lignin or lignan by an ABC membrane transporter, whereas the glucosylated form (coniferin) for storage could only be transported over the vacuolar membrane possibly by another ABC membrane transporter or proton-coupled antiporter [78, 79]. Analyses of transmembrane helices by the TMHMM predictor [80] indicated that DIR has one transmembrane helix. Furthermore, the DIR protein is a glycoprotein with a secretory signal peptide [50]. This indicates that the DIR protein is membrane attached, which is consistent with the findings in *F. suspense* stems. Only the insoluble fraction was capable of stereoselective conversion of coniferyl alcohol to (+)-pinoresinol, whereas soluble enzyme preparations only form racemic pinoresinol [81, 82]. As the DIR protein was found primarily localized within the plant cell wall [83], it might be difficult to target DIR to its natural compartment in bacteria and yeast. However, there is strong indication that monolignol dimerization also occurs intracellular as shown by protoplast experiments in *A. thaliana* and the racemic pinoresinol formation in crude cell-free enzyme preparation of *F. suspense* stems [81, 84]. The disadvantage is the absence of stereoselectivity in the coupling of the two coniferyl alcohols. However, this should not be a problem, if the influx of coniferyl alcohol is large enough. The following proteins lack a transmembrane helix or signal peptide according to the TMHMM predictor and SignalP [85]: PLR, SDH, OMT3, OMT1, and 2-ODD. PLR and 2-ODD are localized to the cytoplasm, and SDH, OMT3, and OMT1 to the chloroplast according to the plant specific localization tool Plant-mPloc [86]. However, the specific chloroplast localization tools ChloroP and PCLR suggest no chloroplast localization, which was confirmed by the localization tools MultiLoc2-LowRes and LocTree3 [87–90]. Therefore, we think that the proteins PLR, SDH, OMT3, OMT1, and 2-ODD are all localized in the cytoplasm. The four cytochromes CYP719A23, CYP71CU1, CYP71BE54, and CYP82D61 contain a targeting peptide and one or two transmembrane helixes. They are probably located in the endoplasmic reticulum (ER) membrane (according to an analysis by Plant-mPloc and MultiLoc2) as most plant cytochromes are anchored in the ER membrane and face the cytosolic side [91]. Our hypothesis is that deoxypodophyllotoxin is converted to podophyllotoxin by a cytochrome that is ER bound (**Figure 2**). Production of podophyllotoxin in *E. coli* would be feasible assuming that PLR, SDH, OMT3, OMT1, and 2-ODD can be actively expressed in the cytosol. As coniferyl alcohol has been produced before in this organism and cytochrome P450 enzymes with modified N-terminus have also been expressed successfully [92], some of the major steps toward podophyllotoxin might be performed in *E. coli*. The disadvantage of *E. coli* is the lack of NAD(P)H P450 reductase, the redox partner of cytochromes necessary for the supply of electrons from the cofactor NAD(P)H [92]. The establishment of a renewable supply has been proven difficult in *E. coli*.

5.3. Conversion of deoxypodophyllotoxin to (epi)podophyllotoxin by engineering

In 2006, Vasilev and coworkers showed that the human liver cytochrome P450 3A4 (CYP3A4) together with human NADPH P450 reductase can convert deoxypodophyllotoxin stereoselectivity into epipodophyllotoxin [93]. The disadvantage of this system is the usage of frozen cells and therefore the need to supply a regenerative system, such as glucose-6-phosphate dehydrogenase and NADP. Changing the system to a resting cell assay or cell-free assay with the usage of a cheaper cofactor and increasing the electron transfer between cytochrome and reductase would greatly increase the usability of this system. As CYP3A4 is quite unspecific, an approach to find a dedicated cytochrome converting deoxypodophyllotoxin into podophyllotoxin could be provided by the systematic analysis of cytochrome encoding genes found by Kumari and coworkers, who analyzed the transcriptome of *P. hexandrum* cultivated at two temperatures. The expression of DIR protein, PLR and SDH were upregulated by at least a factor two at 15°C compared to 25°C [94], accompanied by an increase of podophyllotoxin accumulation at 15°C. Fifteen cytochrome transcripts were upregulated by at least a factor two at 15°C compared to 25°C. These fifteen upregulated cytochrome transcripts would be interesting candidates for future investigation.

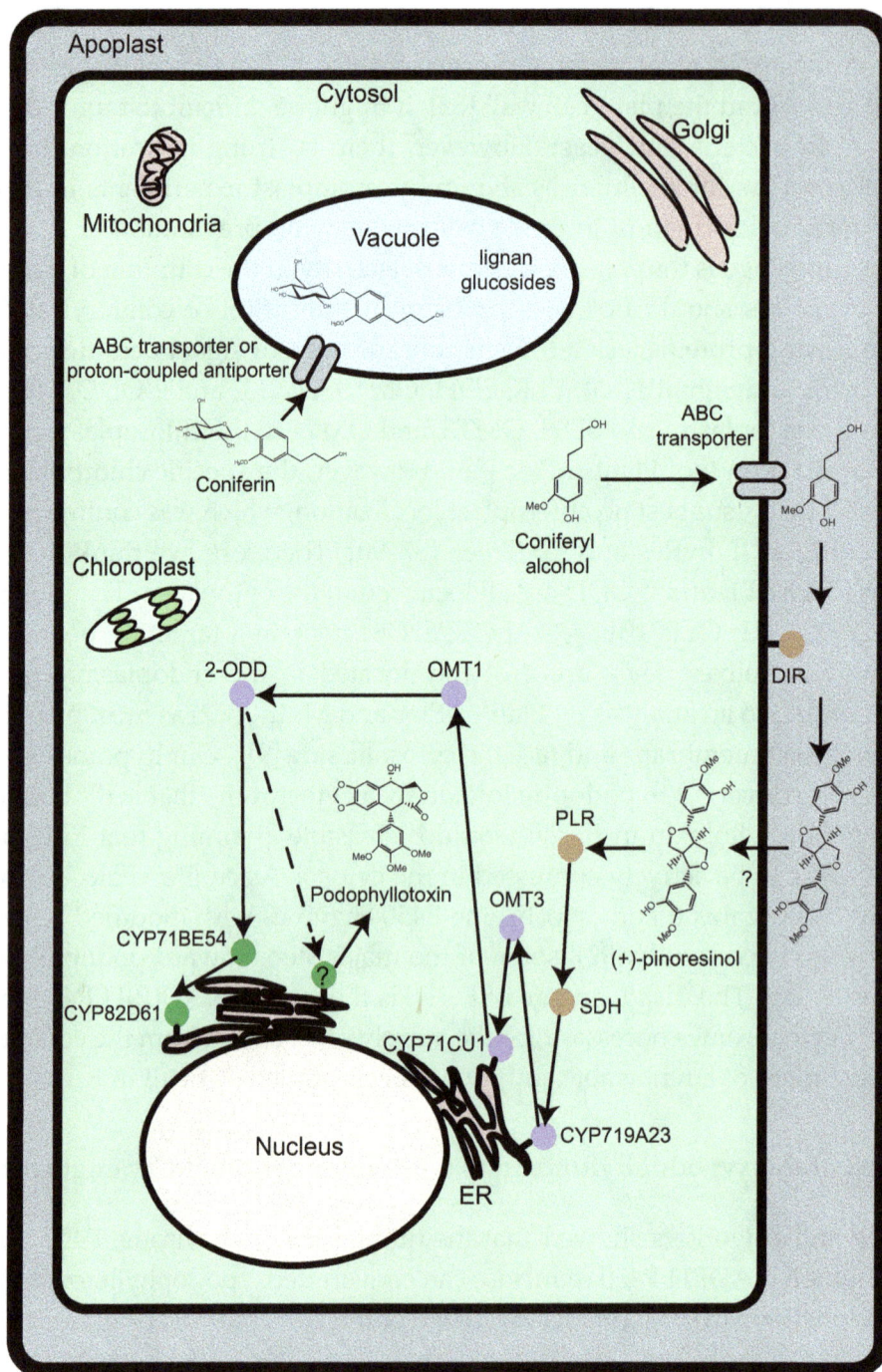

Figure 2. Schematic view of the proposed cellular localization of the enzymes in the lignan pathway in plant cells.

A cytochrome p450 system with high activity toward deoxypodophyllotoxin can form a very interesting production platform in conjunction with a sustainable source of this lignan, as is *A. syl-vestris*, a common wild plant in Europe and temperate Asia, that can be cultivated easily [95, 96].

5.4. Production of etoposide

Industrially, podophyllotoxin is chemically converted to etoposide (**Figure 3**). Podophyllotoxin is converted to 4'-demethyl-epipodophyllotoxin by demethylation and epimerization in two steps with a yield of 52% followed by the protection of the phenolic group by conversion to

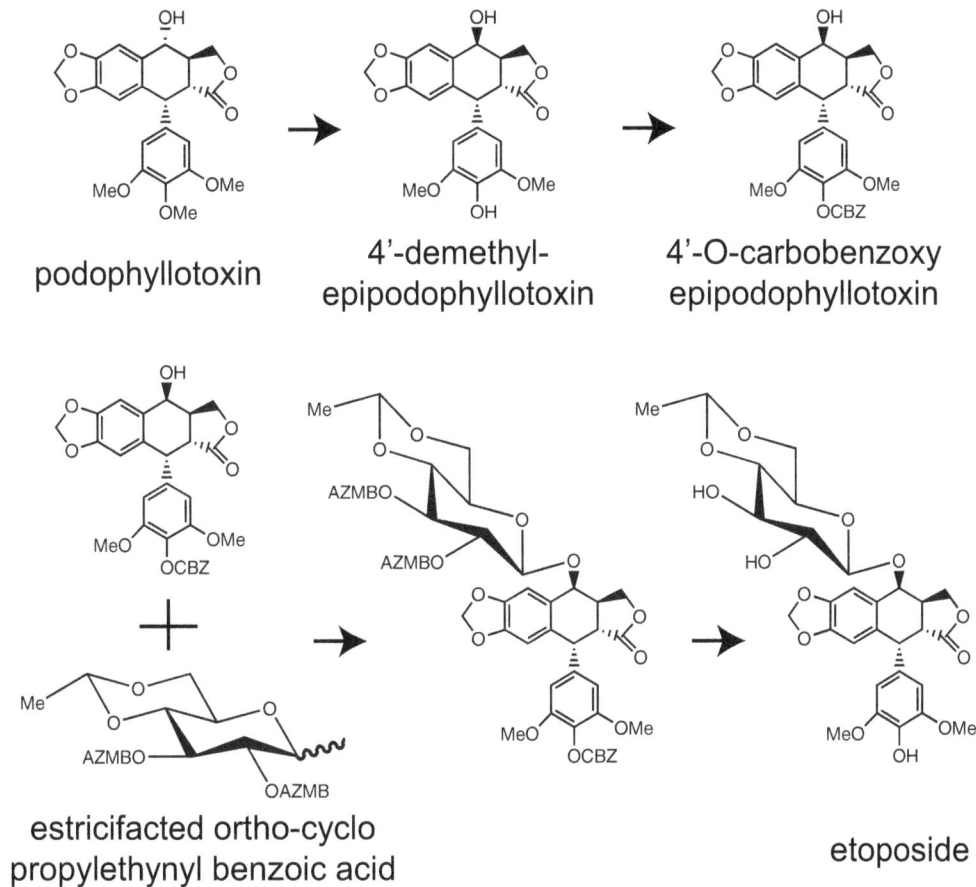

Figure 3. Conversion of podophyllotoxin into etoposide.

4′-O-carbobenzoxy-epipodophyllotoxin in one step with 89% yield [97]. 4′-O-carbobenzoxy-epipodophyllotoxin is then glycosylated to the esterification of *ortho*-cyclopropylethynylbenzoic acid, which is obtained in six steps from β-D-Glucose pentaacetate [98, 99]. After glycosylation, the protective groups are removed in one step with 90% yield [98]. As podophyllotoxin production from deoxypodophyllotoxin is not yet applicable on industrial scale, the chemical conversion of deoxypodophyllotoxin into epipodophyllotoxin is of interest, which can be performed in one step with a yield of 53% [100]. Epipodophyllotoxin can be converted chemically to etoposide in the same manner as podophyllotoxin. The chemical synthesis of etoposide from deoxypodophyllotoxin can be shortened by production of 4′-demethyl-epipodophyllotoxin from deoxypodophyllotoxin by CYP71BE54 and CYP82D61 from *P. hexandrum* (see Section 4.3). As only proof of concept has been shown, optimization is required to make this enzymatic conversion suitable for industrial application. Whether deoxypodophyllotoxin can be converted chemically directly to 4′-demethyl-epipodophyllotoxin still needs to be investigated.

6. Future perspectives

Recent insights in the lignan biosynthetic pathway by Lau and Sattely [69] have progressed the research in the lignan pathway enormously. Engineering of the lignan pathway in a heterologous host will become feasible, if the localization of the enzymes in the pathway has been determined. Depending on this localization, either *E. coli* or *S. cerevisiae* could be a suitable host for production of podophyllotoxin from glucose. The only missing step is the conversion of deoxypodophyllotoxin to podophyllotoxin. Finding this enzyme or replacing this step by the epipodophyllotoxin producing CYP82D61 (with or without CYP71BE54) will advance the development even more. Alternatively, deoxypodophyllotoxin can be chemically converted to etoposide. Considering the huge number of enzymes necessary for conversion of glucose to podophyllotoxin in *E. coli* or *S. cerevisiae*, commercial production in microbial hosts still has a long way to go. Until that time, an alternative approach can be the extraction of deoxy-podophyllotoxin from the easy to cultivate *A. sylvestris* and converting this to (epi)podophyllotoxin. Enzymatic conversion needs to be optimized in order to obtain a system that can be used by the industry. Improvement should focus on engineering a cheap system, by usage of a resting cell assay or the usage of a cheap cofactor in a cell-free system. Furthermore, the deoxypodophyllotoxin conversion should be scaled up to industrial production.

Acknowledgements

This work was supported by EU regional funding. The PhytoSana project in the INTERREG IV A Deutschland-Nederland program: 34- INTERREG IV A I-1-01=193.

Author details

Christel L. C. Seegers, Rita Setroikromo and Wim J. Quax*

*Address all correspondence to: w.j.quax@rug.nl

Department of Chemical and Pharmaceutical Biology, Groningen Research Institute of Pharmacy, University of Groningen, Groningen, The Netherlands

References

[1] Guerram M, Jiang ZZ, Zhang LY. Podophyllotoxin, a medicinal agent of plant origin: past, present and future. Chin J Nat Med. 2012;10:161-9. doi:10.3724/SP.J.1009.2012.00161.

[2] Alam MA, Naik PK. Impact of soil nutrients and environmental factors on podophyllotoxin content among 28 *podophyllum hexandrum* populations of Northwestern Himalayan region using linear and nonlinear approaches. Commun Soil Sci Plant Anal. 2009;40:2485-504. doi:10.1080/00103620903111368.

[3] Convention of International Trade in Endangered Species of Wild Fauna and Flora. n.d. https://www.cites.org/eng/app/appendices.php#hash2 (accessed October 28, 2015).

[4] Canel C, Moraes RM, Dayan FE, Ferreira D. Podophyllotoxin. Phytochemistry. 2000;54:115-20. doi:10.1016/S0031-9422(00)00094-7.

[5] Ting CP, Maimone TJ. CH bond arylation in the synthesis of aryltetralin lignans: a short total synthesis of podophyllotoxin. Angew Chem Int Ed Engl. 2014;53:3115-9. doi:10.1002/anie.201311112.

[6] Petersen M, Alfermann W. The production of cytotoxic lignans by plant cell cultures. Appl Microbiol Biotechnol. 2001;55:135-42. doi:10.1007/s002530000510.

[7] Ionkova I, Antonova I, Momekov G, Fuss E. Production of podophyllotoxin in Linum linearifolium *in vitro* cultures. Pharmacogn Mag. 2010;6:180-5. doi:10.4103/0973-1296.66932.

[8] Turner EE, Hirst EL, Peat S, Haworth RD, Baker W, Linstead RP, et al. Organic chemistry. Annu Reports Prog Chem. 1936;33:228. doi:10.1039/ar9363300228.

[9] Moss GP. Nomenclature of lignans and neolignans (IUPAC Recommendations 2000). Pure Appl Chem. 2000;72:1493-523. doi:10.1351/pac200072081493.

[10] Umezawa T. Diversity in lignan biosynthesis. Phytochem Rev. 2003;2:371-90. doi:10.1023/b:phyt.0000045487.02836.32.

[11] Whiting DA. Ligans and neolignans. Nat Prod Rep. 1985;2:191. doi:10.1039/np9850200191.

[12] Heinonen S, Nurmi T, Liukkonen K, Poutanen K, Wähälä K, Deyama T, et al. *In vitro* metabolism of plant lignans: new precursors of mammalian lignans enterolactone and enterodiol. J Agric Food Chem. 2001;49:3178-86. doi:10.1021/JF010038A.

[13] Peñalvo JL, Heinonen SM, Aura AM, Adlercreutz H. Dietary sesamin is converted to enterolactone in humans. J Nutr. 2005;135:1056-62.

[14] Landete JM. Plant and mammalian lignans: a review of source, intake, metabolism, intestinal bacteria and health. Food Res Int. 2012;46:410-24. doi:10.1016/j.foodres.2011.12.023.

[15] Charlton JL. Antiviral activity of lignans. J Nat Prod. 1998;61:1447-51. doi:10.1021/NP980136Z.

[16] Ayres DC, Loike JD. Lignans: Chemical, Biological and Clinical Properties. vol. 30. Cambridge, NewYork, Port Chester, Melbourne, Sydney: Cambridge University Press; 1990.

[17] Culp OS, Kaplan IW. Condylomata acuminata: two hundred cases treated with podophyllin. Ann Surg. 1944;120:251-6.

[18] von Krogh G, Lacey CJN, Gross G, Barrasso R, Schneider A. European course on HPV associated pathology: guidelines for primary care physicians for the diagnosis and management of anogenital warts. Sex Transm Infect. 2000;76:162-8. doi:10.1136/sti.76.3.162.

[19] Kelly MG, Hart-Well JL. The biological effects and the chemical composition of podophyllin. a review. J Natl Cancer Inst. 1954;14:967-1010. doi:10.1093/jnci/14.4.967.

[20] Stähelin HF, von Wartburg A. The chemical and biological route from podophyllotoxin glucoside to etoposide: ninth cain memorial award lecture. Cancer Res. 1991;51: 5-15.

[21] Imbert TF. Discovery of podophyllotoxins. Biochimie. 1998;80:207-22. doi:10.1016/S0300-9084(98)80004-7.

[22] Liu YQ, Yang L, Tian X. Podophyllotoxin: current perspectives. Curr Bioact Compd. 2007;3:37-66. doi:10.2174/157340707780126499.

[23] Hande K. Etoposide: four decades of development of a topoisomerase II inhibitor. Eur J Cancer. 1998;34:1514-21. doi:10.1016/S0959-8049(98)00228-7.

[24] Senter PD, Saulnier MG, Schreiber GJ, Hirschberg DL, Brown JP, Hellström I, et al. Anti-tumor effects of antibody-alkaline phosphatase conjugates in combination with etopo-side phosphate. Proc Natl Acad Sci U S A. 1988;85:4842-6.

[25] Thompson DS, Greco FA, Miller AA, Srinivas NR, Igwemezie LN, Hainsworth JD, et al. A phase I study of etoposide phosphate administered as a daily 30-minute infusion for 5 days. Clin Pharmacol Ther. 1995;57:499-507. doi:10.1016/0009-9236(95)90034-9.

[26] A to Z List of Cancer Drugs—National Cancer Institute. 2016. https://www.cancer.gov/about-cancer/treatment/drugs.

[27] Cytostatica | Farmacotherapeutisch Kompas. n.d. https://www.farmacotherapeutisch-kompas.nl/bladeren-volgens-boek/inleidingen/inl-cytostatica.

[28] Kalemkerian GP, Akerley W, Bogner P, Borghaei H, Chow LQ, Downey RJ, et al. Small cell lung cancer. J Natl Compr Canc Netw. 2013;11:78-98.

[29] PDQ Pediatric Treatment Editorial Board PPTE. Childhood Acute Myeloid Leukemia/Other Myeloid Malignancies Treatment (PDQ®): Health Professional Version. Bethesda: National Cancer Institute (US); 2002.

[30] Chemotherapy for acute lymphocytic leukemia. n.d. http://www.cancer.org/cancer/leukemia-acutelymphocyticallinadults/detailedguide/leukemia-acute-lymphocytic-treating-chemo therapy.

[31] Kamal A, Hussaini SMA, Rahim A, Riyaz S. Podophyllotoxin derivatives: a patent review (2012-2014). Expert Opin Ther Pat. 2015;25:1025-34.

[32] Liu YQ, Tian J, Qian K, Zhao XB, Morris-Natschke SL, Yang L, et al. Recent progress on C-4-modified podophyllotoxin analogs as potent antitumor agents. Med Res Rev. 2015;35:1-62. doi:10.1002/med.21319.

[33] Mizugaki H, Yamamoto N, Fujiwara Y, Nokihara H, Yamada Y, Tamura T. Current status of single-agent phase I trials in japan: toward globalization. J Clin Oncol. 2015;33:2051-61. doi:10.1200/JCO.2014.58.4953.

[34] Raßmann I, Schrödel H, Schilling T, Zucchetti M, Kaeser-Fröhlich A, Rastetter J, et al. Clinical and pharmacokinetic phase I trial of oral dimethylaminoetoposide (NK611) administered for 21 days every 35 days. Invest New Drugs. 1996;14:379-86. doi:10.1007/BF00180814.

[35] Raβmann I, Thödtmann R, Thödtmann R, Mross M, Hüttmann A, Berdel WE, et al. Phase I clinical and pharmacokinetic trial of the podophyllotoxin derivative NK611 administered as intravenous short infusion. Invest New Drugs. 1998;16:319-24. doi:10.1023/A:1006293830585.

[36] Pagani O, Zucchetti M, Sessa C, de Jong J, D'Incalci M, Fusco M De, et al. Clinical and pharmacokinetic study of oral NK611, a new podophyllotoxin derivative. Cancer Chemother Pharmacol. 1996;38:541-7. doi:10.1007/s002800050524.

[37] Perrin D, van Hille B, Barret JM, Kruczynski A, Etiévant C, Imbert T, et al. F 11782, a novel epipodophylloid non-intercalating dual catalytic inhibitor of topoisomerases I and II with an original mechanism of action. Biochem Pharmacol. 2000;59:807-19. doi:10.1016/S0006-2952(99)00382-2.

[38] Etiévant C, Kruczynski A, Barret JM, Perrin D, van Hille B, Guminski Y, et al. F 11782, a dual inhibitor of topoisomerases I and II with an original mechanism of action in vitro, and markedly superior in vivo antitumour activity, relative to three other dual topoisomerase inhibitors, intoplicin, aclarubicin and TAS-103. Cancer Chemother Pharmacol. 2000;46:101-13. doi:10.1007/s002800000133.

[39] Delord J-P, Bennouna J, Dieras V, Campone M, Lefresne F, Aslanis V, et al. First-in-man study of tafluposide, a novel inhibitor of topoisomerase I and II. Mol Cancer Ther. 2007;6:A138.

[40] Barret JM, Kruczynski A, Vispé S, Annereau JP, Brel V, Guminski Y, et al. F14512, a potent antitumor agent targeting topoisomerase II vectored into cancer cells via the polyamine transport system. Cancer Res. 2008;68:9845-53.

[41] Bahleda R, De Botton S, Quesnel B, Soria JC. 12th TAT congress 5-7 march 2014 Washington DC. Tackling Leuk. Phase I study F14512 relapsed or Refract. AML patients, 2014.

[42] Tierny D, Serres F, Segaoula Z, Bemelmans I, Bouchaert E, Pétain A, et al. Phase I clinical pharmacology study of F14512, a new polyamine-vectorized anticancer drug, in naturally occurring canine lymphoma. Clin Cancer Res. 2015;21:5314-23.

[43] Merzouki A, Buschmann MD, Jean M, Young RS, Liao S, Gal S, et al. Adva-27a, a novel podophyllotoxin derivative found to be effective against multidrug resistant human cancer cells. Anticancer Res. 2012;32:4423-32.

[44] Research programme: type II DNA topoisomerase inhibitors—Sunshine Biopharma—AdisInsight. n.d. http://adisinsight.springer.com/drugs/800032587.

[45] Chen MC, Pan SL, Shi Q, Xiao Z, Lee KH, Li TK, et al. QS-ZYX-1-61 induces apoptosis through topoisomerase II in human non-small-cell lung cancer A549 cells. Cancer Sci. 2012;103:80-7. doi:10.1111/j.1349-7006.2011.02103.x.

[46] Lewis NG, Davin LB, Sarkanen S. Lignin and lignan biosynthesis: distinctions and reconciliations. 1998; 697:pp. 1-27. doi:10.1021/bk-1998-0697.ch001.

[47] Rutledge PJ, Challis GL. Discovery of microbial natural products by activation of silent biosynthetic gene clusters. Nat Rev Microbiol. 2015;13:509-23. doi:10.1038/nrmicro3496.

[48] Davin LB, Wang HB, Crowell AL, Bedgar DL, Martin DM, Sarkanen S, et al. Stereoselective bimolecular phenoxy radical coupling by an auxiliary (dirigent) protein without an active center. Science (80-). 1997;275:362-7. doi:10.1126/science.275.5298.362.

[49] Kim KW, Moinuddin SGA, Atwell KM, Costa MA, Davin LB, Lewis NG. Opposite stereoselectivities of dirigent proteins in arabidopsis and schizandra species. J Biol Chem. 2012;287:33957-72. doi:10.1074/jbc.M112.387423.

[50] Gang DR, Costa MA, Fujita M, Dinkova-Kostova AT, Wang HB, Burlat V, et al. Regiochemical control of monolignol radical coupling: a new paradgm for lignin and lignan biosynthesis. Chem Biol. 1999;6:143-51. doi:10.1016/S1074-5521(99)89006-1.

[51] Seneviratne HK, Dalisay DS, Kim KW, Moinuddin SGA, Yang H, Hartshorn CM, et al. Non-host disease resistance response in pea (Pisum sativum) pods: biochemical function of DRR206 and phytoalexin pathway localization. Phytochemistry. 2015;113:140-8. doi:10.1016/j.phytochem.2014.10.013.

[52] Pickel B, Constantin MA, Pfannstiel J, Conrad J, Beifuss U, Schaller A. An enantiocomplementary dirigent protein for the enantioselective laccase-catalyzed oxidative coupling of phenols. Angew Chemie Int Ed. 2010;49:202-4. doi:10.1002/anie.200904622.

[53] Dalisay DS, Kim KW, Lee C, Yang H, Rübel O, Bowen BP, et al. Dirigent protein-mediated lignan and cyanogenic glucoside formation in flax seed: integrated omics and MALDI mass spectrometry imaging. J Nat Prod. 2015;78:1231-42. doi:10.1021/acs.jnatprod.5b00023.

[54] Kim KW, Smith CA, Daily MD, Cort JR, Davin LB, Lewis NG. Trimeric structure of (+)-pinoresinol-forming dirigent protein at 1.95 Å resolution with three isolated active sites. J Biol Chem. 2015;290:1308-18. doi:10.1074/jbc.M114.611780.

[55] Dinkova-Kostova AT, Gang DR, Davin LB, Bedgar DL, Chu A, Lewis NG. (+)-Pinoresinol/ (+)-Lariciresinol Reductase from Forsythia intermedia: protein purrification, cDNA cloning, heterologous expression and comparision to isoflavone reductase. J Biol Chem. 1996;271:29473-82. doi:10.1074/jbc.271.46.29473.

[56] Katayama T, Davin LB, Chu A, Lewis NG. Novel benzylic ether reductions in lignan biogenesis in Forsythia intermedia. Phytochemistry. 1993;33:581-91. doi:10.1016/0031-9422(93)85452-W.

[57] von Heimendahl CBI, Schäfer KM, Eklund P, Sjöholm R, Schmidt TJ, Fuss E. Pinoresinol–lariciresinol reductases with different stereospecificity from Linum album and Linum usitatissimum. Phytochemistry. 2005;66:1254-63. doi:10.1016/j.phytochem.2005.04.026.

[58] Hemmati S, Heimendahl CBI von, Klaes M, Alfermann AW, Schmidt TJ, Fuss E, et al. Pinoresinol-Lariciresinol reductases with opposite enantiospecificity determine the enantiomeric composition of lignans in the different organs of Linum usitatissimum L. Planta Med. 2010;76:928-34. doi:10.1055/s-0030-1250036.

[59] Bayindir Ü, Alfermann AW, Fuss E. Hinokinin biosynthesis in Linum corymbulosum Reichenb. Plant J. 2008;55:810-20. doi:10.1111/j.1365-313X.2008.03558.x.

[60] Fujita M, Gang DR, Davin LB, Lewis NG. Recombinant pinoresinol-lariciresinol reductases from western Red Cedar (*Thuja plicata*) catalyze opposite enantiospecific conversions. J Biol Chem. 1999;274:618-27. doi:10.1074/jbc.274.2.618.

[61] Hemmati S, Schmidt TJ, Fuss E. (+)-Pinoresinol/(−)-lariciresinol reductase from Linum perenne Himmelszelt involved in the biosynthesis of justicidin B. FEBS Lett. 2007;581:603-10. doi:10.1016/j.febslet.2007.01.018.

[62] Nakatsubo T, Mizutani M, Suzuki S, Hattori T, Umezawa T. Characterization of *Arabidopsis thaliana* pinoresinol reductase, a new type of enzyme involved in lignan biosynthesis. J Biol Chem. 2008;283:15550-7. doi:10.1074/jbc.M801131200.

[63] Min T, Kasahara H, Bedgar DL, Youn B, Lawrence PK, Gang DR, et al. Crystal structures of pinoresinol-lariciresinol and phenylcoumaran benzylic ether reductases and their relationship to isoflavone reductases. J Biol Chem. 2003;278:50714-23. doi:10.1074/jbc.M308493200.

[64] Xia ZQ, Costa M a, Pelissier HC, Davin LB, Lewis NG. Secoisolariciresinol dehydrogenase purification, cloning, and functional expression. Implications for human health protection. J Biol Chem. 2001;276:12614-23. doi:10.1074/jbc.M008622200.

[65] Youn B, Moinuddin SGA, Davin LB, Lewis NG, Kang C. Crystal structures of apo-form and binary/ternary complexes of podophyllum secoisolariciresinol dehydrogenase, an enzyme involved in formation of health-protecting and plant defense lignans. J Biol Chem. 2005;280:12917-26. doi:10.1074/jbc.M413266200.

[66] Kamil WM, Dewick PM. Biosynthetic relationship of aryltetralin lactone lignans to dibenzylbutyrolactone lignans. Phytochemistry. 1986;25:2093-102. doi: 10.1016/0031-9422(86)80072-3.

[67] Jackson DE, Dewick PM. Biosynthesis of *Podophyllum lignans*—II. Interconversions of aryltetralin lignans in *Podophyllum hexandrum*. Phytochemistry. 1984;23:1037-42. doi:10.1016/S0031-9422(00)82604-7.

[68] Marques JV, Kim KW, Lee C, Costa M a, May GD, Crow JA, et al. Next generation sequencing in predicting gene function in podophyllotoxin biosynthesis. J Biol Chem. 2013;288:466-79. doi:10.1074/jbc.M112.400689.

[69] Lau W, Sattely ES. Six enzymes from mayapple that complete the biosynthetic pathway to the etoposide aglycone. Science (80-). 2015;349:1224-8. doi:10.1126/science.aac7202.

[70] Sakakibara N, Suzuki S, Umezawa T, Shimada M. Biosynthesis of yatein in *Anthriscus sylvestris*. Org Biomol Chem. 2003;1:2474-85.

[71] Ragamustari SK, Nakatsubo T, Hattori T, Ono E, Kitamura Y, Suzuki S, et al. A novel O-methyltransferase involved in the first methylation step of yatein biosynthesis from

matairesinol in *Anthriscus sylvestris*. Plant Biotechnol. 2013;30:375-84. doi:10.5511/plantbiotechnology.13.0527b.

[72] Weiss SG, Tin-Wa M, Perdue RE, Farnsworth NR. Potential anticancer agents II: antitumor and cytotoxic lignans from Linum album (Linaceae). J Pharm Sci. 1975;64:95-8. doi:10.1002/jps.2600640119.

[73] Shiraishi A, Murata J, Matsumoto E, Matsubara S, Ono E, Satake H, et al. De novo transcriptomes of *Forsythia koreana* using a novel assembly method: insight into tissue- and species-specific expression of lignan biosynthesis-related gene. PLoS One. 2016;11:e0164805. doi:10.1371/journal.pone.0164805.

[74] Chen Z, Sun X, Li Y, Yan Y, Yuan Q. Metabolic engineering of *Escherichia coli* for microbial synthesis of monolignols. Metab Eng. 2016;39:102-9. doi:10.1016/j.ymben.2016.10.021.

[75] Huang Q, Lin Y, Yan Y. Caffeic acid production enhancement by engineering a phenylalanine over-producing *Escherichia coli* strain. Biotechnol Bioeng. 2013;110:3188-96. doi:10.1002/bit.24988.

[76] Eichenberger M, Lehka BJ, Folly C, Fischer D, Martens S, Simón E, et al. Metabolic engineering of *Saccharomyces cerevisiae* for de novo production of dihydrochalcones with known antioxidant, antidiabetic, and sweet tasting properties. Metab Eng. 2016;39:80-89. doi:10.1016/j.ymben.2016.10.019.

[77] Gidijala L, Kiel JAKW, Douma RD, Seifar RM, van Gulik WM, Bovenberg RAL, et al. An engineered yeast efficiently secreting penicillin. PLoS One. 2009;4:e8317. doi:10.1371/journal.pone.0008317.

[78] Miao YC, Liu CJ. ATP-binding cassette-like transporters are involved in the transport of lignin precursors across plasma and vacuolar membranes. Proc Natl Acad Sci U S A. 2010;107:22728-33. doi:10.1073/pnas.1007747108.

[79] Tsuyama T, Kawai R, Shitan N, Matoh T, Sugiyama J, Yoshinaga A, et al. Proton-dependent coniferin transport, a common major transport event in differentiating xylem tissue of woody plants. Plant Physiol. 2013;162:918-26. doi:10.1104/pp.113.214957.

[80] Krogh A, Larsson B, von Heijne G, Sonnhammer EL. Predicting transmembrane protein topology with a hidden markov model: application to complete genomes. J Mol Biol. 2001;305:567-80. doi:10.1006/jmbi.2000.4315.

[81] Umezawa T, Davin LB, Yamamoto E, Kingston DGI, Lewis NG, Lewis NG, et al. Lignan biosynthesis in forsythia species. J Chem Soc Chem Commun. 1990;41:1405. doi:10.1039/c39900001405.

[82] Davin LB, Bedgar DL, Katayama T, Lewis NG. On the stereoselective synthesis of (+)-pinoresinol in Forsythia suspensa from its achiral precursor, coniferyl alcohol. Phytochemistry. 1992;31:3869-74. doi:10.1016/S0031-9422(00)97544-7.

[83] Burlat V, Kwon M, Davin LB, Lewis NG. Dirigent proteins and dirigent sites in lignifying tissues. Phytochemistry. 2001;57:883-97. doi:10.1016/S0031-9422(01)00117-0.

[84] Dima O, Morreel K, Vanholme B, Kim H, Ralph J, Boerjan W. Small glycosylated lignin oligomers are stored in arabidopsis leaf vacuoles. Plant Cell. 2015;27:695-710. doi:10.1105/tpc.114.134643.

[85] Petersen TN, Brunak S, von Heijne G, Nielsen H. SignalP 4.0: discriminating signal peptides from transmembrane regions. Nat Methods. 2011;8:785-6. doi:10.1038/nmeth.1701.

[86] Chou KC, Shen HB, Ehrlich J, Hansen M, Nelson W, Glory E, et al. Plant-mPLoc: a top-down strategy to augment the power for predicting plant protein subcellular localization. PLoS One. 2010;5:e11335. doi:10.1371/journal.pone.0011335.

[87] Emanuelsson O, Nielsen H, Heijne G Von. ChloroP, a neural network-based method for predicting chloroplast transit peptides and their cleavage sites. Protein Sci. 1999;8:978-84. doi:10.1110/ps.8.5.978.

[88] Schein AI, Kissinger JC, Ungar LH. Chloroplast transit peptide prediction: a peek inside the black box. Nucleic Acids Res. 2001;29:E82.

[89] Blum T, Briesemeister S, Kohlbacher O, Emanuelsson O, Brunak S, Heijne G von, et al. MultiLoc2: integrating phylogeny and gene ontology terms improves subcellular protein localization prediction. BMC Bioinformatics. 2009;10:274. doi:10.1186/1471-2105-10-274.

[90] Goldberg T, Hecht M, Hamp T, Karl T, Yachdav G, Ahmed N, et al. LocTree3 prediction of localization. Nucleic Acids Res. 2014;42:W350-5. doi:10.1093/nar/gku396.

[91] Schuler MA, Werck-Reichhart D. Functional genomics of P450s. Annu Rev Plant Biol. 2003;54:629-67. doi:10.1146/annurev.arplant.54.031902.134840.

[92] Gillam EMJ. Engineering cytochrome P450 enzymes. Chem Res Toxicol. 2007;21:220-31. doi:10.1021/tx7002849.

[93] Vasilev NP, Julsing MK, Koulman A, Clarkson C, Woerdenbag HJ, Ionkova I, et al. Bioconversion of deoxypodophyllotoxin into epipodophyllotoxin in *E. coli* using human cytochrome P450 3A4. J Biotechnol. 2006;126:383-93. doi:10.1016/j.jbiotec.2006.04.025.

[94] Kumari A, Singh HR, Jha A, Swarnkar MK, Shankar R, Kumar S. Transcriptome sequencing of rhizome tissue of Sinopodophyllum hexandrum at two temperatures. BMC Genomics. 2014;15:871. doi:10.1186/1471-2164-15-871.

[95] Magnússen SH. NOBANIS –Invasive Alien Species Fact Sheet -*Anthriscus sylvestris*. Database of the European Network on Invasive Alien Species. 2011.

[96] Hendrawati O, Woerdenbag HJ, Hille J, Quax WJ, Kayser O. Seasonal variations in the deoxypodophyllotoxin content and yield of *Anthriscus sylvestris* L. (Hoffm.) grown in the field and under controlled conditions. J Agric Food Chem. 2011;59:8132-9. doi:10.1021/jf200177q.

[97] Lee KH, Imakura Y, Haruna M, Beers SA, Thurston LS, Dai HJ, et al. Antitumor agents, 107. New cytotoxic 4-alkylamino analogues of 4'-demethyl-epipodophyllotoxin as inhibitors of human DNA topoisomerase II. J Nat Prod. 1989;52:606-13. doi:10.1021/np50063a021.

[98] Liu H, Liao JX, Hu Y, Tu YH, Sun JS. A highly efficient approach to construct (*epi*)-podophyllotoxin-4- *O* -glycosidic linkages as well as its application in concise syntheses of etoposide and teniposide. Org Lett. 2016;18:1294-7. doi:10.1021/acs.orglett.6b00216.

[99] Zong G, Barber E, Aljewari H, Zhou J, Hu Z, Du Y, et al. Total synthesis and biological evaluation of ipomoeassin F and its unnatural 11 *R* -epimer. J Org Chem. 2015;80:9279-91. doi:10.1021/acs.joc.5b01765.

[100] Yamaguchi Hi, Arimoto M, Nakajima S, Tanoguchi M, Fukada Y. Studies on the constituents of the seeds of Hernandia ovigera L. V Syntheses of epipodophyllotoxin and podophyllotoxin from desoxypodophyllotoxin. Chem Pharm Bull (Tokyo). 1986;34:2056-60. doi:10.1248/cpb.34.2056.

2

Recent Progress on the Molecular Mechanisms of Anti-invasive and Metastatic Chinese Medicines for Cancer Therapy

Wei Guo, Ning Wang and Yibin Feng

Abstract

Despite of the recent advances in diagnostic and therapeutic approaches, cancer remains as the leading cause of death worldly with diverse causal factors regarding genes and environment. Invasion and metastasis, as one of the most important hallmarks for cancer, have restrained the successful clinical therapy and are the primary causes of death among cancer patients. So far, most chemotherapeutic drugs are not effective for metastatic cancer due to drug resistance and serious side effects. Therefore, it is urgently essential to develop more effective therapeutic methods. Owing to their diverse biological activities and low toxicity, naturally active compounds derived from Chinese medicines, as a complementary and alternative approach, are reported to promote the therapeutic index and provoked as an excellent source for candidates of anti-metastatic drugs. With the rapid development of molecular biology techniques, the molecular mechanisms of the effects of potential anti-invasive and metastatic Chinese medicines are gradually elucidated. This chapter reviews the potential anti-invasive and metastatic mechanisms of naturally active compounds from Chinese medicines, including suppression of EMT, proteases and cancer-induced angiogenesis, anoikis regulation of circulating tumor cells and regulation of miRNA-mediated gene expression, providing scientific evidence for clinically using Chinese medicines in the field of cancer therapy.

Keywords: Chinese medicines, anti-invasion and metastasis, molecular mechanisms, cancer therapy

1. Introduction

Despite of all the recent advances in diagnostic and therapeutic approaches, cancer remains the leading cause of death and primary public health hazard all over the world [1, 2]. With diverse causal factors (genetic and environmental, physical, psychological and biochemical factors), cancer has a various disease spectrum to more than a hundred different kinds of malignancies, such as lung cancer, breast cancer, renal carcinoma, hepatocellular carcinoma, and so on [3]. It is a progressive disease with multiple pathological processes covering cancer initiation, development, and metastasis. Cancer is characterized by several key hallmarks [4–6], namely uncontrolled replication ability of abnormal cells, resistance to programmed cell death, invasion into the surrounding extracellular matrix (ECM), sustained capability of angiogenesis, and metastatic spread to other sites.

As one of the most important hallmarks for cancer, metastasis is an intricate process concerning the following six steps (as shown in **Figure 1**): (i) detachment of cancer cells through degrading ECM, (ii) local migration and invasion into the surrounding tissues, (iii) intravasation into blood and/or lymphatic vessel systems, (iv) survival and circulation in the circulatory system, (v) extravasation into the targeted secondary organ site, and (vi) multiplication and formation of a secondary tumor [7–9]. During these steps, the metastatic cancer cells should have special properties to overcome the obstacles, such as the capability of invasion, resistance to anoikis, and angiogenesis. Basically, these steps are regulated by multiple factors, including but not limited to changes of expression of related genes, cytoskeleton remodeling, proteolysis degradation of ECM, and so on [10]. Metastasis is a nonrandom process, and different metastatic cancer types possess their corresponding preferred sites of metastasis. For instance, the preferred sites of breast cancer cells are lung, liver, and bone [11]. Since invasion and metastasis restrain the successful clinical therapy and are the primary causes of death among cancer patients, it has been widely accepted that invasion and metastasis become a highlighted topic of research interests, and active efforts are still needed to understand the underlying molecular mechanisms and develop effective anti-metastatic therapies.

At the present day, there are three conventional therapeutic approaches which are used to treat metastatic cancers, namely surgical resection, chemotherapy, and radiotherapy. Though remain as the main treatment approach for metastatic cancer patients, most chemotherapeutic drugs are not effective for metastatic cancer due to drug resistance and serious side effects. Most chemotherapeutic drugs fail to selectively kill cancer cells without destroying normal cells at the sites of metastasis [12] and thus cause severe toxicity, such as appetite loss, weight loss, insomnia, fatigue, even life threat etc [13, 14]. Although chemotherapeutics significantly leads to regression of the primary tumor, some investigations even report that it may also promote and enhance metastatic formation of a secondary tumor [15, 16]. Besides, metastatic cancers are demonstrated to be largely resistant against chemotherapeutics. Despite that various approaches have been applied to treat metastatic cancers, the clinical outcomes of metastatic cancer treatment are still not at a satisfactory level. Therefore, it is urgently essential to develop more effective therapeutic methods with minimal adverse effects for metastatic cancer treatment.

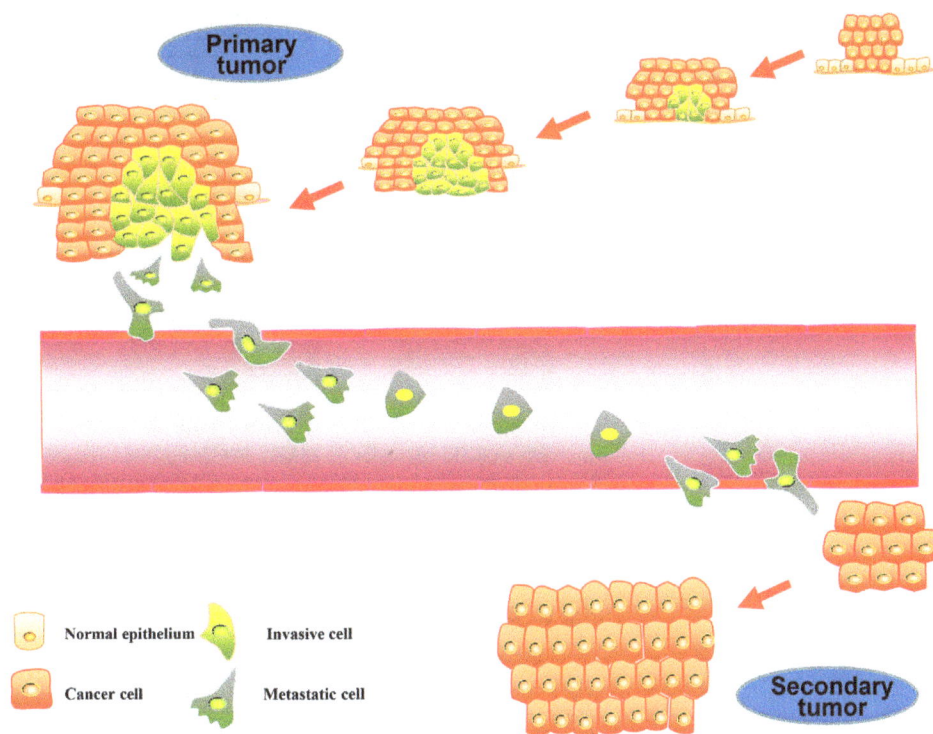

Figure 1. The process involving in cancer metastasis.

Traditional medicine, such as Chinese medicine, has been shown to exhibit various phar-macological activities and used in treatment of various diseases in Asian countries and regions for a long time [17]. The numerous natural compounds obtained from Chinese medicines chemically range from flavonoids and polyphenols to mineral salts, which have been reported to be an excellent source for anti-cancer agents [18]. Owing to their long-lasting efficacy, diversity in biological activities, and low toxicity, natural active products from Chinese medicines, including single compounds and various extracts, are being developed for treatment of metastatic cancer [19, 20]. In line with such a concept, sev-eral natural active products from Chinese medicines have been currently investigated as a complementary and alternative approach, and their anti-metastatic properties have been focused to find newly discovered mechanisms with the hope to promote the therapeutic index of metastatic cancer.

With the rapid development of molecular biology techniques, the molecular mechanisms underlying the effects of potential anti-invasive and metastatic Chinese medicines are gradu-ally elucidated. Understanding of the underlying molecular mechanisms may in turn lead to the discovery of novel anticancer drugs. In summary, this chapter reviews the anti-invasive and metastatic effect of natural active compounds from Chinese medicines and their molecu-lar mechanisms. **Tables 1** and **2** respectively summarized the potential underlying molecular mechanisms of single pure compounds and various extracts from Chinese medicines to sup-press cancer invasion and metastasis.

Single pure compound	Cancer type	Study type	Mechanism of actions	Ref. (PMID)
Arctigenin	Breast cancer	In vitro MCF-7 and MDA-MB-231 cells	Suppress MMP-9 and uPA	28035371
	Colorectal cancer	In vitro CT26, MC38, CCD-18Co and SW620 cells and in vivo BALB/c female mice	Induce anoikis via MAPKs signaling, inhibit EMT through increasing E-cadherin and decreasing N-cadherin, vimentin, β-catenin, and Snail and downregulate MMP-2/9	27618887
Astragaloside IV	Breast cancer	In vitro MDA-MB-231 cells and in vivo athymic Balb/c nude mice	Downregulate Vav3 and MMP-2/9	27930970
Berberine	Hepatocellular carcinoma	In vitro MHCC-97L, Bel-7402, SMMC-7721 cells and in vivo nude mice	Downregulate uPA and suppress Id-1 via HIF-1α/ VEGF pathway	27092498 25496992
	Nasopharyngeal carcinoma	In vitro HONE1 cells	Suppress Rho GTPases including RhoA, Cdc42, and Rac1	19513545
Notoginsenoside R1	Colorectal cancer	In vitro HCT-116 cells	Reduce MMP-9, integrin-1, E-selectin and ICAM-1 expressions	27840961
Matrine	Prostate cancer	In vitro DU145 and PC-3 and male Balb/c nude mice inoculated subcutaneously with cells	Downregulate MMP-2/9	28000853
Bibenzyl 4,5,4'-trihydroxy-3,3'-dimethoxybibenzyl	Lung cancer	In vitro H292 cells	Suppress EMT markers (vimentin and Snail) and increase the level of E-cadherin and induce anoikis by reduction of activated protein kinase B (p-AKT) and activated extracellular signal-regulated kinase (p-ERK)	24692728
Curcumin	Lung cancer	In vitro H460 cells	Sensitize anoikis by down-regulating Bcl-2	20127174
Imperatorin	Lung cancer	In vitro H23, H292 and A549 cells	Sensitize anoikis by down-regulating Mcl-1 protein and up-regulating Bax	23108812
Artonin E	Lung cancer	In vitro H460, A549 and H292 cells	Sensitize anoikis by down-regulating Mcl-1 protein	23225436

Single pure compound	Cancer type	Study type	Mechanism of actions	Ref. (PMID)
Ecteinascidin 770	Lung cancer	In vitro H23 and H460 cells	Sensitize anoikis by down-regulating Mcl-1 protein and up-regulating Bax	23393342
Renieramycin M	Lung cancer	In vitro H460 cells	Sensitize anoikis by down-regulating survival proteins p-ERK and p-AKT and anti-apoptotic proteins BCL2 and MCL1	27069144
Oroxylin A	Lung cancer	In vitro A549 cells and in vivo nude mice	Sensitize anoikis by inactivating the c-Src/AKT/HK II pathway	23500080
Geraniin	Lung cancer	In vitro A549 cells	Inhibit the TGF-β1-induced EMT	26169124
Genipin	Hepatocellular carcinoma	In vitro HepG2 and MHCC97L cells and in vivo male nude mice	Overexpress TIMP-1 and inhibit MMP-2	23029478
Kukoamine A	Glioblastoma	In vitro C6, U251 and WJ1 cells and in vivo nude mice (BALB/C-nu/nu)	Inhibit EMT and induce anoikis by downregulating expressions of C/EBPβ and 5-LOX	27824118
Gigantol	Lung cancer	In vitro H460 cells	Decrease EMT markers including N-cadherin, vimentin, and Slug	26733180
Moscatilin	Lung cancer	In vitro H460 cells	Inhibit EMT by suppressing mesenchymal cell markers (vimentin, Slug, and Snail) and induce anoikis by survival proteins (ERK and Akt) suppression and Cav-1 down-regulation	26384689
2,3,5- Trimethoxy-4-cresol	Lung cancer	In vitro A549 cells	Suppress Akt, MMP-2 and MMP-9 and increase E-cadherin and TIMP-1	25951809
Deoxyelephantopin	Lung cancer	In vitro A549 cells	Suppress MMP-2, MMP-9, uPA, and uPAR	25686703
Bufalin	Lung cancer	In vitro NCI-H460 cells	Suppress MMP-2, MMP-9, MAPKs, and NF-kB	26446205
Epicatechin-3-gallate	Lung cancer	In vitro A549 cells and in vivo BALB/c nude mice	Inhibit the TGF-β1-induced EMT by up-regulating epithelial marker (E-cadherin) and down-regulating mesenchymal markers (fibronectin and p-FAK)	27224248

Single pure compound	Cancer type	Study type	Mechanism of actions	Ref. (PMID)
Rocaglamide-A	Prostate cancer, breast cancer and cervical cancer	In vitro PC-3, MDA- MB-231, HCT116, HeLa, and 293T cells	Inhibit the activity of Rho GTPases RhoA, Rac1 and Cdc42	27340868
Chamaejasmenin B	Breast cancer	In vitro MDA-MB-231, ZR75-1 and 4T1 cells and in vivo BALB/c mice	Block TGF-beta induced EMT	27374079
Artesunate	Cervical cancer	In vitro CaSki and Hela cells	Inhibit HOTAIR and COX-2 expressions	27736969
Ginsenoside Rd	Breast cancer	In vitro 4T1 cells and in vivo BALB/c mice	Derepress miR-18a-mediated Smad2 expression	27641158
Quercetin	Colorectal cancer	In vitro CT26 and MC38 cells and in vivo BALB/c female mice	Induce apoptosis through the MAPKs pathway, regulate EMT markers including E-, N-cadherin, β-catenin, and snail and regulate MMPs and TIMPs	27823633
Sulforaphane	Lung cancer	In vitro H1299, 95C and 95D cells and in vivo male BALB/c nude mice	Inhibit EMT by silencing miR-616-5p	27890917
Tricetin	Osteosarcoma	In vitro U2OS and HOS cells	Repress MMP-9 via p38 and Akt pathways	27860196
Arsenic trioxide	Chondrosarcoma	In vitro HCS-2/8, OUMS-27, SW1353, and JJ012 cells	Inhibit EMT via the miR-125b/Stat3 axis	27576314
Cucurbitacin B	Breast cancer	In vitro MDA-MB-231 and 4T1 cells	Inhibit angiogenesis via downregulating VEGF/FAK/MMP-9 signaling	27210504
2,3,5,4'-Tetrahydroxystilbene-2-O-β-D-glucoside	Colorectal cancer	In vitro HT-29 cells	Suppress MMP-2 and ICAM-1 via NF-κB pathway	27278328
7,7''-Dimethoxyagastisflavone	Melanoma	In vitro B16F10 cells and in vivo female C57BL/6JNarl mice	Down-regulate the polymerization of F-actin via Cdc42/Rac1 pathway and inhibit lamellipodia formation via suppressing CREB phosphorylation	27487150
Nobiletin	Osteosarcoma	In vitro U2OS and HOS cells	Block ERK and JNK-mediated MMPs expression	27144433

Table 1. Summary on the potential underlying molecular mechanisms of single pure compound from Chinese medicines to suppress cancer invasion and metastasis.

Various extracts	Cancer type	Study type	Mechanism of actions	Ref. (PMID)
Ethanol extract of baked Gardeniae Fructus	Melanoma	In vitro B16F10 and in vivo C57BL/6 mice	Inhibiting the release of pro-angiogenic factors from tumor cells	27779658
Mixture of flavonoids extracted from Korean *Citrus aurantium*	Lung cancer	In vitro A549 cells and in vivo NOD/SCID mice	Induce apoptosis through regulating the apoptosis related protein cleaved caspase-3 and p-p53	No
Bibenzyl compounds isolated from *Dendrobium pulchellum*	Lung cancer	In vitro	Induce anoikis	23472473
Aqueous extract of *Andrographis paniculata*	Esophageal cancer	In vitro EC-109 and KYSE-520 cells	Inhibit anoikis resistance	26885447
Methanol extracts of *Euphorbia humifusa* Willd	Breast cancer	In vitro MDA-MB-231 and in vivo Balb/c mice	Reduce TNFα-induced MMP-9 expression	27776550
Ethanol extract of Lophatheri Herba	Fibrosarcoma, breast cancer, prostate carcinoma and melanoma	In vitro HT1080, MDA-MB231, DU145, B16F10 cells and in vivo C57BL/6J mice and ICR mice	Suppress tumor-induced angiogenesis by decreasing the pro-angiogenic factors	27808120
Coptidis Rhizoma aqueous extract	Hepatocellular carcinoma	In vitro Hep G2 and MHCC97-L cells and in vivo nude mice	Suppress Rho/ROCK signaling pathway and inhibit VEGF secretion	21106616 24363282
Methanol extracts and butanol extracts of *Oldenlandia diffusa*	Breast cancer	In vitro MCF-7 cells	Inhibit PMA-induced MMP-9 and ICAM-1 expressions	27876502
Annona muricata leaf aqueous extract	Breast cancer	In vitro 4 T1 cells and in vivo female BALB/c mice	Induce the apoptosis	27558166
Ethanol extract of *Siegesbeckia orientalis*	Endometrial Cancer	In vitro RL95-2 and HEC-1A	Reverse the TGFβ1-induced EMT	27527140
Polyphenols of *Artemisia annua* L.	Breast cancer	In vitro MDA-MB-231 cells	Suppress EMT by inhibiting MMP-2/-9 and vascular cell adhesion molecule-1	27151203
Gegen Qinlian decoction	Renal carcinoma	In vitro ACHN and Caki-1 cells and in vivo male BALB/c nude mice	Suppress neoangiogenesis via MMP-2 inhibition	25228536

Table 2. Summary on the potential underlying molecular mechanisms of various extracts from Chinese medicines to suppress cancer invasion and metastasis.

2. Suppression of epithelial-mesenchymal transition

Recent studies clearly showed that epithelial-mesenchymal transition (EMT) plays an important role in the metastasis of cancers [21]. As the fundamental step during cancer metastasis, EMT is a complex process during which immotile epithelial cells undergo a morphological transformation into motile mesenchymal-appeared cells, triggering cancer cells to detach from the primary site via the loss of cell-to-cell junctions and thus promoting cell migration [22]. There are three different subtypes of EMT, and the third subtype of EMT is associated with the invasion and metastasis of cancers [23]. EMT-phenotypic cells can decrease the level of epithelial marker E-cadherin, a junction protein for cell-cell contact. Besides, they can also increase the level of mesenchymal markers, such as N-cadherin, β-catenin, and vimentin, as well as promote transcription factors of EMT switch, such as Slug and Snail [24, 25]. As EMT has been significantly linked to the metastatic behaviors of cancer cells, natural products obtained from Chinese medicines with the ability to suppress EMT are attracting attention for the development of anti-metastasis therapies.

Among potential natural products, geraniin, a polyphenolic component derived from Phyllanthus amarus, has gained considerable attention over the past decade. Previous study has demonstrated that EMT can be induced by transforming growth factor-beta 1 (TGF-β1) and thus stimulates the migration and invasion of lung adenocarcinoma. Geraniin has been shown to inhibit TGF-β1-induced EMT of lung cancer A549 cells in vitro by inducing the epithelial marker E-cadherin and suppressing Snail and mesenchymal marker N-cadherin and vimentin [26]. A compound derived from *Dendrobium ellipsophyllum*, bibenzyl 4,5,4'-trihydroxy-3,3'-dimethoxybibenzyl was shown to inhibit EMT of lung cancer cells via down-regulating EMT markers (vimentin and Snail) and upregulating E-cadherin [27]. Such EMT suppression was also observed in lung cancer cells treated with other single compounds obtained from Chinese medicine, such as moscatilin [28], gigantol [29], and epicatechin-3-gallate [30]. A flavonoid obtained from *Stellera chamaejasme* L., namely chamaejasmenin B, was also reported to block the TGF-β-induced EMT in breast cancer [31]. 5-lipoxygenase (5-LOX) is an enzyme to convert arachidonic acid to leukotrienes [32] and abrogating its expression can inhibit the migration, invasion, and metastasis of cancer cells by suppressing EMT via inactivating E-cadherin and activating snail [33]. CCAAT/enhancer binding protein β (C/EBPβ) was also reported to be related to the migration, invasion, and metastasis of cancer cells by EMT regulation [34]. Kukoamine A, a spermine alkaloid extracted from Cortex lycii radicis, was demonstrated to suppress the migratory and invasive ability of human glioblastoma cell both in vitro and in vivo, and this action was mediated through EMT attenuation via decreasing the levels of 5-LOX and C/EBPβ [35]. Likewise, similar EMT inhibitory effects have also been observed in various extracts from Chinese medicines. *Siegesbeckia orientalis* Linne is a traditionally used Chinese medicinal herb that exhibits various pharmacological activities. Its ethanol extract (SOE) has been reported as a potential anti-metastatic agent by reversing the TGFβ1-induced EMT via ERK1/2, JNK1/2, and Akt pathways [36]. SOE can inhibit the migration and invasion of endometrial cancer RL95-2 and HEC-1A cells in a dose-dependent manner. *Artemisia annua* L. is a traditional medicine which has been applied for treating multiple diseases. The polyphenolic compounds from *Artemisia annua* L. (pKAL) were found to exhibit anti-metastatic property on highly metastatic breast cancer cells MDA-MB-231 [37]. This anti-metastatic property of pKAL was achieved through suppressing EMT by inhibiting MMP-2/-9 and vascular cell adhesion molecule-1 (VCAM-1).

3. Suppression of proteases expression

Matrix metalloproteinases (MMPs) is regarded as primary factors to trigger metastasis [38]. As extracellular zinc-dependent endopeptidases, they can degrade the basement membrane and ECM and thus play an important role in the migration and invasion of cancers. There are 23 members in MMPs family, among which MMP-2 and MMP-9 are considered to be the key enzymes and play crucial roles in cancer metastasis [39, 40]. The activities of MMPs are finely mediated by tissue inhibitors of metalloproteinases (TIMPs) via their non-covalent binding to the active zinc-binding sites of MMPs [41]. In addition, as a serine-specific protease, uro-kinase-type plasminogen activator (uPA) can also degrade ECM via binding to uPA receptor (uPAR) and activating plasmin [42]. It is well-known that reorganization of the actin cyto-skeleton plays an important role in the migration of cancer cell [43]. This process is mainly regulated by the Rho family GTPases, such as RhoA, Rac1, and Cdc42 via a shuttle between an inactive GDP-bound form and an active GTP-bound form [44, 45]. Since these proteases play an important role in cancer invasion and metastasis via proteolysis, natural products obtained from Chinese medicines with the ability to suppress these proteases are attracting attention for the development of anti-metastasis therapies.

As a phytoestrogen-botanical lignan derived from Arctium lappa, arctigenin was shown to exert its anti-metastatic property through suppressing MMP-9 and uPA of breast cancer cells via inhibiting the upstream signaling pathways including Akt, NF-κB, and MAPK (ERK 1/2 and JNK 1/2), which is dependent to the modulation on estrogen receptor (ER) expression [46]. Such protease regulation was also observed in breast cancer cells treated with astragaloside IV [47]. Notoginsenoside R1 (NGR1) is a primary compound in Panax notoginseng, and its anti-metastatic property has also been revealed [48]. NGR1 can inhibit the migration, invasion, and adhesion of cultured human colorectal cancer cells (HCT-116) via suppressing MMP-9, integrin-1, E-selectin, and ICAM-1 expressions. Such inhibition on colorectal cancer cells was also observed when treated with 2,3,5,4'-tetrahydroxystilbene-2-O-β-D-glucoside [49]. As an alkaloid derived from Sophora flavescens, matrine can inhibit the invasion and migration of castration-resistant prostate cancer DU145 and PC3 cells by suppressing MMP-9 and MMP-2 expressions through NF-κB pathway [50]. The phenol derived from Taiwanese edible fungus *Antrodia cinnamomea*, 2,3,5-trimethoxy-4-cresol, was recently described as an effective anti-metastatic agent against lung cancer via suppressing Akt, MMP-2 and MMP-9, and increasing E-cadherin and TIMP-1[51]. Such protease regulation was also observed in lung cancer cells treated with other single compounds derived from Chinese medicine, such as deoxyelephan-topin [52] and bufalin [53]. Genipin, a natural compound obtained from the fruit of Gardenia jasminoides, was reported to exhibit anti-metastatic effect on hepatocellular carcinoma both in cell and animal model. This effect may be related with TIMP-1 overexpression and MMP-2 inhibition of genipin [54]. As an isoquinoline alkaloid isolated from Coptidis rhizome and other medicinal plants, berberine has been shown to exhibit multiple pharmacological actions in treating human diseases, including cancers [55]. Recently, it was reported to inhibit naso-pharyngeal carcinoma cell migration and invasion in vitro through suppressing Rho GTPases including RhoA, Rac1, and Cdc42 [56]. The anti-metastatic ability of Rocaglamide-A was also recently described via inhibiting the activity of Rho GTPases RhoA, Rac1, and Cdc42 [57]. As a dietary flavonoid in Eucalyptus honey and Myrtaceae pollen, tricetin was shown to attenu-ate osteosarcoma cell migration via suppressing MMP-9 via p38 and Akt pathways [58]. Such inhibition on osteosarcoma cells was also observed when treated with nobiletin [59]. The com-pound obtained from Taxus x media cv. Hicksii, 7,7"-Dimethoxyagastisflavone (DMGF) has been reported to inhibit the invasion and metastasis of melanoma cells in vivo and in vitro

[60]. The mechanism study provided evidence that DMGF can downregulate the polymerization of F-actin via Cdc42/Rac1 pathway and inhibit lamellipodia formation via suppressing cAMP response element-binding protein (CREB) phosphorylation. Likewise, similar protease inhibitory effects have also been observed in various extracts from Chinese medicines. The methanol extracts of *Euphorbia humifusa* Willd was reported to have anti-metastatic effects on breast cancer both in vitro and in vivo via reducing TNFα-induced MMP-9 expression [61]. In addition, the methanol extracts and butanol extracts of *Oldenlandia diffusa* were also shown to block the metastasis of breast cancer via inhibiting PMA-induced MMP-9 and ICAM-1 expressions [62].

4. Suppression of cancer-induced angiogenesis

Angiogenesis is a normal physiological process to sprout new vessels during the development of embryogenesis. To the contrary, pathological angiogenesis is associated with multiple diseases including cancers [63]. Highly malignant tumors can induce angiogenesis to provide sufficient oxygen and nutrients for themselves [64]. Additionally, angiogenesis also provides paths for cancer cells to metastasize distant tissues [65]. In tumor microenvironment, tumor and host cells release pro-angiogenic and anti-angiogenic factors. The pro-angiogenic factors include transforming growth factor (TGF), vascular endothelial growth factor (VEGF), tumor necrosis factor (TNF), epidermal growth factor (EGF), and so on, and there is a fine balance between them. When the balance is skewed to the pro-angiogenic state, tumor shifts from a dormant state to a hyper-vascularized state [66]. Since angiogenesis plays an important role in the metastatic behaviors of cancer cells, natural products obtained from Chinese medicines targeting on tumor-induced angiogenesis have been regarded as promising agents to metastatic cancers.

Berberine has been shown to exhibit a significant inhibition on the migratory and invasive ability of hepatocellular carcinoma cells. Except for downregulation of uPA, berberine also inhibits angiogenesis through suppressing inhibitor of differentiation/DNA binding (Id-1) via HIF-1α/VEGF pathway [67, 68]. Cucurbitacin B (CuB), a plant triterpenoid, obtained from Cucurbitaceae family has been shown to inhibit the metastasis and angiogenesis of breast cancer MDA-MB-231 and 4T1 cells via downregulating VEGF/FAK/MMP-9 signaling [69]. Recently, a study of artesunate, a normal traditional Chinese medicine, has been conducted to investigate the anti-metastatic effects of artesunate on cervical cancer. The results demonstrated that artesunate inhibits cancer cell migration and invasion in vitro through suppressing HOTAIR and COX-2-mediated angiogenesis [70]. Likewise, similar inhibitory effects have also been observed in various extracts from Chinese medicines. The aqueous extract of Coptidis Rhizoma, a traditional Chinese medicinal herb with a long history, was observed to inhibit hepatocellular carcinoma cell migration both in vitro and in vivo through suppressing Rho/ROCK signaling pathway and inhibiting VEGF secretion [71, 72]. Gardeniae Fructus, a fruit obtained from *Gardenia jasminoides* Ellis, has been applied as traditional medicine and possesses various health benefits against multiple diseases. A recent study has shown that the ethanol extract of baked Gardeniae Fructus has an inhibitory effect on the angiogenic and metastatic ability of melanoma cells both in vitro and in vivo via inhibiting the release of pro-angiogenic factors [73]. Lophatheri Herba, a dried leaf obtained from Lophatherum gracile Brongn, possesses inhibitory effects on the metastasis and angiogenesis of malignant cancer cells at noncytotoxic doses. It has been shown that ethanol extract of Lophatheri Herba (ELH) can inhibit the cancer cell metastasis both in vitro and in vivo through suppressing tumor-induced angiogenesis via decreasing the pro-angiogenic factors [74]. As an ancient Chinese medicine formula, Gegen Qinlian decoction was reported to suppress the neoangiogenesis in xenografted renal carcinoma cell tumor through inhibiting the enzyme activity of MMP-2 [75].

5. Anoikis regulation of circulating tumor cells

Anoikis, known as detachment-induced apoptosis, is a process of programmed cell death [76]. It can block metastasis by eliminating circulating cancer cells. However, in highly metastatic cancer cells, anoikis can be overcome and cancer cells can survive in a circulating condition until reaching a proper secondary site [77]. Anoikis is controlled by Bcl-2 family proteins. The pro-apoptotic proteins, such as Bax and the anti-apoptotic proteins, such as Bcl-2 and Bcl-xL, interact during anoikis [78]. In addition, anti-apoptotic protein myeloid leukemia cell sequence-1 (MCL-1) and caveolin-1 (CAV-1) have also been demonstrated to suppress anoikis [79]. Anoikis has become potential therapeutic target, and discovering new natural products obtained from Chinese medicines targeting anoikis is of great interest [80].

The anti-metastatic study of arctigenin on colorectal cancer has been recently conducted. Arctigenin can induce anoikis via MAPKs signaling, inhibit EMT through increasing E-cadherin and decreasing N-cadherin, vimentin, β-catenin, and Snail, and downregulate MMP-2/9, so that inhibition on the tumor cell migration and invasion both in vitro and in vivo was achieved [81]. Imperatorin, an active furanocoumarin component obtained from the root of *Angelica dahurica*, has been demonstrated to sensitize anoikis by downregulating Mcl-1 protein and upregulating Bax in lung cancer [82]. As a major dietary flavonoid, quercetin was reported to induce apoptosis through the MAPKs pathway, regulate EMT markers including E-, N-cadherin, β-catenin, and snail and modulate MMPs and TIMPs in colorectal cancer [83]. Curcumin, a compound derived from the rhizome of turmeric, was reported to inhibit the migratory and invasive ability of lung cancer cells through sensitizing anoikis, which was associated with downregulation of Bcl-2 [84]. Such anoikis regulation was also observed in lung cancer cells challenged other single compounds obtained from Chinese medicine, such as artonin E [85], ecteinascidin 770 [86], renieramycin M [87], Oroxylin A [88], and so on. In addition, regulation on anoikis was also observed in tumor cells treated with various extracts from Chinese medicines. Annona muricata Linn from Annonaceae family has long been applied to treat different diseases. Recently, its leaf aqueous extract (B1 AMCE) has been reported to exhibit anti-metastatic property in breast cancer [89]. B1 AMCE can significantly suppress the metastasis of 4T1 breast cancer cells in vitro and in vivo via inducing their apoptosis. The aqueous extract of *Andrographis paniculata* was demonstrated to inhibit anoikis resistance in esophageal cancer [89]. The bibenzyl compounds from *Dendrobium pulchellum*

[90] and the mixture of flavonoids extracted from Korean *Citrus aurantium* have been shown to induce apoptosis and inhibit metastasis of lung cancer cells [91].

6. Regulation of miRNA-mediated gene expression

As negative regulators of gene expression, microRNAs (miRNAs) have been shown to modulate multiple biological functions, such as immune response, metabolism, and metastasis [92]. miRNAs mediate the expression of target protein through degrading its mRNA or inhibiting the translation of mRNA via binding to mRNA three prime untranslated region (3'UTR). There is a dual action of miRNAs in cancers, either functioning as cancer promoters or inhibitors. Nearly, all human tumors have the characteristic of miRNAs dysregulation [93]. Since miRNAs play an important role in the metastatic behaviors of cancer cells, developing natural products obtained from Chinese medicines targeting miRNAs may be a promising strategy to treat metastatic cancers.

Recently, the anti-metastatic property of arsenic trioxide (ATO) in chondrosarcoma has been elucidated. It was reported that ATO attenuate the metastasis of chondrosarcoma cells through inhibit miR-125b/Stat3 axis [94]. As a common antioxidant obtained from cruciferous plants, sulforaphane has been reported to inhibit the migratory and invasive ability of lung cancer both in vitro and in vivo. This action is mediated by miR-616-5p [95]. In addition, ginsenoside Rd (Rd), one of the chemical compounds in Panax Notoginseng Saponins, has been investigated for its anti-metastatic property recently. The results showed that Rd treatment inhibited the migratory and invasive ability of breast cancer both in vitro and in vivo via suppressing miR-18a-mediated Smad2 expression [96].

7. Conclusion and future challenges

Accumulating evidence has demonstrated that Chinese medicine is an excellent source for the development of novel therapies for metastatic cancer. As mentioned above, the molecular mechanisms underlying the effects of potential anti-invasive and metastatic Chinese medicines include suppression of EMT (e.g., epithelial and mesenchymal markers), suppression of proteases expression (e.g., MMPs, uPA and Rho GTPases), suppression of cancer-induced angiogenesis (e.g., pro-angiogenic and anti-angiogenic factors), anoikis regulation of circulating tumor cells (e.g., pro-apoptotic and anti-apoptotic proteins), and regulation of miRNA-mediated gene expression (e.g., miR-125b, miR-616-5p and miR-18a). The chapter summarized the potential anti-invasive and metastatic drug candidates, which provided scientific evidence for clinically used Chinese medicines in the field of cancer therapy. Understanding of the underlying molecular mechanisms may in turn lead to discovery and development of novel anticancer drugs. Although these findings show the anti-metastatic potential of Chinese medicines, studies to evaluating the marked efficacies and determining the appropriate therapeutic doses of anti-metastatic Chinese medicines in animal models and clinical trials are still badly necessary in the future. In addition, the modern techniques such as nanoparticles which may improve the anti-cancer properties via better cellular uptake, enhanced bioavailability, and localization to targeted sites should also be studied in the future.

Acknowledgements

The study was financially supported by grants from the research council of the University of Hong Kong (Project Codes: 104003422, 104004092, 104004460), the Research Grants Committee (RGC) of Hong Kong, HKSAR (Project Codes: 764708, 766211, 17152116), Wong's Donation on Modern Oncology of Chinese Medicine (Project code: 200006276), Gala Family Trust (Project Code: 200007008), Government-Matching Grant Scheme (Project Code: 207060411) and Donation of Vita Green Health Products Co., Ltd. (Project cord: 200007477).

Author details

Wei Guo, Ning Wang and Yibin Feng*

*Address all correspondence to: yfeng@hku.hk

School of Chinese Medicine, Li Ka Shing Faculty of Medicine, The University of Hong Kong, China

References

[1] Siege RL, Miller KD and Jemal A. Cancer statistics. CA: A Cancer Journal for Clinicians. 2016;**66**:7-30. DOI: 10.3322/caac.21332

[2] Miller KD, Siegel RL, Lin CC, Mariotto AB, Kramer JL, Rowland JH, Stein KD, Alteri R and Jemal A. Cancer treatment and survivorship statistics. CA: A Cancer Journal for Clinicians. 2016;**66**:271-289. DOI: 10.3322/caac.21349

[3] Weiss RA and McMichael AJ. Social and environmental risk factors in the emergence of infectious diseases. Nature Medicine. 2004;**10**:S70-S76. DOI: 10.1038/nm1150

[4] Hanahan D and Weinberg RA. The hallmarks of cancer. Cell. 2000;**100**:57-70. DOI: 10.1016/S0092-8674(00)81683-9

[5] Hanahan D and Weinberg RA. Hallmarks of cancer: The next generation. Cell. 2011;**144**:646-674. DOI: 10.1016/j.cell.2011.02.013

[6] Kumar S and Weaver VM. Mechanics, malignancy, and metastasis: The force journey of a tumor cell. Cancer and Metastasis Reviews. 2009;**28**:113-127. DOI: 10.1007/s10555-008-9173-4

[7]   Chambers AF, Groom AC and MacDonald IC. Dissemination and growth of cancer cells in metastatic sites. Nature Reviews Cancer. 2002;**2**:563-572. DOI: 10.1038/nrc865

[8]   Sahai E. Mechanisms of cancer cell invasion. Current Opinion in Genetics & Development. 2005;**15**:87-96. DOI: 10.1016/j.gde.2004.12.002

[9]   Coghlin C and Murray GI. Current and emerging concepts in tumour metastasis. Journal of Pathology. 2010;**222**:1-15. DOI: 10.1002/path.2727

[10]   Brooks SA, Lomax-Browne HJ, Carter TM, Kinch CE and Hall DM. Molecular inter-actions in cancer cell metastasis. Acta Histochemica. 2010;**112**:3-25. DOI: 10.1016/j.acthis.2008.11.022

[11]   Helbig G, Christopherson KW, 2nd, Bhat-Nakshatri P, Kumar S, Kishimoto H, Miller KD, Broxmeyer HE and Nakshatri H. NF-kappaB promotes breast cancer cell migration and metastasis by inducing the expression of the chemokine receptor CXCR4. Journal of Biological Chemistry. 2003;**278**:21631-21638. DOI: 10.1074/jbc.M300609200

[12]   Liotta LA. An attractive force in metastasis. Nature. 2001;**410**:24-25. DOI: 10.1038/35065180

[13]   Mohammad NH, ter Veer E, Ngai L, Mali R, van Oijen MG and van Laarhoven HW. Optimal first-line chemotherapeutic treatment in patients with locally advanced or met-astatic esophagogastric carcinoma: Triplet versus doublet chemotherapy: A systematic literature review and meta-analysis. Cancer and Metastasis Reviews. 2015;**34**:429-441. DOI: 10.1007/s10555-015-9576-y

[14]   Liou SY, Stephens JM, Carpiuc KT, Feng W, Botteman MF and Hay JW. Economic bur-den of haematological adverse effects in cancer patients: A systematic review. Clinical Drug Investigation. 2007;**27**:381-396. DOI: 10.2165/00044011-200727060-00002

[15]   Park SI, Liao J, Berry JE, Li X, Koh AJ, Michalski ME, Eber MR, Soki FN, Sadler D, Sud S, Tisdelle S, Daignault SD, Nemeth JA, Snyder LA, Wronski TJ, Pienta KJ and McCauley LK. Cyclophosphamide creates a receptive microenvironment for prostate cancer skeletal metastasis. Cancer Research. 2012;**72**:2522-2532. DOI: 10.1158/0008-5472.CAN-11-2928

[16]   Daenen LG, Roodhart JM, van Amersfoort M, Dehnad M, Roessingh W, Ulfman LH, Derksen PW and Voest EE. Chemotherapy enhances metastasis formation via VEGFR-1-expressing endothelial cells. Cancer Research. 2011;**71**:6976-6985. DOI: 10.1158/0008-5472.CAN-11-0627

[17]   Feng Y, Wang N, Zhu M, Feng Y, Li H and Tsao S. Recent progress on anticancer can-didates in patents of herbal medicinal products. Recent Patents on Food, Nutrition & Agriculture. 2011;**3**:30-48. DOI: 10.2174/2212798411103010030

[18]   Cragg GM and Newman DJ. Plants as a source of anti-cancer agents. Journal of Ethnopharmacology. 2005;**100**:72-79. DOI: 10.1016/j.jep.2005.05.011

[19]   Liu TG, Xiong SQ, Yan Y, Zhu H and Yi C. Use of chinese herb medicine in cancer patients: A survey in southwestern china. Evidence-based Complementary and Alternative Medicine. 2012;**2012**:769042. DOI: 10.1155/2012/769042

[20] Yang G, Li X, Li X, Wang L, Li J, Song X, Chen J, Guo Y, Sun X, Wang S, Zhang Z, Zhou X and Liu J. Traditional chinese medicine in cancer care: A review of case series published in the chinese literature. Evidence-based Complementary and Alternative Medicine. 2012;**2012**:751046. DOI: 10.1155/2012/751046

[21] Kalluri R and Weinberg RA. The basics of epithelial-mesenchymal transition. Journal of Clinical Investigation. 2009;**119**:1420-1428. DOI: 10.1172/JCI39104

[22] Yang J and Weinberg RA. Epithelial-mesenchymal transition: At the crossroads of development and tumor metastasis. Developmental Cell. 2008;**14**:818-829. DOI: 10.1016/j.devcel.2008.05.009

[23] Iwatsuki M, Mimori K, Yokobori T, Ishi H, Beppu T, Nakamori S, Baba H and Mori M. Epithelial-mesenchymal transition in cancer development and its clinical significance. Cancer Science. 2010;**101**:293-299. DOI: 10.1111/j.1349-7006.2009.01419.x

[24] Thiery JP, Acloque H, Huang RY and Nieto MA. Epithelial-mesenchymal transitions in development and disease. Cell. 2009;**139**:871-890. DOI: 10.1016/j.cell.2009.11.007

[25] De Craene B and Berx G. Regulatory networks defining EMT during cancer initiation and progression. Nature Reviews Cancer. 2013;**13**:97-110. DOI: 10.1038/nrc3447

[26] Ko H. Geraniin inhibits TGF-beta1-induced epithelial-mesenchymal transition and suppresses A549 lung cancer migration, invasion and anoikis resistance. Bioorganic & Medicinal Chemistry Letters. 2015;**25**:3529-3534. DOI: 10.1016/j.bmcl.2015.06.093

[27] Chaotham C, Pongrakhananon V, Sritularak B and Chanvorachote P. A Bibenzyl from *Dendrobium ellipsophyllum* inhibits epithelial-to-mesenchymal transition and sensitizes lung cancer cells to anoikis. Anticancer Research. 2014;**34**:1931-1938

[28] Busaranon K, Plaimee P, Sritularak B and Chanvorachote P. Moscatilin inhibits epithelial-to-mesenchymal transition and sensitizes anoikis in human lung cancer H460 cells. Journal of Natural Medicines. 2016;**70**:18-27. DOI: 10.1007/s11418-015-0931-7

[29] Unahabhokha T, Chanvorachote P and Pongrakhananon V. The attenuation of epithelial to mesenchymal transition and induction of anoikis by gigantol in human lung cancer H460 cells. Tumour Biology. 2016;**37**:8633-8641. DOI: 10.1007/s13277-015-4717-z

[30] Huang SF, Horng CT, Hsieh YS, Hsieh YH, Chu SC and Chen PN. Epicatechin-3-gallate reverses TGF-beta1-induced epithelial-to-mesenchymal transition and inhibits cell invasion and protease activities in human lung cancer cells. Food and Chemical Toxicology. 2016;**94**:1-10. DOI: 10.1016/j.fct.2016.05.009

[31] Li Q, Wang Y, Xiao H, Li Y, Kan X, Wang X, Zhang G, Wang Z, Yang Q, Chen X, Weng X, Chen Y, Zhou B, Guo Y, Liu X and Zhu X. Chamaejasmenin B, a novel candidate, inhibits breast tumor metastasis by rebalancing TGF-beta paradox. Oncotarget. 2016;**7**:48180-48192. DOI: 10.18632/oncotarget.10193

[32] Venugopala KN, Govender R, Khedr MA, Venugopala R, Aldhubiab BE, Harsha S and Odhav B. Design, synthesis, and computational studies on dihydropyrimidine scaffolds

as potential lipoxygenase inhibitors and cancer chemopreventive agents. Drug Design, Development and Therapy. 2015;**9**:911-921. DOI: 10.2147/DDDT.S73890

[33] Shin VY, Jin HC, Ng EK, Sung JJ, Chu KM and Cho CH. Activation of 5-lipoxygenase is required for nicotine mediated epithelial-mesenchymal transition and tumor cell growth. Cancer Letters. 2010;**292**:237-245. DOI: 10.1016/j.canlet.2009.12.011

[34] Homma J, Yamanaka R, Yajima N, Tsuchiya N, Genkai N, Sano M and Tanaka R. Increased expression of CCAAT/enhancer binding protein beta correlates with prognosis in glioma patients. Oncology Reports. 2006;**15**:595-601. DOI: 10.3892/or.15.3.595

[35] Wang Q, Li H, Sun Z, Dong L, Gao L, Liu C and Wang X. Kukoamine A inhibits human glioblastoma cell growth and migration through apoptosis induction and epithelial-mesenchymal transition attenuation. Scientific Reports. 2016;**6**:36543. DOI: 10.1038/srep36543

[36] Chang CC, Ling XH, Hsu HF, Wu JM, Wang CP, Yang JF, Fang LW and Houng JY. *Siegesbeckia orientalis* extract inhibits TGFbeta1-induced migration and invasion of endometrial cancer cells. Molecules. 2016;**21**. DOI: 10.3390/molecules21081021

[37] Ko YS, Lee WS, Panchanathan R, Joo YN, Choi YH, Kim GS, Jung JM, Ryu CH, Shin SC and Kim HJ. Polyphenols from Artemisia annua L Inhibit Adhesion and EMT of Highly Metastatic Breast Cancer Cells MDA-MB-231. Phytotherapy Research. 2016;**30**:1180-1188. DOI: 10.1002/ptr.5626

[38] Leeman MF, Curran S and Murray GI. New insights into the roles of matrix metalloproteinases in colorectal cancer development and progression. Journal of Pathology. 2003;**201**:528-534. DOI: 10.1002/path.1466

[39] Lu S, Zhu Q, Zhang Y, Song W, Wilson MJ and Liu P. Dual-Functions of miR-373 and miR-520c by Differently Regulating the Activities of MMP2 and MMP9. Journal of Cellular Physiology. 2015;**230**:1862-1870. DOI: 10.1002/jcp.24914

[40] Huang Q, Lan F, Wang X, Yu Y, Ouyang X, Zheng F, Han J, Lin Y, Xie Y, Xie F, Liu W, Yang X, Wang H, Dong L, Wang L and Tan J. IL-1beta-induced activation of p38 promotes metastasis in gastric adenocarcinoma via upregulation of AP-1/c-fos, MMP2 and MMP9. Molecular Cancer. 2014;**13**:18. DOI: 10.1186/1476-4598-13-18

[41] Gomis-Ruth FX, Maskos K, Betz M, Bergner A, Huber R, Suzuki K, Yoshida N, Nagase H, Brew K, Bourenkov GP, Bartunik H and Bode W. Mechanism of inhibition of the human matrix metalloproteinase stromelysin-1 by TIMP-1. Nature. 1997;**389**:77-81. DOI: 10.1038/37995

[42] Raghu H, Sodadasu PK, Malla RR, Gondi CS, Estes N and Rao JS. Localization of uPAR and MMP-9 in lipid rafts is critical for migration, invasion and angiogenesis in human breast cancer cells. BMC Cancer. 2010;**10**:647. DOI: 10.1186/1471-2407-10-647

[43] Gardel ML, Schneider IC, Aratyn-Schaus Y and Waterman CM. Mechanical integration of actin and adhesion dynamics in cell migration. Annual Review of Cell and Developmental Biology. 2010;**26**:315-333. DOI: 10.1146/annurev.cellbio.011209.122036

[44] Vega FM and Ridley AJ. Rho GTPases in cancer cell biology. FEBS Letters. 2008;**582**:2093-2101. DOI: 10.1016/j.febslet.2008.04.039

[45] Ridley AJ. Rho GTPases and cell migration. Journal of Cell Science. 2001;**114**:2713-2722

[46] Maxwell T, Chun SY, Lee KS, Kim S and Nam KS. The anti-metastatic effects of the phytoestrogen arctigenin on human breast cancer cell lines regardless of the status of ER expression. International Journal of Oncology. 2017;**50**:727-735. DOI: 10.3892/ijo.2016.3825

[47] Jiang K, Lu Q, Li Q, Ji Y, Chen W and Xue X. Astragaloside IV inhibits breast cancer cell invasion by suppressing Vav3 mediated Rac1/MAPK signaling. International Immunopharmacology. 2017;**42**:195-202. DOI: 10.1016/j.intimp.2016.10.001

[48] Lee CY, Hsieh SL, Hsieh S, Tsai CC, Hsieh LC, Kuo YH and Wu CC. Inhibition of human colorectal cancer metastasis by notoginsenoside R1, an important compound from Panax notoginseng. Oncology Reports. 2017;**37**:399-407. DOI: 10.3892/or.2016.5222

[49] Lin CL, Hsieh SL, Leung W, Jeng JH, Huang GC, Lee CT and Wu CC. 2,3,5,4'-tetra-hydroxystilbene-2-O-beta-D-glucoside suppresses human colorectal cancer cell metastasis through inhibiting NF-kappaB activation. International Journal of Oncology. 2016;**49**:629-638. DOI: 10.3892/ijo.2016.3574

[50] Huang H, Du T, Xu G, Lai Y, Fan X, Chen X, Li W, Yue F, Li Q, Liu L and Li K. Matrine suppresses invasion of castration-resistant prostate cancer cells by downregulating MMP-2/9 via NF-kappaB signaling pathway. International Journal of Oncology. 2017;**50**:640-648. DOI: 10.3892/ijo.2016.3805

[51] Lin CC, Chen CC, Kuo YH, Kuo JT, Senthil Kumar KJ and Wang SY. 2,3,5-Trimethoxy-4-cresol, an anti-metastatic constituent from the solid-state cultured mycelium of Antrodia cinnamomea and its mechanism. Journal of Natural Medicines. 2015;**69**:513-521. DOI: 10.1007/s11418-015-0916-6

[52] Farha AK, Dhanya SR, Mangalam SN and Remani P. Anti-metastatic effect of deoxyelephantopin from *Elephantopus scaber* in A549 lung cancer cells in vitro. Natural Product Research. 2015;**29**:2341-2345. DOI: 10.1080/14786419.2015.1012165

[53] Wu SH, Hsiao YT, Kuo CL, Yu FS, Hsu SC, Wu PP, Chen JC, Hsia TC, Liu HC, Hsu WH and Chung JG. Bufalin inhibits NCI-H460 human lung cancer cell metastasis in vitro by inhibiting MAPKs, MMPs, and NF-kappaB pathways. American Journal of Chinese Medicine. 2015;**43**:1247-1264. DOI: 10.1142/S0192415X15500718

[54] Wang N, Zhu M, Tsao SW, Man K, Zhang Z and Feng Y. Up-regulation of TIMP-1 by genipin inhibits MMP-2 activities and suppresses the metastatic potential of human hepatocellular carcinoma. PLoS One. 2012;**7**:e46318. DOI: 10.1371/journal.pone.0046318

[55] Wang N, Tan HY, Li L, Yuen MF and Feng Y. Berberine and Coptidis Rhizoma as potential anticancer agents: Recent updates and future perspectives. Journal of Ethnopharmacology. 2015;**176**:35-48. DOI: 10.1016/j.jep.2015.10.028

[56] Tsang CM, Lau EP, Di K, Cheung PY, Hau PM, Ching YP, Wong YC, Cheung AL, Wan TS, Tong Y, Tsao SW and Feng Y. Berberine inhibits Rho GTPases and cell migration at low doses but induces G2 arrest and apoptosis at high doses in human cancer cells. International Journal of Molecular Medicine. 2009;24:131-138. DOI: 10.3892/ijmm_00000216

[57] Becker MS, Muller PM, Bajorat J, Schroeder A, Giaisi M, Amin E, Ahmadian MR, Rocks O, Kohler R, Krammer PH and Li-Weber M. The anticancer phytochemical rocaglamide inhibits Rho GTPase activity and cancer cell migration. Oncotarget. 2016;7:51908-51921. DOI: 10.18632/oncotarget.10188

[58] Chang PY, Hsieh MJ, Hsieh YS, Chen PN, Yang JS, Lo FC, Yang SF and Lu KH. Tricetin inhibits human osteosarcoma cells metastasis by transcriptionally repressing MMP-9 via p38 and Akt pathways. Environmental Toxicology. 2016;Nov 8. DOI: 10.1002/tox.22380

[59] Cheng HL, Hsieh MJ, Yang JS, Lin CW, Lue KH, Lu KH and Yang SF. Nobiletin inhibits human osteosarcoma cells metastasis by blocking ERK and JNK-mediated MMPs expression. Oncotarget. 2016;7:35208-35223. DOI: 10.18632/oncotarget.9106

[60] Lin CM, Lin YL, Ho SY, Chen PR, Tsai YH, Chung CH, Hwang CH, Tsai NM, Tzou SC, Ke CY, Chang J, Chan YL, Wang YS, Chi KH and Liao KW. The inhibitory effect of 7, 7″-dimethoxyagastisflavone on the metastasis of melanoma cells via the suppression of F-actin polymerization. Oncotarget. 2016;Jul 30. DOI: 10.18632/oncotarget.10960

[61] Shin SY, Kim CG, Jung YJ, Jung Y, Jung H, Im J, Lim Y and Lee YH. *Euphorbia humifusa* Willd exerts inhibition of breast cancer cell invasion and metastasis through inhibition of TNFalpha-induced MMP-9 expression. BMC Complementary and Alternative Medicine. 2016;16:413. DOI: 10.1186/s12906-016-1404-6

[62] Chung TW, Choi H, Lee JM, Ha SH, Kwak CH, Abekura F, Park JY, Chang YC, Ha KT, Cho SH, Chang HW, Lee YC and Kim CH. *Oldenlandia diffusa* suppresses metastatic potential through inhibiting matrix metalloproteinase-9 and intercellular adhesion molecule-1 expression via p38 and ERK1/2 MAPK pathways and induces apoptosis in human breast cancer MCF-7 cells. Journal of Ethnopharmacology. 2017;195:309-317. DOI: 10.1016/j.jep.2016.11.036

[63] Carmeliet P and Jain RK. Angiogenesis in cancer and other diseases. Nature. 2000;407:249-257. DOI: 10.1038/35025220

[64] Tonini T, Rossi F and Claudio PP. Molecular basis of angiogenesis and cancer. Oncogene. 2003;22:6549-6556. DOI: 10.1038/sj.onc.1206816

[65] Eichhorn ME, Kleespies A, Angele MK, Jauch KW and Bruns CJ. Angiogenesis in cancer: Molecular mechanisms, clinical impact. Langenbeck's Archives of Surgery. 2007;392:371-379. DOI: 10.1007/s00423-007-0150-0

[66] Baeriswyl V and Christofori G. The angiogenic switch in carcinogenesis. Seminars in Cancer Biology. 2009;19:329-337. DOI: 10.1016/j.semcancer.2009.05.003

[67] Wang X, Wang N, Li H, Liu M, Cao F, Yu X, Zhang J, Tan Y, Xiang L and Feng Y. Up-regulation of PAI-1 and down-regulation of uPA are involved in suppression of invasiveness and motility of hepatocellular carcinoma cells by a natural compound berberine. International Journal of Molecular Sciences. 2016;**17**:577. DOI: 10.3390/ijms17040577

[68] Tsang CM, Cheung KC, Cheung YC, Man K, Lui VW, Tsao SW and Feng Y. Berberine suppresses Id-1 expression and inhibits the growth and development of lung metastases in hepatocellular carcinoma. Biochimica et Biophysica Acta. 2015;**1852**:541-551. DOI: 10.1016/j.bbadis.2014.12.004

[69] Sinha S, Khan S, Shukla S, Lakra AD, Kumar S, Das G, Maurya R and Meeran SM. Cucurbitacin B inhibits breast cancer metastasis and angiogenesis through VEGF-mediated suppression of FAK/MMP-9 signaling axis. International Journal of Biochemistry & Cell Biology. 2016;**77**:41-56. DOI: 10.1016/j.biocel.2016.05.014

[70] Zhang L, Qian H, Sha M, Luan Z, Lin M, Yuan D, Li X, Huang J and Ye L. Downregulation of HOTAIR expression mediated anti-metastatic effect of artesunate on cervical cancer by inhibiting COX-2 expression. PLoS One. 2016;**11**:e0164838. DOI: 10.1371/journal.pone.0164838

[71] Wang N, Feng Y, Lau EP, Tsang C, Ching Y, Man K, Tong Y, Nagamatsu T, Su W and Tsao S. F-actin reorganization and inactivation of rho signaling pathway involved in the inhibitory effect of Coptidis Rhizoma on hepatoma cell migration. Integrative Cancer Therapies. 2010;**9**:354-364. DOI: 10.1177/1534735410379121

[72] Tan HY, Wang N, Tsao SW, Zhang Z and Feng Y. Suppression of vascular endothelial growth factor via inactivation of eukaryotic elongation factor 2 by alkaloids in Coptidis rhizome in hepatocellular carcinoma. Integrative Cancer Therapies. 2014;**13**:425-434. DOI: 10.1177/1534735413513635

[73] Im M, Kim A and Ma JY. Ethanol extract of baked Gardeniae Fructus exhibits in vitro and in vivo anti-metastatic and anti-angiogenic activities in malignant cancer cells: Role of suppression of the NF-kappaB and HIF-1alpha pathways. International Journal of Oncology. 2016;**49**:2377-2386. DOI: 10.3892/ijo.2016.3742

[74] Kim A, Im M, Gu MJ and Ma JY. Ethanol extract of Lophatheri Herba exhibits anti-cancer activity in human cancer cells by suppression of metastatic and angiogenic potential. Scientific Reports. 2016;**6**:36277. DOI: 10.1038/srep36277

[75] Wang N, Feng Y, Cheung F, Wang X, Zhang Z and Feng Y. A Chinese medicine formula Gegen Qinlian decoction suppresses expansion of human renal carcinoma with inhibition of matrix metalloproteinase-2. Integrative Cancer Therapies. 2015;**14**:75-85. DOI: 10.1177/1534735414550036

[76] Chiarugi P and Giannoni E. Anoikis: A necessary death program for anchorage-dependent cells. Biochemical Pharmacology. 2008;**76**:1352-1364. DOI: 10.1016/j.bcp.2008.07.023

[77] Guadamillas MC, Cerezo A and Del Pozo MA. Overcoming anoikis--pathways to anchorage-independent growth in cancer. Journal of Cell Science. 2011;**124**:3189-3197. DOI: 10.1242/jcs.072165

[78] Fulda S and Debatin KM. Extrinsic versus intrinsic apoptosis pathways in anticancer chemotherapy. Oncogene. 2006;**25**:4798-4811. DOI: 10.1038/sj.onc.1209608

[79] Chunhacha P, Pongrakhananon V, Rojanasakul Y and Chanvorachote P. Caveolin-1 regulates Mcl-1 stability and anoikis in lung carcinoma cells. American Journal of Physiology. Cell Physiology. 2012;**302**:C1284-C1292. DOI: 10.1152/ajpcell.00318.2011

[80] Wang N and Feng Y. Elaborating the role of natural products-induced autophagy in cancer treatment: Achievements and artifacts in the state of the art. BioMed Research International. 2015;**2015**:934207. DOI: 10.1155/2015/934207

[81] Han YH, Kee JY, Kim DS, Mun JG, Jeong MY, Park SH, Choi BM, Park SJ, Kim HJ, Um JY and Hong SH. Arctigenin inhibits lung metastasis of colorectal cancer by regulating cell viability and metastatic phenotypes. Molecules. 2016;**21**. DOI: 10.3390/molecules21091135

[82] Choochuay K, Chunhacha P, Pongrakhananon V, Luechapudiporn R and Chanvorachote P. Imperatorin sensitizes anoikis and inhibits anchorage-independent growth of lung cancer cells. Journal of Natural Medicines. 2013;**67**:599-606. DOI: 10.1007/s11418-012-0719-y

[83] Kee JY, Han YH, Kim DS, Mun JG, Park J, Jeong MY, Um JY and Hong SH. Inhibitory effect of quercetin on colorectal lung metastasis through inducing apoptosis, and suppression of metastatic ability. Phytomedicine. 2016;**23**:1680-1690. DOI: 10.1016/j.phymed.2016.09.011

[84] Pongrakhananon V, Nimmannit U, Luanpitpong S, Rojanasakul Y and Chanvorachote P. Curcumin sensitizes non-small cell lung cancer cell anoikis through reactive oxygen species-mediated Bcl-2 downregulation. Apoptosis. 2010;**15**:574-585. DOI: 10.1007/s10495-010-0461-4

[85] Wongpankam E, Chunhacha P, Pongrakhananon V, Sritularak B and Chanvorachote P. Artonin E mediates MCL1 down-regulation and sensitizes lung cancer cells to anoikis. Anticancer Research. 2012;**32**:5343-5351

[86] Powan P, Saito N, Suwanborirux K and Chanvorachote P. Ecteinascidin 770, a tetrahydroisoquinoline alkaloid, sensitizes human lung cancer cells to anoikis. Anticancer Research. 2013;**33**:505-512

[87] Sirimangkalakitti N, Chamni S, Suwanborirux K and Chanvorachote P. Renieramycin M sensitizes anoikis-resistant H460 lung cancer cells to anoikis. Anticancer Research. 2016;**36**:1665-1671

[88] Wei L, Dai Q, Zhou Y, Zou M, Li Z, Lu N and Guo Q. Oroxylin A sensitizes non-small cell lung cancer cells to anoikis via glucose-deprivation-like mechanisms: c-Src and hexokinase II. Biochimica et Biophysica Acta. 2013;**1830**:3835-3845. DOI: 10.1016/j.bbagen.2013.03.009

[89] Syed Najmuddin SU, Romli MF, Hamid M, Alitheen NB and Nik Abd Rahman NM. Anti-cancer effect of Annona Muricata Linn Leaves Crude Extract (AMCE) on breast cancer cell line. BMC Complement Altern Med. 2016;**16**:311. DOI: 10.1186/s12906-016-1290-y

[90] Chanvorachote P, Kowitdamrong A, Ruanghirun T, Sritularak B, Mungmee C and Likhitwitayawuid K. Anti-metastatic activities of bibenzyls from *Dendrobium pulchellum*. Natural Products Communications. 2013;**8**:115-118

[91] Park KI, Park HS, Kim MK, Hong GE, Nagappan A, Lee HJ, Yumnam S, Lee WS, Won CK, Shin SC and Kim GS. Flavonoids identified from Korean *Citrus aurantium* L. inhibit non-small cell lung Cancer growth in vivo and in vitro. Journal of Functional Foods. 2014;**7**:287-297. DOI: 10.1016/j.jff.2014.01.032

[92] Chen PS, Su JL and Hung MC. Dysregulation of microRNAs in cancer. Journal of Biomedical Science. 2012;**19**:90. DOI: 10.1186/1423-0127-19-90

[93] Tili E, Michaille JJ and Croce CM. MicroRNAs play a central role in molecular dysfunctions linking inflammation with cancer. Immunology Reviews. 2013;**253**:167-184. DOI: 10.1111/imr.12050

[94] Bao X, Ren T, Huang Y, Wang S, Zhang F, Liu K, Zheng B and Guo W. Induction of the mesenchymal to epithelial transition by demethylation-activated microRNA-125b is involved in the anti-migration/invasion effects of arsenic trioxide on human chondro-sarcoma. Journal of Experimental & Clinical Cancer Research. 2016;**35**:129. DOI: 10.1186/s13046-016-0407-y

[95] Wang DX, Zou YJ, Zhuang XB, Chen SX, Lin Y, Li WL, Lin JJ and Lin ZQ. Sulforaphane suppresses EMT and metastasis in human lung cancer through miR-616-5p-mediated GSK3beta/beta-catenin signaling pathways. Acta Pharmacologica Sinica. 2017;**38**:241-251. DOI: 10.1038/aps.2016.122

[96] Wang P, Du X, Xiong M, Cui J, Yang Q, Wang W, Chen Y and Zhang T. Ginsenoside Rd attenuates breast cancer metastasis implicating derepressing microRNA-18a-regulated Smad2 expression. Scientific Reports. 2016;**6**:33709. DOI: 10.1038/srep33709

3

Computational Studies and Biosynthesis of Natural Products with Promising Anticancer Properties

Aurélien F.A. Moumbock, Conrad V. Simoben,

Ludger Wessjohann, Wolfgang Sippl,

Stefan Günther and Fidele Ntie-Kang

Abstract

We present an overview of computational approaches for the prediction of metabolic pathways by which plants biosynthesise compounds, with a focus on selected very promising anticancer secondary metabolites from floral sources. We also provide an overview of databases for the retrieval of useful genomic data, discussing the strengths and limitations of selected prediction software and the main computational tools (and methods), which could be employed for the investigation of the uncharted routes towards the biosynthesis of some of the identified anticancer metabolites from plant sources, eventually using specific examples to address some knowledge gaps when using these approaches.

Keywords: anticancer, biosynthesis, computational prediction, natural products, plant metabolism

1. Introduction

An immense number of secondary metabolites (SMs) exist in nature, originating from plants, bacteria, fungi and marine life forms, serving as drugs for the treatment of many life-threatening diseases, including cancer [1–4]. Taxol, vinblastine, vincristine, podophyllotoxin and camptothecin, for example, are typically well-known drugs used in cancer treatment, which are of plant origin. The search for drugs against cancer has often resorted to plants and marine life for lead compounds. To illustrate this, Newmann and Cragg published a recent study in which it was shown that ~49% of drugs used in cancer treatment were either natural products

(NPs) or their derivatives [5]. We would henceforth refer to SMs and NPs interchangeably, since NPs are the products of secondary (or specialised) metabolism, as opposed to primary metabolism, which results in molecules playing a key role in physiological processes of the organism and are thus necessary for the plant's survival. It should be mentioned that SMs are important for the plant's defence against attacks by other organisms. Several efforts have also been made towards the collection of data on naturally occurring plant metabolites showing anticancer properties. As an example, Mangal and co-workers published the naturally occurring plant-based anti-cancer compound activity-target database (NPACT), containing about 1,500 NPs [6]. In addition to the experimentally verified *in vitro* and *in vivo* data for these NPs, the authors also include biological activities (in the form of IC_{50}s, ED_{50}s, EC_{50}s, GI_{50}s, etc.), along with physical, elemental and topological properties of the NPs, the tested cancer types, cell lines, protein targets, commercial suppliers and drug likeness of the NPACT compounds. A similar effort was published the following year, for NPs from African flora, resulting in a dataset of about 400 compounds, named AfroCancer [7]. A further study showed that the NPACT and AfroCancer datasets showed little intersection, thus providing us a combined dataset of about 2,000 NPs [8]. The anticancer properties of some of the most promising AfroCancer compounds have been described in detail in recent reviews [9–12]. Further curation of data from Northern African species has recently resulted in the Northern African Natural Products Database (NANPDB), a web accessible and completely downloadable vast database of NPs, with a significant proportion of anticancer metabolites [13]. The NANPDB effort was founded on the observation that the Northern Africa region is particularly highly endowed with diverse vegetation types, serving as a huge reservoir of bioactive natural products [14–16].

For decades, NPs were identified exclusively by using chemical identification based on bio-activity-guided screening approaches. Recently, it has been postulated that genomics and bioinformatics would transform the approach of natural products discovery, even though genome mining has had only little influence on the advancement of natural product discovery until now [17]. Several algorithms have been developed for the mining of the (meta)genomic data, which continue to be generated. Computational methods and tools for the identification of biosynthetic gene clusters (BGCs, which are physically clustered groups of a few genes in a particular genome that together encode a biosynthetic pathway for the production of a specialised metabolite) in genome sequences and the prediction of chemical structures of their products have been developed [18]. BGCs for SM biosynthetic pathways are important in bacteria and filamentous fungi, with examples being recently discovered in plants [19, 20], although some metabolic processes in plants, for example, the thalianol pathway for triterpene synthesis in *Arabidopsis thaliana* has been suggested to be controlled by operon-like (clusters of unrelated) gene clusters [21]. This, coupled with the rapid progress in sequencing technologies has led to the development of new screening methods, which focus on whole genome sequences of the organisms producing the NPs. Genome mining approaches for NP discovery basically focus on:

- identifying the genes of the organism involved in the biosynthesis of the NPs,

- identifying the metabolic pathways by which the NPs are biosynthesised and

- predicting the products of the identified pathways (**Figure 1A**).

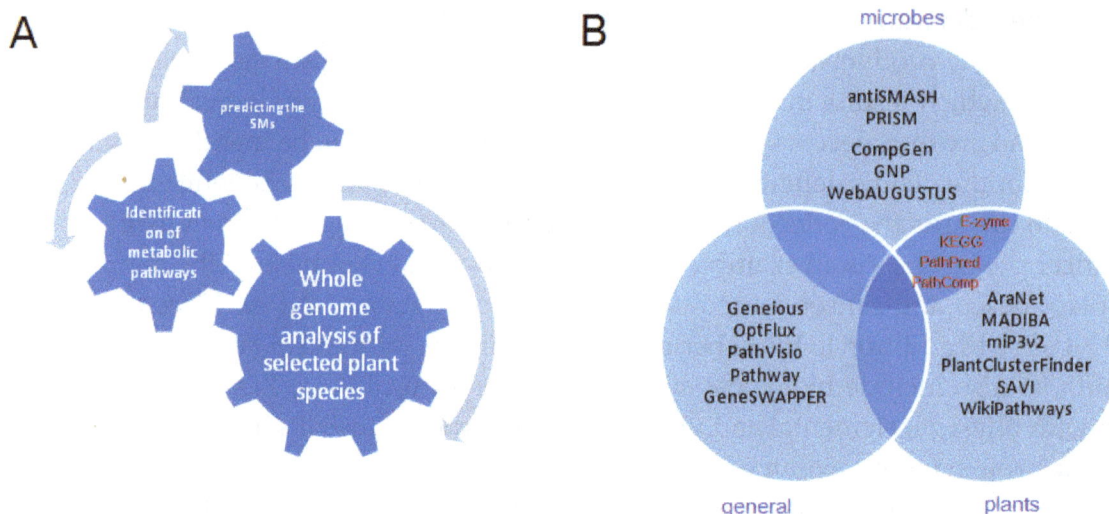

Figure 1. (A) Summary of genome mining approaches for the discovery of SMs and (B) classification of tools by applicability domain.

The four main strategies that are mostly employed to identify such pathways are based on processes involved in the production of plant secondary metabolites, for example, physical clustering, co-expression, evolutionary co-occurrence and epigenomic co-regulation of the genes [22–25]. Such approaches have been successfully applied for the investigation of fungal and microbial metabolites [26–28]. Since the discovery of the first gene cluster for secondary metabolism in *Zea mays*, the corn species [29], BGCs for plant secondary metabolism have become an emerging theme in plant biology [30]. It is even believed that synthetic biology technologies will eventually lead to the effective functional reconstitution of candidate pathways using a variety of genetic systems [25]. A knowledge of BGCs and their manipulation is therefore important in understanding how to activate a number of 'silent' gene clusters observed from the investigation of whole-genome sequencing of organisms. This would make available a wealth of new chemical entities (NCEs), which could be evaluated as drug leads and biologically active compounds [20].

This chapter aims at discussing the metabolic pathways by which plants biosynthesise compounds with anticancer activities, with a focus on selected very promising anticancer SMs from the African flora. We also aim to provide an overview of computational tools, which have been used to predict metabolic pathways and eventually address knowledge gaps when using the former. Additionally, we will present some databases for the retrieval of useful genomic data, discuss the strengths and limitations of selected computational (prediction) tools, which could be employed for the investigation of the uncharted routes towards the biosynthesis of some of the identified anticancer metabolites from plant sources, with specific examples. It is believed that properly addressing knowledge gaps that exist would lay the foundation for proper future investigations.

2. Natural products and plant genomic data

Genome data mining indicates that the vast majority of plant-based NPs have not yet been discovered [24, 25]. In addition, SMs are normally produced only at later growth stages of plant metabolism and are frequently found only at low concentrations within complex mixtures in plant extracts, due to several factors. Some of these factors include physiological variations, geographic variations, environmental conditions and genetic factors [25, 31, 32]. The aforementioned factors are the main drawbacks in the isolation and purification of NPs in meaningful quantities for either research or commercial aims. Nowadays, BGCs can be investigated using computational methodologies and used to predict the NPs present in microbial, fungal and floral matter [18, 20, 33, 34]. It is current knowledge that more than 70 genome sequences for several plant species have been made available, along with a wealth of transcriptome data [25]. However, the interpretation of such data, for example, the translation of predicted sequences into enzymes, pathways and SMs remains challenging. Advances in bioinformatics and synthetic biology have permitted the cheap and efficient overproduction of secondary metabolites of medicinal interest in heterologous (non-native) host organisms by reengineering of BGCs [35]. This is carried out through reengineering of BGCs as well as the activation of silent BGCs to yield unreported natural products of the target chemical space [17, 36], for example, an engineered *Escherichia coli* strain was used as the heterologous host organism for the production of taxadiene (a vital precursor of paclitaxel, an anticancer agent isolated from the bark of *Taxus brevifolia*), a precursor of the anticancer agent taxol [37]. In this way, quite a number of interesting SMs of plant origin (e.g. resveratrol, vanillin, conolidin, etc.) have been objects of pathway engineering in bacteria, yeast and other plants [38]. Thus, chemical libraries of diverse and novel hybrid natural products analogues can now be generated through combinatorial biosynthesis by manipulation of biosynthetic enzymes [39], for example, several analogues of the antibiotic erythromycin were obtained *via* combinatorial biosynthesis [40]. Such bioengineered libraries of 'unnatural' natural products show promises in drug discovery campaigns against multidrug-resistant cancer cells.

3. Some database resources for retrieving secondary metabolism prediction information

A summary of databases for retrieving information on BGCs is provided in **Table 1**. A majority of them focus on microbial BGCs, for example, ClusterMine360, ClustScan, DoBISCUIT, IMG-ABC and the Recombinant ClustScan Database. Details on the utility of the aforementioned databases have been provided in excellent recent reviews [26–28, 53]. Further efforts towards the construction of plant-based BGC and genomic databases include those of the Medicinal Plants Genomics and Metabolomics Resource consortium [47]. This effort has been focused on 14 medicinal plants and includes a BLAST search module, a genome browser, a genome putative search function tool and transcriptome search tools. While the entire database is available for download, similar efforts from the Plant Metabolic Network (PMN) have the advantage of having included several plant metabolic pathway databases, mostly among food crops [49, 50]. The PMN, for example, currently houses one multi-species reference database called PlantCyc and 22 species/taxon-specific databases, providing access to manually curated and/or computationally predicted information about enzymes, pathways, and more for individual species.

Database	Description	Web accessibility	Advantages	Disadvantages	Reference
ClusterMine360	A database of microbial polyketide and non-ribosomal peptide gene clusters.	http://www.clustermine360.ca/	Users can make contributions. Automation leads to high data consistency and quality data.	Focuses only on microbial PKS/NRPS biosynthesis	[41, 42]
ClustScan Database	A database for *in silico* detection of promising new compounds.	http://csdb.bioserv.pbf.hr/csdb/ClustScanWeb.html	Allows easy extraction of DNA and protein sequences of polypeptides, modules, and domains.	Currently includes data for only 57 SMs (PKS), 51 SMs (NRPS) and 62 SMs (PKS-NRPS hybrid) biosynthesis.	[43, 44]
DoBISCUIT	A database of secondary metabolite biosynthetic gene clusters.	http://www.bio.nite.go.jp/pks/	Provides standardised gene/module/domain descriptions related to the gene clusters. Available for download	Contains mostly data relating to bacterial species, mostly of the genus *Streptomyces*.	[45]
GenomeNet	A network of databases and computational services for genome research and related research areas in biomedical sciences.	http://www.genome.jp/	Provides several web accessible tools, e.g. KEGG, E-zyme, etc. See **Table 2**.		
IMG-ABC	A knowledge base for biosynthetic gene clusters for the discovery of novel SMs.	https://img.jgi.doe.gov/cgi-bin/abc-public/main.cgi	Integrates structural and functional genomics with annotated BGCs and associated SMs.	Not available for download. Limited to data on microbes	[46]
Medicinal Plants Genomics Resource	A database for medicinal plants genome sequence data.	http://medicinalplantgenomics.msu.edu/	Available for download	Only genomic data for 14 species are currently available.	[47]
Medicinal Plants Metabolomics Resource	A database for medicinal plants metabolomics data.	http://metnetweb.gdcb.iastate.edu/mpmr_public/	Available for download	Currently limited to metabolite data for 2 medicinal plant species.	[48]

Database	Description	Web accessibility	Advantages	Disadvantages	Reference
Minimum Information about a Biosynthetic Gene cluster (MIBiG)	A community standard for annotations and metadata on biosynthetic gene clusters and their molecular products.	http://mibig. secondarymetabolites.org/ index.html	Facilitates the standardised deposition and retrieval of biosynthetic gene cluster data. Useful for the development of comprehensive comparative analysis tools. Available for download		[18]
Plant Metabolic Network (PMN)	Several plant metabolic pathway databases.	http://www.plantcyc.org/	Includes species/taxon-specific data for more than 22 plant species.		[49, 50]
Plant Reactome/"Cyc" Pathways	A pathway database for several crops and model plant species.	http://gramene.org/ pathways	Currently includes gene homology-based pathway projections to 62 plant species.		[51]
Recombinant ClustScan Database	A database of gene cluster recombinants and their corresponding chemical structures.	http://csdb.bioserv.pbf.hr/ csdb/RCSDB.html	Provides a virtual compound library, which could be a useful resource for computer-aided drug design of pharmaceutically relevant chemical entities.	Currently contains only 47 cluster combinations	[44, 52]
SMBP	Secondary metabolites bioinformatics portal.	http://www. secondarymetabolites.org/	Includes hand-curated links to all major tools and databases commonly used in the field		[53]

Table 1. Summary of currently available database resources for retrieving genomic data for biosynthesis prediction.

It provides a broad network of plant metabolic pathway databases that contain curated information from the literature and computational analyses about the genes, enzymes, compounds, reactions and pathways involved in primary and secondary metabolism in the included plant species. The PlantCyc database also provides access to manually curated or reviewed information about shared and unique metabolic pathways present in over 350 plant species. On the other hand, Plant Reactome is a pathway database for several crops and model plant species, making use of a framework of a eukaryotic cell model. Currently, it uses rice as a reference species and gene homology-based pathway projections have been made to 62 plant species [51].

4. Some computational tools for the analysis of genomic data and specialised metabolism prediction

Some computational tools for biochemical pathway prediction have been summarised in excellent reviews [54]. We have provided a more detailed summary of the main tools that could be useful in analysing plant and microbial genomic data for metabolism prediction in **Table 2**. Some of the tools are designed for the detection and analysis of specialised metabolism in microbes (e.g. antiSMASH, CompGen, GNP, PRISM and WebAUGUSTUS). Others are specially designed for plant metabolism prediction or may only include data for some specific organisms (e.g. AraNet, MADIBA, miP3v2, PlantClusterFinder, SAVI and WikiPathways for plants), while others are more general tools, useful for both microbial and plant metabolism prediction and BGC analysis (e.g. E-zyme, KEGG, PathPred and PathComp) and others are more useful for developers (e.g. Geneious, OptFlux, PathVisio and Pathway GeneSWAPPER), **Figure 1B**. We could also classify the tools according to their respective tasks; prediction and analysis of BGCs (e.g. antiSMASH, MADIBA, Pathway GeneSWAPPER, WebAUGUSTUS), searching, visualisation and prediction of biosynthetic pathways and reaction paths (e.g. BioCyc, CycSim, FMM, GNP, KEGG, MetaCyc, PathComp, PathPred, PathSearch, PathVisio, Pathway GeneSWAPPER, PlantClusterFinder, SAVI, WikiPathways for plants), prediction of SMs (PRISM), metabolic engineering (OptFlux), other functions (miP3v2). Among the tools for specialised metabolism in plants, AraNet is a probabilistic functional gene network (with currently a total of 27,029 protein-encoding genes) of *A. thaliana*. It is based on a modified Bayesian integration of data from multiple organisms, each data type being weighted based on how well it links genes that are known to function together in *A. thaliana*. Each interaction is associated with a log-likelihood score (LLS), which is a measure of the probability of an interaction representing a true functional linkage between two genes [56]. On the other hand, MADIBA facilitates the interpretation of *Plasmodium* and plant (data currently available for *Oryza sativa* and *A. thaliana*) gene clusters [64]. This tool eases the task by automating the post-processing stage during the assignment of biological meaning to gene expression clusters. MADIBA is designed as a relational database and has stored data from gene to pathway for the aforementioned species. Tools within the GUI allow the rapid analyses of each cluster with the view of identifying the Gene Ontology terms, as well as visualising the metabolic pathways where the genes are implicated, their genomic localisations, putative common

Tool	Utility	Web accessibility	Advantage	Disadvantage	Reference
antiSMASH*	A web server and tool for the automatic genomic identification and analysis of biosynthetic gene clusters.	http://antismash. secondarymetabolites.org.	Detects putative gene clusters of unknown types. Identifies similarities of identified clusters to any of 1172 clusters with known end products, etc.	Designed for analysis of BGCs in microbes.	[55]
AraNet	Gene function identification and genetic dissection of plant traits.	http://www.functionalnet. org/aranet/	Had greater precision than literature-based protein interactions (21%) for 55% of tested genes. Is highly predictive for diverse biological pathways.	Applicability is limited to one species - *A. thaliana*.	[56]
BioCyc/CycSim/ MetaCyc	Online tools for genome-scale metabolic modelling.	https://biocyc.org/http:// www.genoscope.cns.fr/ cycsim https://metacyc.org/	Support the design and simulation of knockout experiments, e.g. deletions mutants on specified media, etc.		[57, 58]
CompGen	Carry out *in silico* homologous recombination between gene clusters.	http://csdb.bioserv.pbf.hr/ csdb/RCSDB.html		Focuses on gene clusters encoding PKSs in *Streptomyces* sp. and related bacterial genera.	[52]
E-zyme	Assignment of EC numbers.	http://www.genome.jp/ tools/e-zyme/	Classifies enzymatic reactions and links the enzyme genes or proteins to reactions in metabolic pathways.		[59]
From Metabolite to metabolite (FMM)	A web server to find biosynthetic routes between two metabolites within the KEGG database.	http://FMM.mbc.nctu.edu.tw/	Both local and global graphical views of the metabolic pathways are designed.		[60]
Geneious	Organisation and analysis of sequence data.	http://www.geneious.com/ basic	Includes a public application programming interface (API) available for developers. Freely available for download.		[61]
Genomes-to-Natural Products platform (GNP)	Prediction, combinatorial design and identification of PKs and NRPs from biosynthetic assembly lines.	http://magarveylab.ca/gnp/	Uses LC–MS/MS data of crude extracts to make predictions in a high-throughput manner.	Focuses on bacterial NPs.	[62]

Tool	Utility	Web accessibility	Advantage	Disadvantage	Reference
Gene Regulatory network inference ACcuracy Enhancement (GRACE)	An algorithm to enhance the accuracy of transcriptional gene regulatory networks.	https://dpb.carnegiescience.edu/labs/rhee-lab/software	Focuses on plant species. Available for download.	Only algorithm is available. Lacks a graphical user interface	
KEGG Mapper	A tool to search a biosynthetic pathway.	http://www.kegg.jp/kegg tool/map_pathway1.html?rn	KEGG is applicable to all organisms and enables interpretation of high-level functions from genomic and molecular data.		[63]
MicroArray Data Interface for Biological Annotation (MADIBA)	A webserver toolkit for biological interpretation of *Plasmodium* and plant gene clusters.	http://www.bi.up.ac.za/ MADIBA	It allows rapid gene cluster analyses and the identification of the relevant Gene Ontology terms, visualisation of metabolic pathways, genomic localisations, etc.	Only 2 plant species are currently considered [rice (*Oryza sativa*), and *A. thaliana*].	[64]
miP3v2	Predicts microproteins in a sequenced genome.	https://github.com/npklein/miP3	Sheds light on the prevalence, biological roles, and evolution of microProteins.	Only the algorithm is available. Lacks a graphical user interface	[65]
OptFlux	A software platform for *in silico* metabolic engineering.	http://www.optflux.org/	Open source platform. Integrates visualisation tools. Allows users to load a genome-scale model of a given organism. Wild type and mutants can be simulated. Available for download.		[66]
PathComp	Possible reaction path computation.	http://www.genome.jp/tools/pathcomp/			
PathPred	Prediction of biodegradation and/or biosynthetic pathways.	http://www.genome.jp/tools/pathpred/	Specifically designed for biosynthesis of SMs (in plants) and xenobiotics biodegradation of environmental compounds (by bacteria).		[67]
PathSearch	Search for similar reaction pathways.	http://www.genome.jp/tools/pathsearch/			

Tool	Utility	Web accessibility	Advantage	Disadvantage	Reference
PathVisio	A biological pathway analysis software that allows users to draw, edit and analyse biological pathways.	http://www.pathvisio.org/	Plugins are included, which provide advanced analysis methods, visualisation options or additional import/export functionality. Available for download.		[68, 69]
Pathway GeneSWAPPER	Maps homologous genes from one species onto the PathVisio pathway diagram of another species.	http://jaiswallab.cgrb. oregonstate.edu/software/PGS	Improves the functionalities of PathVisio and WikiPathways for plants.		[70]
PlantClusterFinder	Predicts metabolic gene clusters from plant genomes.	https://dpb.carnegiescience. edu/labs/rhee-lab/software	Focuses on plant species. Available for download.	Only the algorithm is available. Lacks a graphical user interface	
Prediction informatics for secondary metabolomes (PRISM)	Genomes to natural products prediction informatics for secondary metabolomes.	http://magarveylab.ca/prism/	Open-source, user-friendly web available application.	Focuses on microbial SMs.	[71]
RetroPath	A webserver for retrosynthetic pathway design.	http://www.jfaulon.com/bioretrosynth/	Integrates pathway prediction and ranking, prediction of compatibility with host genes, toxicity prediction and metabolic modeling.		[72, 73]
Semi-Automated Validation Infrastructure (SAVI)	Predicts metabolic pathways using pathway metadata (e.g. taxonomic distribution, key reactions, etc.).	https://dpb.carnegiescience. edu/labs/rhee-lab/software	Decides which pathways to keep, remove or validate manually. Available for download.	Only the algorithm is available. Lacks a graphical user interface.	
WebAUGUSTUS	Gene prediction tool.	http://bioinf.uni-greifswald. de/webaugustus	One of the most accurate tools for eukaryotic gene prediction.	Focuses on eukaryotes.	[74]
WikiPathways for plants	A community pathway curation portal.	http://plants.wikipathways. org	Freely available.	Currently limited to rice and *Arabidopsis* sp.	[70, 75, 76]

*Currently provided detection rules for 44 classes and subclasses of SMs.

Table 2. Summary of current computational tools which could be useful for the plant genomic data analysis.

transcriptional regulatory elements in the upstream sequences, and an analysis specific to the organism being studied.

PlantClusterFinder, SAVI and WikiPathways for plants are all purpose tools designed to assist in the prediction of metabolic gene cluster from plant genomes, although WikiPathways for plants has currently included mostly data for rice and *Arabidopsis* sp. SAVI has the added advantage of offering the user the possibility of including pathway metadata (e.g. taxonomic distribution, key reactions, etc.) and offering the possibility to decide which pathway(s) to keep and which to remove or validate manually.

5. Some computational methods for efficient production and the *de novo* engineering of natural products

Two main areas for computational tools can be distinguished: on the one hand the rational modification of genomes for the production of molecules by host organisms, and on the other hand the modification or the *de novo* design of gene clusters for the biosynthesis of novel NPs. For both genetic engineering approaches, the already known genomes of bacteria, fungi and more and more plants provide the basic datasets. A very important computational approach for a rational modification of NP-producing host organisms is the genome-scale metabolic modelling [77, 78].

Automatic assignments of functional annotations of all genes in a genome are ideally proven by manual curation and enriched by current knowledge about the metabolic network of subjected organisms. The curated genomes are then applied to a complete automatic reconstruction of the metabolic pathways of the cell. These metabolic models are normally encoded in the Systems Biology Markup Language (SBML) and are compatible with various software tools, for example, Cytoscape [79], which can be applied for static network analyses. For instance, missing enzymes (gaps) within the network become apparent by substrates that are not taken up or have not been produced by the cell, as well as products that are not consumed by other reactions and are not secreted from cell. The RAST annotation pipeline provides a full automatic server for predicting all gene functions and discovering new pathways in microbial genomes of bacteria [80]. Such models can then be used to predict the turnover rate of each reaction in a Flux Balance Analysis (FBA) [81]. Several tools have been built, which apply FBA to identify enzymes that should be either introduced or knocked-out in the organism to increase production rate in the host organisms. A widely used FBA package is the MATLAB-based COBRA Toolbox [82]. With CycSim [58], BioMet [83] and FAME [84] powerful web-based FBA applications were published that do not require any software installation.

Within the last 10 years, FBA was applied to support numerous genetic engineering approaches, for example, for the determination of minimal media in *Helicobacter pylori* [85], for growth rate predictions in *Bacillus subtilis* [86] or for the development of metabolic engineering strategies in *Pseudomonas putida* [87]. Based on FBA, it was possible to increase vanillin production in baker's yeast by twofold and enhance sesquiterpene production in the same species [88, 89].

The rational modification of a given genome to design novel molecules needs a detailed understanding of the producing gene clusters. Well-studied gene clusters such as polyketide synthases consist of specific domain types that can be identified by trained hidden Markov models that are stored in related databases, for example, PFAM [90]. Gene cluster analysis tools such as antiSMASH [55, 91] or PRISM [71] analyse a given gene cluster to predict the specific domains and to describe the architecture of a gene cluster. However, the prediction of the structure of the resulting natural products is a difficult task because substrate recognition of active sites and the correct ordering of enzymatic reactions has to be predicted. If subjected enzymes are catalysing multiple substrates, the availability of each substrate has to be predicted. Most frequently, the automatic analysis of a cluster is based on the deduction of information from gene clusters similar to the queried one. If well-annotated similar gene clusters do not exist, the prediction of the structure of the biosynthesised NP is challenging. With more and more knowledge about the structure of natural products and the encoding sequences, the relation between the composition of the active sites and substrate binding will be better understood. Existing algorithms are often based on machine-learning approaches and predict the correct substrates for a selected set of enzyme families [92]. For the prediction of NPs synthesised by non-ribosomal peptide synthetases, such a sequence-based prediction method is integrated in the related web-server NRPSpredictor2 [93]. Rational substitution of residues to generate novel molecules still requires a detailed manual analysis of the encoding gene cluster, and new software tools that propose mutations leading to novel molecules might accelerate this approach considerably in future.

6. Selected natural products with promising anticancer properties from African sources

Recent reviews on the anticancer potential of African flora have discussed the anticancer, cytotoxic, antiproferative and antitumour activities of about 500 NPs [9–12]. In this section, we focus on the most promising (recent) results for anticancer SMs from African flora (**Table 3, Figure 2**), published after the last reviews. The isolation of two new lignans; 3α-O-(β-D-glucopyranosyl) desoxypodophyllotoxin (**1**) and 4-O-(β-D-glucopyranosyl) dehydropodophyllotoxin (**2**), alongside other known lignans (**3** and **4**), have been reported from the species, *Cleistanthus boivinianus* (Phyllanthaceae), collected in Madagascar (coordinates 13°06′37″S 049°09′39″E) [94]. These compounds showed potent to moderate antiproliferative activities against the A2780 ovarian cancer cell line, with compound **1** showing potent antiproliferative activity against the HCT-116 human colon carcinoma cell line (IC$_{50}$ = 0.03 μM). The known compounds with promising activities from this species included the lignans; (±)-β-apopicropodophyllin (**3**, PubChem CID: 6452099), (−)-desoxypodophyllotoxin (**4**, PubChem CID: 345501). The same authors also isolated a new butanolide, macrocarpolide A (**5**, PubChem CID: 122372160) and two new secobutanolides; macrocarpolides B (**6**, PubChem CID: 122372161) and C (**7**, PubChem CID: 122372162), together with other known compounds from the ethanol extract of the roots of the Madagascan

Cpd. No.*	Molecule class	Source species (Family)	Cancer cell line	IC_{50} (µM)	Biosynthetic pathway	References
1	lignan	*Cleistanthus boivinianus* (Phyllanthaceae)	HCT-116 human colon carcinoma cell line	0.03	shikimic acid pathway, via phenylalanine	[94]
2	"	"	A2780 ovarian cancer cell line	0.02	"	"
3	"	"	"	2.10	"	"
4	"	"	"	0.06	"	"
	"	"	"	0.23	"	
5	butanolide	*Ocotea macrocarpa* (Lauraceae)	"	2.57		[95]
6	secobutanolide	"	"	1.98		"
7	"	"	"	1.67		"
8	butanolide	"	"	2.43		"
9	"	"	"	1.65		"
10	polyoxygenated cyclohexene derivative	*Cleistochlamys kirkii* (Annonaceae)	MDA-MB-231 triple-negative human breast cancer cell line	0.03	Shikimic acid pathway	[96]
11	"	"	"	0.29	"	"
12	"	"	"	0.29	"	"
13	"	"	"	0.12	"	"
14	"	"	"	0.45	"	"
15	"	"	"	2.10	"	"
16	"	"	"	0.09	"	"
17	"	"	"	2.70	"	"
18	"	"	"	0.24	"	"

*Compound number.

Table 3. Summary of recently published selected promising anticancer SMs from African flora.

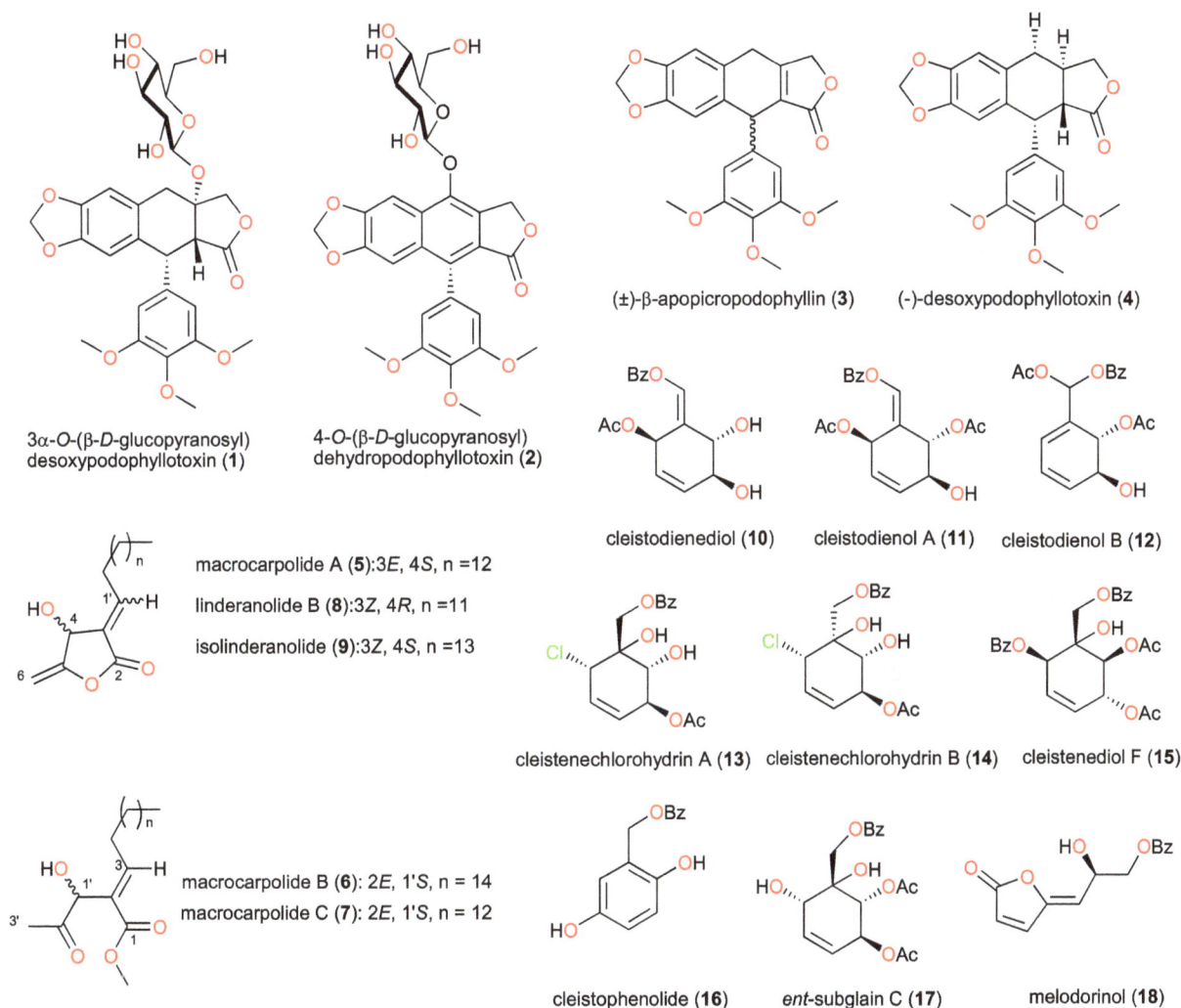

Figure 2. Chemical structures of selected anticancer SMs from African flora.

species *Ocotea macrocarpa* (Lauraceae), which showed antiproliferative activities against the A2780 ovarian cell line [95]. The known isolates included the butanolides; linderano- lide B (**8**, PubChem CID: 53308122) and isolinderanolide (**9**, PubChem CID: 44576054). The anticancer activities showed IC_{50} values of 2.57 (**5**), 1.98 (**6**), 1.67 (**7**), 2.43 (**8**) and 1.65 μM (**9**) against A2780 ovarian cancer cell lines. Additionally, the leaves of *Cleistochlamys kirkii* (Annonaceae) from Tanzania have been recently shown to be a rich source of polyoxygen- ated cyclohexene derivatives with antiplasmodial activities, along with very potent activi- ties against MDA-MB-231 triple-negative human breast cancer cell line [96]. The isolates; cleistodienediol (**10**), cleistodienol A (**11**), cleistodienol B (**12**), cleistenechlorohydrin A (**13**), cleistenechlorohydrin B (**14**), cleistenediol F (**15**), cleistophenolide (**16**), *ent*-subglain C (**17**) and melodorinol (**18**, PubChem CID: 6438687) showed some activities as low as $IC_{50} = 0.09$ μM against the aforementioned cancer cell lines. To the best of our knowledge, mode of action studies have not yet been conducted for the SMs **1** to **18** and *in vivo* activity data is currently unavailable.

7. Case studies

In this section, we shall discuss specific examples of the investigation of biosynthesis of anti-cancer plant-based SMs by (computational) analysis of genomic data.

7.1. Biogenesis of several anticancer metabolites by *Ocimum tenuiflorum* (Lamiaceae)

Species from the genus *Ocimum* are well known for their high medicinal values and are therefore used to cure a variety of ailments in Ayurveda, an Indian system of medicine [97, 98]. About 30 SMs have been reported from the genus *Ocimum*, with a variety of biological properties [99]. Only 14 of these SMs belong to the five basic groups of compounds having a complete biosynthetic pathway information in the PMN database [49, 50], thereby leaving us with ~15 medicinally relevant metabolites from *Ocimum* sp. with unknown pathways. This has prompted further investigation on SMs with uncharted biosynthetic pathways. Several bioactive SMs, including the anticancer compounds; apigenin (**19**, PubChem CID: 5280443), rosmarinic acid (**20**, PubChem CID: 5281792), taxol (**21**, PubChem CID: 36314), ursolic acid (**22**, PubChem CID: 64945), oleanolic acid (**23**, PubChem CID: 10494) and the plant steroid sitosterol (**24**, PubChem CID: 222284) have been identified from the herb Krishna Tulsi (*O. tenuiflorum*, Lamiaceae), with the mature leaves retaining the medicinally relevant metabolites [100]. Upadhyay et al. carried out a draft genome analysis of the species and generated paired-end and mate-pair sequence libraries for the whole sequenced genome, together with transcriptomic analysis (RNA-Seq) of two subtypes of *O. tenuiflorum* (Krishna and Rama Tulsi) and reporting the relative expression of genes in the both varieties. The authors further investigated the pathways, which lead to the biosynthesis of the identified SMs, with respect to similar pathways in *A. thaliana* and other model plants (e.g. *Oryza sativa japonica*). Six important genes (including *Q8RWT0* and *F1T282*) were expressed and identified from analysis of genome data. These were validated by q-RT-PCR on the different studied tissues (e.g. roots, mature leaves, etc.) of five closely related species (e.g. *O. gratissimum, O. sacharicum, O. kilmund, Solanum lycopersicum* and *Vitis vinifera*), which showed a high extent of urosolic acid-producing genes in young leaves. The other identified anticancer metabolites included eugenol and ursolic acid. As an example, the authors employed sequence search algorithms to search for the three enzymes of the three-step synthetic pathway of ursolic acid from squalene in the Tulsi genome. Each of these enzymes in Tulsi (squalene epoxidase, α-amyrin synthase and α-amyrin 2,8 monoxygenase) were queried from the PlantCyc database, starting from their protein sequences. The search for analogous enzymes in the model plants *O. sativa japonica* and *A. thaliana*, showed sequence identity covering from 50 to 80% of the query length. The whole genome and sequence analysis of *O. tenuiflorum* suggested that small amino acid changes at the functional sites of genes involved in metabolite synthesis pathways could confer special medicinal (particularly anticancer) properties to this herb.

7.2. Biosynthesis of the anticancer alkaloid noscapine by *Papaver somniferum* (Papaveraceae)

Noscapine (**25**, PubChem CID: 275196) is an antitumour phthalideisoquinoline alkaloid from opium poppy (*Papaver somniferum*, Papaveraceae). Compound **25** is known to bind stoichiometrically to tubulin, alters its conformation, affects microtubule assembly (promotes microtubule polymerisation), hence arresting metaphase and inducing apoptosis in many cell types [101]. It has been demonstrated that the compound has potent antitumour activity against solid murine lymphoid tumours (even when the drug was administered orally). This drug has also shown potency against human breast, ovarian and bladder tumours implanted in nude mice and in dividing human cells [102, 103]. Although the compound is water-soluble and absorbed after oral administration, its chemotherapeutic potential in human cancer could not be fully exploited for drug discovery projects because, like most SMs, this has been limited by the typically small amounts produced in the slow-growing plant species [104]. The quest to improve production levels of the NP is essential for drug discovery. However, such would require a proper understanding biological processes underlying the biosynthesis of this SM, known from isotope-labelling experiments to be derived from scoulerine since the 1960s [105]. Winzer et al. have carried out a transcriptomic analysis, with the aim of elucidating the biosynthetic pathway of this important metabolite for the improvement of its commercial production in both poppy and other systems [106]. The analysis of a high noscapine-producing poppy variety, HN1, showed the exclusive expression of 10 genes encoding five distinct enzyme classes, whereas five functionally characterised genes (*BBE, TNMT, SalR, SalAT* and *T6ODM*) were present in all three of the studied poppy varieties, respectively, rich in morphine, thebaine and noscapine (HM1, HN1 and HT1). The authors analysed the expressed sequence tag (EST) abundance and discovered some previously uncharacterised genes expressed in HN1, which were completely absent from the other (HM1 and HT1) EST libraries. This led to the identification of the corresponding enzymes as three *O*-methyltransferases (*PSMT1, PSMT2, PSMT3*), four cytochrome P450s (*CYP82X1, CYP82X2, CYP82Y1* and *CYP719A21*), an acetyltransferase (*PSAT1*), a carboxylesterase (*PSCXF1*) and a short-chain dehydrogenase/reductase (*PSSDR1*). Further analysis of an F2 mapping population, using HN1 and HM1 as parents, indicated that these genes are tightly linked in HN1. Moreover, bacterial artificial chromosome sequencing confirmed the existence of a complex BGC for plant alkaloids. Based on the knowledge derived from the investigation, the authors could make suggestions for the improved production of noscapine and related bioactive molecules by the molecular breeding of commercial poppy varieties or engineering of new production systems, for example, by virus-induced gene silencing, which resulted in the accumulation of pathway intermediates, thus allowing gene function to be linked to noscapine synthesis [104, 106].

7.3. Biosynthesis of vinblastine and vincristine by *Catharanthus roseus* (Apocynaceae)

Vinblastine (**26**, PubChem CID: 13342) and vincristine (**27**, PubChem CID: 5978) are chemotherapy drugs used to treat a number of cancer types. These are among the >120 known terpenoid indole alkaloids from the medicinal plant *C. roseus*, also known as the Madagascar periwinkle [107]. Since these two very important anticancer compounds have only been produced in very low amounts in *C. roseus*, as opposed to the fairly high levels of several monomeric alkaloids (e.g. ajmalicine and serpentine) [108], attempts to improve the yields of compounds **26** and **27** have led to the genome-wide transcript profiling of elicited *C. roseus* cell cultures, by cDNA-amplified fragment-length polymorphism combined with metabolic profiling [107]. This resulted in the identification of several gene-to-gene and gene-to-metabolite networks obtained by an attempt to establish correlations between the expression profiles of 417 gene tags and the accumulation profiles of 178 metabolite peaks. The results proved that different branches of terpenoid indole alkaloid biosynthesis and various other metabolic pathways are affected by differences in hormonal regulation. Thus, the investigations of Rischer et al. provided the foundations for a proper understanding of secondary metabolism in *C. roseus*, thereby enhancing the applicability of metabolic engineering of Madagascar periwinkle. This study provided the possibility of exploring a select number of genes (e.g. *STR*, *10HGO*, *T16H* and *DAT*) involved in biosynthesis of terpenoid indole alkaloids [107].

8. The way forward

The case studies show that the detailed computational analysis of the transcriptomic and metabolomic data of a plant species could reveal its metabolic capacity and hence help identify candidate genes involved in the biosynthesis of the important SMs it contains. Thus, modifying the plant genes could represent a premise for improving metabolite yield. It should be mentioned that other compounds from some of the aforementioned compound classes (**Table 3**), from both floral and microbial sources, have shown promising anticancer activities [109–113], e.g. isolinderanolide B (**28**, PubChem CID: 53308122) (**Figure 3**), a butanolide from the stems of *Cinnamomum subavenium* (Lauraceae) had shown antiproliferative activity in T24 human bladder cancer cells by blocking cell cycle progression and inducing apoptosis [112]. In addition, subamolide B (**29**, PubChem CID: 16104907), another butanolide from this same species, is known to induce cytotoxicity in human cutaneous squamous cell carcinoma through mitochondrial and CHOP-dependent cell death pathways [113]. Meanwhile, obtusilactone B (**30**, PubChem CID: 101286261), from *Machilus thunbergii* (Lauraceae), is known to target barrier-to-autointegration factor to treat cancer [111].

From the African flora, apart from the Lauraceae, Phyllanthaceae and Annonaceae, known to be rich in anticancer metabolites, the genus *Tacca* of the yam family (Dioscoreaceae) is known for the abundant presence of taccalonolides, which are microtubule stabilisers with clinical potential for cancer treatment [114]. Additionally, the genus *Tamarix* (e.g. *T. aphylla*

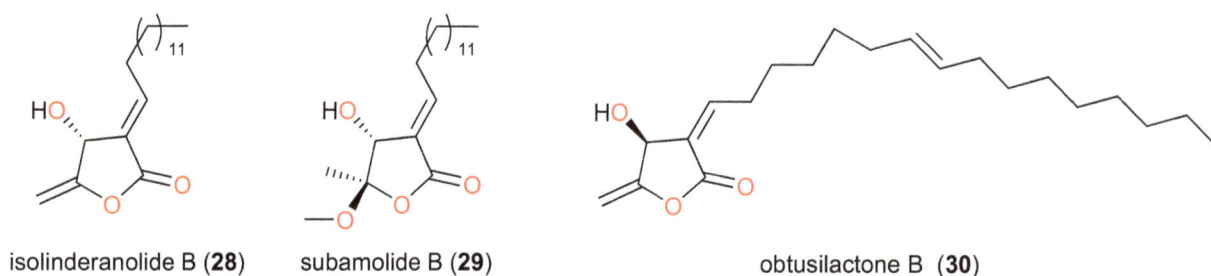

isolinderanolide B (**28**)   subamolide B (**29**)   obtusilactone B (**30**)

Figure 3. Chemical structures of selected anticancer butanolides from Lauraceae.

and *T. nilotica* from Northern Africa), together with the genus *Reaumuria* (Tamaricaceae) are known for the abundant presence of tannins (gallo-ellagitannin, gallotannins) with remarkable cytotoxic effects. The high salt content of the leaves of *Tamarix* species, rendering them useful locally as a fire barrier, and their adaptability to drought and high salinity are of equal interest. It therefore becomes urgent to investigate the genomics of some of the aforementioned plant species, particularly those from the *Cinnamomum* sp., *Ocotea* sp. and *Machilus* sp. (Lauraceae), *Tacca* sp. (Dioscoreaceae), *Cleistanthus* sp. (Phyllanthaceae), *Cleistochlamys* sp. (Annonaceae), *Tamarix* sp. (Tamaricaceae) and so on, and hence further investigate the genes or BGCs responsible for secondary metabolism with the view of understanding and better exploring the biosynthetic pathways of the anticancer SMs.

9. Conclusions

It has been our intention in this chapter to provide a detailed overview of the important computational tools and resources for the analysis of plant genomic data and for the prediction of biosynthetic pathways in plants. We have taken a few case studies of anticancer SMs to illustrate this. Even though it is unclear how widespread plant genes are clusters, genes that encode the biosynthesis of several small plant SMs are well known, including the vital genes for the production of some highly potent anticancer drugs. With the use of the tools and databases described, along with the drop in the cost of whole genome sequencing in plant species, the future for the discovery of new plant-based anticancer metabolites would involve the identification of one or more genes or BGCs encoding the enzymes in the biosynthetic pathway for the target compound(s), followed by the co-expression analysis, also exploiting the knowledge of the chemical structure of the target compound, for the identification of other enzymes that might be involved in this pathway. As an example, the exploration of the pathway for podophyllotoxin biosynthesis by the use transcriptome mining in *Podophyllum hexandrum* led to the identification biosynthetic genes, 29 of which were combinatorially expressed in the tobacco plant (*Nicotiana benthamiana*), leading to the identification of six pathway enzymes, among which is oxoglutarate-dependent dioxygenase responsible for closing the core cyclohexane ring of the aryltetralin scaffold [115]. An alternative approach could be, if the metabolic pathway and nature of SMs are unknown, then the identified co-expressed genes encoding the enzymes for secondary metabolism could be subjected to untargeted metabolomics for the elucidation of unknown pathways and chemical structures. As an example, a single pathogen-induced P450 enzyme, CYP82C2, with a combination of untargeted metabolomics and co-expression analysis was used to uncover the complete biosynthetic pathway, which leads to the metabolite 4-hydroxyindole-3-carbonyl nitrile, previously unknown to *Arabidopsis* sp. This rare and hitherto unprecedented plant metabolite, with a cyanogenic functionality revealed a hidden capacity of *Arabidopsis* sp. for cyanogenic glucoside biosynthesis. This was confirmed by expressing 4-OH-ICN engineering biosynthetic enzymes in *Saccharomyces cerevisiae* and *Nicotiana benthamiana*, to reconstitute the complete pathway *in vitro* and *in vivo*, thus validating the functions of the enzymes involved in the pathway [116].

Acknowledegments

FNK acknowledges a Georg Forster fellowship from the Alexander von Humboldt Foundation, Germany. CVS is currently a doctoral candidate financed by the German Academic Exchange Services (DAAD), Germany.

Competing interests

The authors declare that they have no competing interests.

Abbreviations

AfroCancer	African Anticancer Natural Products Database
BGC	Biosynthetic gene clusters
EC_{50}	Half maximal effective concentration, that is, the concentration of a drug, antibody or toxicant, which induces a response halfway between the baseline and maximum after a specified exposure time
ED_{50}	The median effective dose, a dose that produces the desired effect in 50% of a population
FBA	Flux Balance Analysis
GI_{50}	The growth inhibition of 50%, drug concentration resulting in a 50% reduction in the net protein increase.
IC_{50}	The drug concentration causing 50% inhibition of the desired activity
IMG-ABC	The Integrated Microbial Genomes Atlas of Biosynthetic gene Clusters
NANPDB	Northern African Natural Products Database
NP	Natural product
NPACT	Naturally Occurring Plant-based Anti-cancer Compound Activity-Target Database
NRP	Nonribosomal peptide
NRPS	Nonribosomal peptide synthase
PK	Polyketide
PKS	Polyketides synthase
PMN	Plant Metabolic Network
PRISM	PRediction Informatics for Secondary Metabolomes
SM	Secondary metabolite

Author details

Aurélien F.A. Moumbock[1], Conrad V. Simoben[2], Ludger Wessjohann[3], Wolfgang Sippl[2], Stefan Günther[4,] and Fidele Ntie-Kang[1,2]*

*Address all correspondence to: ntiekfidele@gmail.com

1 Department of Chemistry, University of Buea, Buea, Cameroon

2 Department of Pharmaceutical Chemistry, Martin-Luther University of Halle-Wittenberg, Halle, Germany

3 Leibniz Institute of Plant Biochemistry, Halle, Germany

4 Pharmaceutical Bioinformatics, Albert-Ludwig-University Freiburg, Freiburg, Germany

References

[1] Cragg GM, Newman DJ. Plants as a source of anti-cancer and anti-HIV agents. Ann Appl Biol. 2003;143:127-133. doi:10.1111/j.1744-7348.2003.tb00278.x

[2] Cragg GM, Grothaus PG, Newman DJ. Impact of natural products on developing new anti-cancer agents. Chem Rev. 2009;109:3012-3043. doi:10.1021/cr900019j

[3] Lamari FN, Cordopatis P. Exploring the potential of natural products in cancer treatment. In: Missailidis S, editor. *Anticancer therapeutics*. West Sussex: Wiley-Blackwell; 2008, pp. 3-16.

[4] Pan L, Chai HB, Kinghorn AD. Discovery of new anticancer agents from higher plants. Front Biosci (Schol Ed). 2013;4:142-156.

[5] Newman DJ, Cragg GM. Natural products as sources of new drugs from 1981 to 2014. J Nat Prod. 2016;79:629-661. doi:10.1021/acs.jnatprod.5b01055

[6] Mangal M, Sagar P, Singh H, Raghava GPS, Agarwal SM. NPACT: naturally occurring plant-based anti-cancer compound activity-target database. Nucleic Acids Res. 2013;41:D1124-D1129. doi:10.1093/nar/gks1047

[7] Ntie-Kang F, Nwodo JN, Ibezim A, Simoben CV, Karaman B, et al. Molecular modeling of potential anticancer agents from African medicinal plants. J Chem Inf Model. 2014;54:2433-2450. doi:10.1021/ci5003697

[8] Ntie-Kang F, Simoben CV, Karaman B, Ngwa VF, Judson PN, et al. Pharmacophore modeling and *in silico* toxicity assessment of potential anticancer agents from African medicinal plants. Drug Des Dev Ther. 2016;10:2137-2154. doi:10.2147/DDDT.S108118

[9] Beutler JA, Cragg GM, Iwu M, Newman DJ, Okunji C. Anticancer potential of African plants: the experience of the United States National Cancer Institute and National

Institutes of Health. In: Gurib-Fakim A, editor. Novel plant bioresources: applications in food, medicine and cosmetics, 1st ed. Oxford: John Wiley & Sons Ltd; 2014, pp. 133-149. doi:10.1002/9781118460566.ch10

[10] Nwodo JN, Ibezim A, Simoben CV, Ntie-Kang F. Exploring cancer therapeutics with natural products from African medicinal plants, part II: alkaloids, terpenoids and flavonoids. Anticancer Agents Med Chem. 2016;16:108-127. doi:10.2174/187152061566615 0520143827

[11] Simoben CV, Ibezim A, Ntie-Kang F, Nwodo JN, Lifongo LL. Exploring cancer therapeutics with natural products from African medicinal plants, part I: xanthones, quinones, steroids, coumarins, phenolics and other classes of compounds. Anticancer Agents Med Chem. 2015;15:1092-1111. doi:10.2174/1871520615666150113110241

[12] Simoben CV, Ntie-Kang F. African medicinal plants: an untapped reservoir of potential anticancer agents. In: Prasad S, Tyagi AK, editors. Cancer preventive and therapeutic compounds: gift from mother nature. Beijing: Bentham Science Publishers; 2016. p. 78-95.

[13] Ntie-Kang F, Telukunta KK, Döring K, Simoben CV, Moumbock, et al. The Northern African Natural Products Database (NANPDB), 2016. www.african-compounds.org/nanpdb

[14] Ntie-Kang F, Yong JN. The chemistry and biological activities of natural products from Northern African plant families: from Aloaceae to Cupressaceae. RSC Adv. 2014;4:61975-61991. doi:10.1039/C4RA11467A

[15] Yong JN, Ntie-Kang F. The chemistry and biological activities of natural products from Northern African plant families: from Ebenaceae to Solanaceae. RSC Adv. 2015;5:26580-26595. doi:10.1039/C4RA15377D

[16] Ntie-Kang F, Njume LE, Malange YI, Günther S, Sippl W, et al. The chemistry and biological activities of natural products from Northern African plant families: from Taccaceae to Zygophyllaceae. Nat Prod Bioprospect. 2016;6:63-96. doi:10.1007/s13659-016-0091-9

[17] Medema MH, Fischbach M. Computational approaches to natural product discovery. Nat Chem Biol. 2015;11:639-648. doi:10.1038/nchembio.1884

[18] Medema MH, Kottmann R, Yilmaz P, Cummings M, Biggins JB, et al. Minimum information about a biosynthetic gene cluster. Nat Chem Biol. 2015;11:625-631. doi:10.1038/nchembio.1890

[19] Nützmann HW, Osbourn A. Gene clustering in plant specialized metabolism. Curr Opin Biotechnol. 2014;26:91-99. doi:10.1016/j.copbio.2013.10.009

[20] Osbourn A. Secondary metabolic gene clusters: evolutionary toolkits for chemical innovation. Trends Genet. 2010;26:449-457. doi:10.1016/j.tig.2010.07.001

[21] Osbourn AE, Field B. Operons. Cell Mol Life Sci. 2009;66:3755-3775. doi:10.1007/s00018-009-0114-3

[22] Rhee SY, Mutwil M. Towards revealing the functions of all genes in plants. Trends Plant Sci. 2014;19:212-221. doi:10.1016/j.tplants.2013.10.006

[23] Xu M, Rhee SY. Becoming data-savvy in a big-data world. Trends Plant Sci. 2014;19:619-622. doi:10.1016/j.tplants.2014.08.003

[24] Chae L, Lee I, Shin J, Rhee SY. Towards understanding how molecular networks evolve in plants. Curr Opin Plant Biol. 2012;15:177-184. doi:10.1016/j.pbi.2012.01.006

[25] Medema MH, Osbourn A. Computational genomic identification and functional reconstitution of plant natural product biosynthetic pathways. Nat Prod Rep. 2016;33:951-962. doi:10.1039/c6np00035e

[26] Weber T. *In silico* tools for the analysis of antibiotic biosynthetic pathways. Int J Med Microbiol. 2014;304:230-235. doi:10.1016/j.ijmm.2014.02.001

[27] Li YF, Tsai KJ, Harvey CJ, Li JJ, Ary BE, et al. Comprehensive curation and analysis of fungal biosynthetic gene clusters of published natural products. Fungal Genet Biol. 201689:18-28. doi:10.1016/j.fgb.2016.01.012

[28] van der Lee TA, Medema MH. Computational strategies for genome-based natural product discovery and engineering in fungi. Fungal Genet Biol. 2016;89:29-36. doi:10.1016/j.fgb.2016.01.006

[29] Frey M, Chomet P, Glawischnig E, Stettner C, Grun S, et al. Analysis of a chemical plant defense mechanism in grasses. Science. 1997;277:696-699. doi:10.1126/science.277.5326.696

[30] Osbourn A. Gene clusters for secondary metabolic pathways: an emerging theme in plant biology. Plant Physiol. 2010;154:531-535. doi:10.1104/pp.110.161315

[31] Figueiredo AC, Barroso JG, Pedro LG, Scheffer JJC. Factors affecting secondary metabolite production in plants: volatile components and essential oils. Flavour Fragr J. 2008;23:213-226. doi:10.1002/ffj.1875

[32] Leal MC, Hilario A, Munro MHG, Blunt JW, Calado R. Natural products discovery needs improved taxonomic and geographic information. Nat Prod Rep. 2016;33:747-750. doi:10.1039/c5np00130g

[33] Luo Y, Enghiad B, Zhao H. New tools for reconstruction and heterologous expression of natural product biosynthetic gene clusters. Nat Prod Rep. 2016;33:174-182. doi:10.1039/c5np00085h

[34] Carbonell P, Currin A, Jervis AJ, Rattray NJW, Swainston N, et al. Bioinformatics for the synthetic biology of natural products: integrating across the Design-Build-Test cycle. Nat Prod Rep. 2016;33:925-932. doi:10.1039/c6np00018e

[35] Song MC, Kim EJ, Kim E, Rathwell K, Nama SJ, et al. Microbial biosynthesis of medicinally important plant secondary metabolites. Nat Prod Rep. 2014;31:1497-1509. doi:10.1039/c4np00057a

[36] Zhao H, Medema MH. Standardization for natural product synthetic biology. Nat Prod Rep. 2016;33:920-924. doi:10.1039/c6np00030d

[37] Ajikumar PK, Xiao WH, Tyo KE, Wang Y, Simeon F, et al. Isoprenoid pathway optimization for Taxol precursor overproduction in *Escherichia coli*. Science. 2010;330:70-74. doi:10.1126/science.1191652

[38] De Luca V, Salim V, Atsumi SM, Yu F. Mining the biodiversity of plants: a revolution in the making. Science. 2012;336:1658-1661. doi:10.1126/science.1217410

[39] Kim E, Moore BS, Yoon YJ. Reinvigorating natural product combinatorial biosynthesis with synthetic biology. Nat Chem Biol. 2015;11:639-659. doi:10.1038/nchembio.1893

[40] Menzella HG, Reid R, Carney JR, Chandran SS, Reisinger SJ, et al. Combinatorial polyketide biosynthesis by *de novo* design and rearrangement of modular polyketide synthase genes. Nat Biotechnol. 2005;23:1171-1176. doi:10.1038/nbt1128

[41] Conway KR, Boddy CN. ClusterMine360: a database of microbial PKS/NRPS biosynthesis. Nucleic Acids Res. 2013;41:D402-D407. doi:10.1093/nar/gks993

[42] Tremblay N, Hill P, Conway KR, Boddy CN. The use of ClusterMine360 for the analysis of polyketide and nonribosomal peptide biosynthetic pathways. Methods Mol Biol. 2016;1401:233-252. doi:10.1007/978-1-4939-3375-4_15

[43] Starcevic A, Zucko J, Simunkovic J, Long PF, Cullum J, et al. ClustScan: an integrated program package for the semi-automatic annotation of modular biosynthetic gene clusters and *in silico* prediction of novel chemical structures. Nucleic Acids Res. 2008;36:6882-6892. doi:10.1093/nar/gkn685

[44] Diminic J, Zucko J, Ruzic IT, Gacesa R, Hranueli D, et al. Databases of the thiotemplate modular systems (CSDB) and their *in silico* recombinants (r-CSDB). J Ind Microbiol Biotechnol. 2013;40:653-659. doi:10.1007/s10295-013-1252-z

[45] Ichikawa N, Sasagawa M, Yamamoto M, Komaki H, Yoshida Y, et al. DoBISCUIT: a database of secondary metabolite biosynthetic gene clusters. Nucleic Acids Res. 2013;41:D408-D414. doi:10.1093/nar/gks1177

[46] Hadjithomas M, Chen IA, Chu K, Ratner A, Palaniappan K, et al. IMG-ABC: a knowledge base to fuel discovery of biosynthetic gene clusters and novel secondary metabolites. mBio. 2015;6:e00932-15. doi:10.1128/mBio.00932-15

[47] Kellner F, Kim J, Clavijo BJ, Hamilton JP, Childs KL, et al. Genome-guided investigation of plant natural product biosynthesis. Plant J. 2015;82:680-692. doi:10.1111/tpj.12827

[48] Hur M, Campbell AA, Almeida-de-Macedo M, Li L, Ransom N, et al. A global approach to analysis and interpretation of metabolic data for plant natural product discovery. Nat Prod Rep. 2013;30:565-583. doi:10.1039/c3np20111b

[49] Chae L, Kim T, Nilo-Poyanco R, Rhee SY. Genomic signatures of specialized metabolism in plants. Science. 2014;344: 510-513. doi:10.1126/science.1252076

[50] Dreher K. Putting the plant metabolic network pathway databases to work: going offline to gain new capabilities. Methods Mol Biol. 2014;1083:151-171. doi:10.1007/978-1-62703 -661-0_10

[51] Naithani S, Preece J, D'Eustachio P, Gupta P, Amarasinghe V, et al. Plant Reactome: a resource for plant pathways and comparative analysis. Nucleic Acids Res. 2017;45:D1029-D1039. doi:10.1093/nar/gkw932

[52] Starcevic A, Wolf K, Diminic J, Zucko J, Ruzic IT, et al. Recombinatorial biosynthesis of polyketides. J Ind Microbiol Biotechnol. 2012;39:503-511. doi:10.1007/s10295-011-1049-x

[53] Weber T, Kim HU. The secondary metabolite bioinformatics portal: computational tools to facilitate synthetic biology of secondary metabolite production. Synth Syst Biotechnol. 2016;1:69-79. doi:10.1016/j.synbio.2015.12.002

[54] Medema MH, van Raaphorst R, Takano E, Breitling R. Computational tools for the synthetic design of biochemical pathways. Nat Rev Microbiol. 2012;10:191-202. doi:10.1038/ nrmicro2717

[55] Weber T, Blin K, Duddela S, Krug D, Kim HU, et al. antiSMASH 3.0—a comprehensive resource for the genome mining of biosynthetic gene clusters. Nucleic Acids Res. 2015;43:W237-W243. doi:10.1093/nar/gkv437

[56] Lee I, Ambaru B, Thakkar P, Marcotte EM, Rhee SY. Rational association of genes with traits using a genome-scale gene network for *Arabidopsis thaliana*. Nat Biotechnol. 2010;28:149-156. doi:10.1038/nbt.1603

[57] Caspi R, Billington R, Ferrer L, Foerster H, Fulcher CA, et al. The MetaCyc database of metabolic pathways and enzymes and the BioCyc collection of pathway/genome databases. Nucleic Acids Res. 2016;44:D471-D480. doi:10.1093/nar/gkv1164

[58] Le Fèvre F, Smidtas S, Combe C, Durot M, d'Alché-Buc F, et al. CycSim—an online tool for exploring and experimenting with genome-scale metabolic models. Bioinformatics. 2009;25:1987-1988. doi:10.1093/bioinformatics/btp268

[59] Yamanishi Y, Hattori M, Kotera M, Goto S, Kanehisa M. E-zyme: predicting potential EC numbers from the chemical transformation pattern of substrate-product pairs. Bioinformatics. 2009;25:i179-i186. doi:10.1093/bioinformatics/btp223

[60] Chou CH, Chang WC, Chiu CM, Huang CC, Huang HD. FMM: a web server for metabolic pathway reconstruction and comparative analysis. Nucleic Acids Res. 2009;37:W129-W134. doi:10.1093/nar/gkp264

[61] Kearse M, Moir R, Wilson A, Stones-Havas S, Cheung M, et al. Geneious basic: an integrated and extendable desktop software platform for the organization and analysis of sequence data. Bioinformatics. 2012;28:1647-1649. doi:10.1093/bioinformatics/bts199

[62] Johnston CW, Skinnider MA, Wyatt MA, Li X, Ranieri MRM, et al. An automated Genomes-to-Natural Products platform (GNP) for the discovery of modular natural products. Nat Commun. 2015;6:8421. doi:10.1038/ncomms9421

[63] Kanehisa M. KEGG bioinformatics resource for plant genomics and metabolomics. Methods Mol Biol. 2016;1374:55-70. doi:10.1007/978-1-4939-3167-5_3

[64] Law PJ, Claudel-Renard C, Joubert F, Louw AI, Berger DK. MADIBA: a web server toolkit for biological interpretation of *Plasmodium* and plant gene clusters. BMC Genomics. 2008;9:105. doi:10.1186/1471-2164-9-105

[65] de Klein N, Magnani E, Banf M, Rhee SY. microProtein Prediction Program (miP3): a software for predicting microProteins and their target transcription factors. Int J Genomics. 2015;2015:734147. doi:10.1155/2015/734147

[66] Rocha I, Maia P, Evangelista P, Vilaça P, Soares S, et al. OptFlux: an open-source software platform for *in silico* metabolic engineering. BMC Syst Biol. 2010;4:45. doi:10.1186/1752-0509-4-45

[67] Moriya Y, Shigemizu D, Hattori M, Tokimatsu T, Kotera M, et al. PathPred: an enzyme-catalyzed metabolic pathway prediction server. Nucleic Acids Res. 2010;38:W138-W143. doi:10.1093/nar/gkq318

[68] Kutmon M, van Iersel MP, Bohler A, Kelder T, Nunes N, et al. PathVisio 3: an extendable pathway analysis toolbox. PLoS Comput Biol. 2015;11:e1004085. doi:10.1371/journal.pcbi.1004085

[69] van Iersel MP, Kelder T, Pico AR, Hanspers K, Coort S, et al. Presenting and exploring biological pathways with PathVisio. BMC Bioinformat. 2008;9:399. doi:10.1186/1471-2105-9-399

[70] Hanumappa M, Preece J, Elser J, Nemeth D, Bono G, et al. WikiPathways for plants: a community pathway curation portal and a case study in rice and *Arabidopsis* seed development networks. Rice. 2013;6:14. doi:10.1186/1939-8433-6-14

[71] Skinnider MA, Dejong CA, Rees PN, Johnston CW, Li H, et al. Genomes to natural products PRediction Informatics for Secondary Metabolomes (PRISM). Nucleic Acids Res. 2015;43:9645-9662. doi:10.1093/nar/gkv1012

[72] Carbonell P, Planson AG, Fichera D, Faulon JL. A retrosynthetic biology approach to metabolic pathway design for therapeutic production. BMC Syst Biol. 2011;5:122. doi:10.1186/1752-0509-5-122

[73] Planson AG, Carbonell P, Grigoras I, Faulon JL. A retrosynthetic biology approach to therapeutics: from conception to delivery. Curr Opin Biotechnol. 2012;23:948-956. doi:10.1016/j.copbio.2012.03.009

[74] Hoff KJ, Stanke M. WebAUGUSTUS - a web service for training AUGUSTUS and predicting genes in eukaryotes. Nucleic Acids Res. 2013;41:W123-W128. doi:10.1093/nar/gkt418

[75] Kelder T, van Iersel MP, Hanspers K, Kutmon M, Conklin BR, et al. WikiPathways: building research communities on biological pathways. Nucleic Acids Res. 2012,40:D1301-D1307. doi:10.1093/nar/gkr1074

[76] Kutmon M, Riutta A, Nunes N, Hanspers K, Willighagen EL, et al. WikiPathways: capturing the full diversity of pathway knowledge. Nucleic Acids Res. 2016;44:D488-D494. doi:10.1093/nar/gkv1024

[77] Durot M, Bourguignon PY, Schachter V. Genome-scale models of bacterial metabolism: reconstruction and applications. FEMS Microbiol Rev. 2009;33:164-190. doi:10.1111/j.1574-6976.2008.00146.x

[78] Feist AM, Herrgård MJ, Thiele I, Reed JL, Palsson BØ. Reconstruction of biochemical networks in microorganisms. Nat Rev Microbiol. 2009;7:129-143. doi:10.1038/nrmicro1949

[79] Shannon P, Markiel A, Ozier O, Baliga NS, Wang JT, et al. Cytoscape: a software environment for integrated models of biomolecular interaction networks. Genome Res. 2003;13:2498-2504. doi:10.1101/gr.1239303

[80] Overbeek R, Olson R, Pusch GD, Olsen GJ, Davis JJ, et al. The SEED and the Rapid Annotation of microbial genomes using Subsystems Technology (RAST). Nucleic Acids Res. 2014;42:D206-D214. doi:10.1093/nar/gkt1226

[81] Orth JD, Thiele I, Palsson BØ. What is flux balance analysis? Nat Biotechnol. 2010;28:245-248. doi:10.1038/nbt.1614

[82] Schellenberger J, Que R, Fleming RM, Thiele I, Orth JD, et al. Quantitative prediction of cellular metabolism with constraint-based models: the COBRA Toolbox v2.0. Nat Protoc. 2011;6:1290-1307. doi:10.1038/nprot.2011.308

[83] Garcia-Albornoz M, Thankaswamy-Kosalai S, Nilsson A, Väremo L, Nookaew I, Nielsen J. BioMet Toolbox 2.0: genome-wide analysis of metabolism and omics data. Nucleic Acids Res. 2014;42:W175-W181. doi:10.1093/nar/gku371

[84] Boele J, Olivier BG, Teusink B. FAME, the flux analysis and modeling environment. BMC Syst Biol. 2012;6:8. doi:10.1186/1752-0509-6-8

[85] Schilling CH, Covert MW, Famili I, Church GM, Edwards JS, Palsson BO. Genome-scale metabolic model of *Helicobacter pylori* 26695. J Bacteriol. 2002;184:4582-4593. doi:10.1128/JB.184.16.4582-4593.2002

[86] Oh YK, Palsson BO, Park SM, Schilling CH, Mahadevan R. Genome-scale reconstruction of metabolic network in *Bacillus subtilis* based on high-throughput phenotyping and gene essentiality data. J Biol Chem. 2007;282:28791-28799. doi:10.1074/jbc.M703759200

[87] Puchałka J, Oberhardt MA, Godinho M, Bielecka A, Regenhardt D, et al. Genome-scale reconstruction and analysis of the *Pseudomonas putida* KT2440 metabolic network facilitates applications in biotechnology. PLoS Comput Biol. 2008;4:e1000210. doi:10.1371/journal.pcbi.1000210

[88] Henry CS, Broadbelt LJ, Hatzimanikatis V. Thermodynamics-based metabolic flux analysis. Biophys J. 2007;92:1792-1805. doi:10.1529/biophysj.106.093138

[89] Asadollahi MA, Maury J, Patil KR, Schalk M, Clark A, Nielsen J. Enhancing sesquiter-pene production in *Saccharomyces cerevisiae* through *in silico* driven metabolic engineer-ing. Metab Eng. 2009;11:328-334. doi:10.1016/j.ymben.2009.07.001

[90] Finn RD, Coggill P, Eberhardt RY, Eddy SR, Mistry J, et al. The Pfam protein families database: towards a more sustainable future. Nucleic Acids Res. 2016;44:D279-D285. doi:10.1093/nar/gkv1344

[91] Blin K, Medema MH, Kottmann R, Lee SY, Weber T. The antiSMASH database, a com-prehensive database of microbial secondary metabolite biosynthetic gene clusters. Nucleic Acids Res. 2017;45:D555-D559. doi:10.1093/nar/gkw960

[92] Röttig M, Rausch C, Kohlbacher O. Combining structure and sequence information allows automated prediction of substrate specificities within enzyme families. PLoS Comput Biol. 2010;6:e1000636. doi:10.1371/journal.pcbi.1000636

[93] Röttig M, Medema MH, Blin K, Weber T, Rausch C, et al. NRPSpredictor2: a web server for predicting NRPS adenylation domain specificity. Nucleic Acids Res. 2011;39:W362-W367. doi:10.1093/nar/gkr323

[94] Liu Y, Young K, Rakotondraibe LH, Brodie PJ, Wiley JD, et al. Antiproliferative com-pounds from *Cleistanthus boivinianus* from the Madagascar dry forest. J Nat Prod. 2015;78:1543-1547. doi:10.1021/np501020m

[95] Liu Y, Cheng E, Rakotondraibe LH, Brodie PJ, Applequist W, et al. Antiproliferative compounds from *Ocotea macrocarpa* from the Madagascar dry forest. Tetrahedron Lett. 2015;56:3630-3632. doi:10.1016/j.tetlet.2015.01.172

[96] Nyandoro SS, Munissi JJE, Gruhonjic A, Duffy S, Pan F, et al. Polyoxygenated cyclohex-enes and other constituents of *Cleistochlamys kirkii* leaves. J Nat Prod. 2016. doi:10.1021/acs.jnatprod.6b00759. PMID: 28001067

[97] Prakash P, Gupta N. Therapeutic uses of *Ocimum sanctum* Linn (Tulsi) with a note on eugenol and its pharmacological actions: a short review. Indian J Physiol Pharmacol. 2005;49:125-131. PMID: 16170979

[98] Willis JC. A dictionary of the flowering plants and ferns. Cambridge: The University Press; 1919

[99] Khare CP. Indian medicinal plants: an illustrated dictionary. Heidelberg: Springer; 2007, p. 443

[100] Upadhyay AK, Chacko AR, Gandhimathi A, Ghosh P, Harini K, et al. Genome sequenc-ing of herb Tulsi (*Ocimum tenuiflorum*) unravels key genes behind its strong medicinal properties. BMC Plant Biol. 2015;15:212. doi:10.1186/s12870-015-0562-x

[101] Ke Y, Ye K, Grossniklaus HE, Archer DR, Joshi HC, et al. Noscapine inhibits tumor growth with little toxicity to normal tissues or inhibition of immune responses. Cancer Immunol Immunother. 2000;49:217-225. PMID: 10941904

[102] Ye K, Ke Y, Keshava N, Shanks J, Kapp JA, et al. Opium alkaloid noscapine is an antitumor agent that arrests metaphase and induces apoptosis in dividing cells. Proc Natl Acad Sci USA. 1998;95:1601-1606. PMID: 9465062

[103] Zhou J, Gupta K, Yao J, Ye K, Panda D, et al. Paclitaxel-resistant human ovarian cancer cells undergo c-Jun NH_2-terminal kinase-mediated apoptosis in response to noscapine. J Biol Chem. 2002;277:39777-39785. doi:10.1074/jbc.M203927200

[104] DellaPenna D, O'Connor SE. Plant gene clusters and opiates. Science. 2012;336:1648-1649. doi:10.1126/science.1225473

[105] Battersby AR, Hirst M, McCaldin DJ, Southgate R, Staunton J. Alkaloid biosynthesis. XII. The biosynthesis of narcotine. J Chem Soc Perkin 1. 1968;17:2163-2172. PMID: 5691486

[106] Winzer T, Gazda V, He Z, Kaminski F, Kern M, et al. A *Papaver somniferum* 10-gene cluster for synthesis of the anticancer alkaloid noscapine. Science. 336:1704-1708. doi:10.1126/science.1220757

[107] Rischer H, Oresic M, Seppänen-Laakso T, Katajamaa M, Lammertyn F, et al. Gene-to-metabolite networks for terpenoid indole alkaloid biosynthesis in *Catharanthus roseus* cells. Proc Natl Acad Sci USA. 2006;103:5614-5619. doi:10.1073/pnas.0601027103

[108] Noble RL. The discovery of the vinca alkaloids-chemotherapeutic agents against cancer. Biochem Cell Biol. 1990;68:1344-1351. doi:10.1139/o90-197

[109] Dong HP, Wu HM, Chen SJ, Chen CY. The effect of butanolides from *Cinnamomum tenuifolium* on platelet aggregation. Molecules. 2013;18:11836-11841. doi:10.3390/molecules181011836

[110] Hoshino S, Wakimoto T, Onaka H, Abe I. Chojalactones A-C, cytotoxic butanolides isolated from *Streptomyces* sp. cultivated with mycolic acid containing bacterium. Org Lett. 2015;17:1501-1504. doi:10.1021/acs.orglett.5b00385

[111] Kim W, Lyu HN, Kwon HS, Kim YS, Lee KH, et al. Obtusilactone B from *Machilus thunbergii* targets barrier-to-autointegration factor to treat cancer. Mol Pharmacol. 2013;83:367-376. doi:10.1124/mol.112.082578

[112] Shen KH, Lin ES, Kuo PL, Chen CY, Hsu YL. Isolinderanolide B, a butanolide extracted from the stems of *Cinnamomum subavenium*, inhibits proliferation of T24 human bladder cancer cells by blocking cell cycle progression and inducing apoptosis. Integr Cancer Ther. 2011;10:350-358. doi:10.1177/1534735410391662

[113] Yang SY, Wang HM, Wu TW, Chen YJ, Shieh JJ, et al. Subamolide B isolated from medicinal plant *Cinnamomum subavenium* induces cytotoxicity in human cutaneous squamous cell carcinoma cells through mitochondrial and CHOP-dependent cell death pathways. Evid Based Complement Alternat Med. 2013;2013:630415. doi:10.1155/2013/630415

[114] Risinger AL, Mooberry SL. Taccalonolides: novel microtubule stabilizers with clinical potential. Cancer Lett. 2010;291:14-19. doi:10.1016/j.canlet.2009.09.020

[115] Lau W, Sattely ES. Six enzymes from mayapple that complete the biosynthetic pathway to the etoposide aglycone. Science. 2015;349:1224-1228. doi:10.1126/science.aac7202

[116] Rajniak J, Barco B, Clay NK, Sattely ES. A new cyanogenic metabolite in *Arabidopsis* required for inducible pathogen defence. Nature. 2015;525:376-379. doi:10.1038/nature14907

4

Annexin Proteins: Novel Promising Targets for Anticancer Drug Development

Filiz Bakar

Abstract

Intracellular Ca^{2+} signaling and Ca^{2+} homeostasis have long been an important subject area of cell biology. Several intracellular Ca^{2+} binding proteins have been demonstrated until now, and among these, annexins are characterized by their ability to interact with membrane phospholipids and they form an evolutionary conserved multigene family with the members being expressed throughout animal and plant kingdoms. Annexin proteins are defined by different structural and biochemical criteria, and this multigene family has several biological features. In certain clinical conditions, the alterations on the localization or expression levels of annexin proteins are considered as the causes of pathological results and/or sequelae of disease. So, annexin proteins are indirectly linked to severe human diseases such as cardiovascular disease and cancer. Since annexin proteins are known to play roles in cancer, the researches are focused on defining the clinical significance of certain annexin proteins in cancer development and by the way anticancer treatments in the last decades. This chapter presents detailed information about annexin proteins and the studies on anticancer drug development targeting certain annexins. The studies denominate that targeting of certain annexin proteins reduces tumorigenesis and therapeutic resistance. So, annexin proteins have growing importance for anticancer drug development.

Keywords: annexin, cancer, anticancer, drug development, treatment

1. Introduction

Annexins are commonly known to be a large multigene family of Ca^{2+}-dependent phospholipid-binding proteins. They were discovered in the late 1970s and before the name "annexin", they were first introduced in diverse names which in Greek means "hold together" [1].

Over a hundred annexin proteins have been discovered in various species. Among these, 12 proteins are found in humans referred as A1–A13 (leaving A2 unassigned) [2], each having a differently positioned calcium/membrane-binding site within the core domain and a different N-terminal domain [3].

Annexins have a unique structure that allows them to locate onto membranes reversibly. They contain a conserved calcium and membrane-binding unit, which constitutes the core domain. It consists of four annexin repeats of about 70–80 amino acids. Its alfa-helical shape forms a slightly curved disc. The convex surface of it carries the calcium and membrane-binding sites as well as binding sites for phospholipids, heparin, and F-actin. The concave side on the other hand is responsible for other interactions. Ahead of the core domain comes the N-terminal region which differs in length and in sequence. It mediates regulatory interactions with protein ligands and annexin-membrane association [2]. It has been recently demonstrated that a part of N-terminal region integrates into the folded core, allowing the N-terminal region to be exposed for additional interactions upon calcium binding [4].

2. Functions of annexins

Annexins are responsible for calcium-regulated endocytotic and exocytotic events along with stabilizing organelle membranes and the plasma membrane [3]. One of the major roles of annexins is acting as scaffold proteins through calcium-regulated binding to phospholipids on the membranes. This allows the cytoplasm and the cytoplasmic side of the cell membrane to interact accordingly [5]. Mobilization of intracellular calcium triggers annexins to be recruited by cell membranes. However, some annexins can bind to membranes in the absence of calcium as well, such as annexins A9 and A10 [2].

Some annexin members specifically engage with certain sites of actin assembly at cellular membranes. For instance, the organization of raft and non-raft microdomains of smooth muscle cell membranes is regulated by annexins A2 and A6 through mediating interactions with the cytoskeleton [6].

2.1. Intracellular activities of annexins

Annexins are able to engage with cytoskeleton components reversibly. However, under certain circumstances, some annexins (A2 and A11) are found to be working together in the nucleus in the cell cycle [7]. Especially, annexin A11 plays an essential role in the terminal phase of cytokinesis. Without it, cells cannot form a midbody and hence end up in apoptosis [8]. Additionally, some annexins can be present on the cell surface. For instance, when cells are exposed to glucocorticoids, annexin A1 is found to be translocating from the cytosol to the cell surface [9]. It has also been demonstrated that annexin A2 functions as a co-receptor for plasminogen in several cell types including tumor cells, macrophages, and endothelial cells. There is also evidence that annexin A2 might be taking part in preserving vascular patency [10].

2.2. Extracellular activities of annexins

Annexins are typically known to be cytosolic proteins. However, some annexins can be found in extracellular fluids as well. There are binding sites on the outer side of cell membranes for these annexins, and they take part in several extracellular functions such as the role of annexin A5 as an anticoagulant protein, annexin A2 as an endothelial cell surface receptor for plasminogen, and the role of annexin A1 with anti-inflammatory activities on leukocytes [11]. As it is mentioned, annexin A2 functions as a receptor for plasminogen through its activities in fibrinolytic cascade as a positive modulator [12]. As a result, overexpression of annexin A2 on the surface of acute promyelocytic leukemia cells could lead to occurrence of bleeding [13].

Annexin A1 is the first member of the annexin family known to be present extracellularly. There are several findings about the extracellular activity of annexin A1. It can be found in human serum, particularly in inflammatory events such as colitis and myocard infarctus [14]. Even though annexins A1 and A4 are both present in ductal prostate epithelium cells, only annexin A1 is present extracellularly [15]. Several studies have shown that annexin A1 strongly inhibits the transendothelial migration of leukocytes, hence limiting the extent of inflammation [16].

3. Association of annexin proteins with diseases

The absence of annexin proteins can cause several abnormalities in the body. Altered expression of annexin A1 has led to a change in the inflammatory response of glucocorticoids and an increase in leukocyte migration. Additionally, it has been demonstrated that expression of other annexin proteins was affected by the loss of annexin A1 as well [17].

Recent studies have revealed that there are single-nucleotide polymorphisms (SNPs) in the genome of annexin proteins. According to studies, annexin A2 gene SNP exists in a higher level in sickle cell patients compared to control groups and is associated with osteonecrosis [18], and annexin A5 gene polymorphism has a role in recurrent pregnancy loss [19].

Annexins also take part in autoimmune diseases such as rheumatoid arthritis and type 1 diabetes. High levels of annexin V cause annexin V autoantibodies to be produced more than necessary, which may play a role in pathogenesis of these diseases [20, 21]. On the other hand, annexin A11 gene polymorphism is found to be associated with sarcoidosis, which is another autoimmune disease characterized by accumulation of epithelioid granulomas in many organs such as kidney and lungs [22].

4. Role of annexins in cancer

Annexin proteins generally exhibit diverse functions in coagulation, inflammation, signal transduction, cell proliferation, apoptosis, tumor development, angiogenesis, invasion/metastasis, and drug resistance. Several studies have revealed that annexins might be playing an important role in the process of tumor differentiation and tumor development through various mechanisms.

4.1. Annexin A1 and cancer

Annexin A1 also known as lipocortin is a member of annexin family [23], expressed in many cell types such as prostate, brain, epithelial cells, and phagocytes. It participates in various intracellular events such as cell growth, migration, cell differentiation, and mediating anti-inflammatory effects of glucocorticoids [24].

Up-regulation of annexin A1 functions as a tumor progression marker in hepatic, pancreatic, breast, and stomach carcinomas [25]. In contrast, it is down-regulated in head and neck cancers, prostate cancer, and esophageal cancers [26]. Increased annexin A1 levels have been correlated with various multidrug-resistant tumor cells as well. Annexin A1 regulates the expression of metastatic matrix metalloproteinase-9 (MMP-9) and its activity and induces the activation of NF-kB as well as promoting migration and invasion in MDA-MD-231 cells [27]. The studies have reported a significant correlation between annexin A1 levels and pathological differentiation of oral squamous cell carcinoma (OSCC) tissues [28]. According to data, the presence of annexin A1 also promotes small cell lung cancer (SCLC) cells adherence to brain endothelium leading to transendothelial migration [29]. These findings suggest that annexin A1 plays an important role in the regulation of tumor cell behavior and can be used as a potential target in breast cancer therapy.

4.2. Annexin A2 and cancer

Annexin A2, also known as Calpactin I or Lipocortin II, is a 36 kDa member of annexin family expressed by various cell types such as endothelial cells, tumor cells, and macrophages [30]. The N-terminal region of annexin A2 contains tissue plasminogen activator (tPA) [31] as well as S100A10 protein binding site [32]. On the other hand, the C-terminal region contains heparin [33], F-actin [3], and plasminogen binding sites [34].

Like the other members of annexin family, intracellular annexin A2 participates in endocytotic and exocytotic events. The down-regulation of annexin A2 inhibits cell proliferation and cell division [35], and degradation of this protein has been linked with apoptosis promoted by p53-induced pathways [36]. Annexin A2 can also function as an antioxidant. Down-regulation of annexin A2 leads tumor cells to apoptosis through pro-apoptotic p38MAPK/JNK/Akt signaling pathways upon hydrogen peroxide exposure [37].

Annexin A2 interacts with tPA which transforms plasminogen into plasmin, hence leading to extracellular matrix degradation and cell invasion. However, blocking off the surface of annexin A2 can prevent tumor cell growth and metastasis [38]. Overexpression of annexin A2 is observed in a wide range of cancer cells such as acute lymphoblastic leukemia (ALL), breast cancer, colorectal cancer (CRC), lung cancer, and many others.

In acute lymphoblastic leukemia (ALL) cells, annexin A2 has been linked with drug resistance. Experiments revealed that phosphorylated annexin A2 expression (and not annexin A2) is higher in prednisolone-resistant cells than in drug-sensitive cell lines, suggesting that preventing annexin A2 phosphorylation can bring therapeutic benefit to the treatment of drug-resistant ALL cells [39].

In pancreatic tumors, annexin A2 levels were observed to be 2- to 8-folds higher than in normal pancreas cells [40]. On the other hand, higher annexin A2 immunoreactivity is observed in lung and squamous cell carcinoma compared to control group [41]. The studies also suggest that annexin A2-dependent plasmin in human breast cancer cells may participate in angiogenesis and metastasis through ubiquitination in breast cancer tissue [42]. Recent studies have demonstrated that annexin A2 is a receptor for gastrin and progastric peptides, which are associated with growth-stimulatory effects on intestinal epithelial and colon cancer cells [43]. Annexin A2 expression is strongly correlated with disease recurrence. Hence, it could be regarded as a potential biomarker for CRC patients.

4.3. Annexin A3 and cancer

The absence of annexin A3 is believed to play an important role in drug resistance and tumor development. According to available data, there is a correlation between up-regulation of annexin A3 and increased drug resistance in ovarian carcinoma. It also increases the metastasis of lung adenocarcinoma and hepatocarcinoma. On the other hand, development of prostatic and renal carcinoma was observed with the down-regulation of annexin A3 [44].

Among digestive tract cancers, colorectal cancer (CRC) is seen very commonly. Since it bears no clinical symptoms at early stages, discovering a biomarker that will aid in diagnosis has become necessary. Annexin A3 is considered to be a potential biomarker for colorectal cancer. The higher level of annexin A3 expression has been determined in blood samples of patients with CRC, indicating the importance of annexin A3 as a biomarker in CRC [45].

4.4. Annexin A4 and cancer

Annexin A4 is a member of annexin family, also known as lipocortin IV with a size of 35.9 kDa [46]. It consists of four annexin repeats, and each region includes 5 alfa-helixes with a calcium-binding motif [47].

Annexin A4 plays an important role in membrane repair, promoting vesicle aggregation and regulation of passive membrane permeability [48]. It also takes part in calcium signaling, anticoagulation, and resistance to apoptosis [49]. Accumulated data show that annexin A4 also involves in tumor progression, invasion, metastasis, and drug resistance in various cancer types [50].

Experiments revealed that there is a positive correlation between annexin A4 and colorectal cancer progression [51]. Moreover, annexin A4 was found to be directly binding to HPA (one of the markers of CRC metastasis), which indicates that it can be considered an important marker for CRC progression [52]. Annexin A4 is also overexpressed in *Helicobacter pylori*-infected gastric cancer tissues compared to not infected ones [53]. The suggested mechanism is that *H. pylori* infection promotes gastric cancer progression through increasing annexin A4 levels in order to induce the expression of IL-8. Hence, annexin A4 can be regarded as a potential marker in gastric cancer development. The studies also showed the relation of annexin A4 with malignant mesothelioma [54], breast, laryngeal, and hepatocellular carcinoma [55, 56].

4.5. Annexin A5 and cancer

Annexin A5, also known as Endonexin II, Lipocortin V, or thromboplastin inhibitor V, plays an important role in cell membrane repair during anti-inflammatory, profibrinolytic, and anti-thrombotic activities. Intracellular annexin A5 participates in calcium channel activity on plasma membrane interacting with actin in platelets during the coagulation process [57]. On the other hand, extracellular annexin A5 plays an important role in apoptosis and phagocytosis [58].

As the most studied member of annexin family, annexin A5 also plays important role in cancer development and progression.

Experiments on tumor samples obtained from patients with hepatocellular carcinoma revealed that annexin A5 was up-regulated by 134% [59]. Hence, it could be a novel biomarker for portal vein tumor thrombus formation. Annexin A5 was also correlated with hepatocarcinoma lymphatic metastasis. Half of tumor metastasis occurs through lymphatic system leading to poor prognosis. Studies showed that in metastatic hepatocarcinoma, annexin A5 was increased by 216%, which indicates that annexin A5 levels could be used in diagnosing lymphatic metastasis of tumors [60]. Annexin A5 has been found overexpressed in human cutaneous SCC cell lines. Experiments showed that annexin A5 is mainly present in growing tumor areas [61], suggesting that annexin A5 may involve in cell proliferation and metastasis. On the other hand, knockdown of annexin A5 by siRNA decreased the invasion capability of human oral carcinoma cells while up-regulating a metastasis suppressor gene KISS-1 [62].

Annexin A5 is significantly up-regulated in pancreatic cancer cells under hypoxia condition, indicating that it may be a significant reference value in pancreatic ductal adenocarcinoma [63]. Results obtained from studies suggest that annexin A5 is involved in breast cancer since up-regulation of this protein suppressed Raf-1, MEK1/2, and ERK1/2 phosphorylation of breast cancer cells [64].

Additionally, the studies revealed that annexin A5 is also involved in cervical, colorectal, bladder carcinomas, and inflammation-associated carcinogenesis of fibrosarcoma by different mechanisms.

4.6. Annexin A7 and cancer

Annexin A7 (also known as synexin) is a member of annexin family. On human chromosome, it is located where several tumor-suppressor genes are present [65]. Although it can be found in the nucleus, it is mostly found in membranes [66].

Available data indicate that annexin A7 might function as a tumor-suppressor gene in prostate cancer, melanoma, and glioblastoma; however, it might act as a tumor promoter in gastric cancer, liver cancer, colorectal cancer, and breast cancer. Additionally, down-regulation of annexin A7 could participate in tumor invasion and metastasis [65].

5. Annexin-targeted studies

The certain members of annexin family have important functions in the development and prognosis of several carcinomas mentioned above. Thus, the studies are focused on targeting these proteins to prevent or treat the disease. The recent findings on annexin-targeted treatments are summarized hereafter.

Prostate cancer is the most common malignant cancer diagnosed in men. It accounts for 10% of all male cancers and is difficult to detect at early stages. Therefore, it is necessary to discover a novel biomarker that will aid in early diagnosis [67]. To investigate the effect of Simvastatin and annexin A10 in human PC-3 prostate cancer cells, a nude mouse tumor xenograft model was used. Simvastatin was administered with 5 and 50 mg/kg doses. According to results obtained, Simvastatin up-regulated the expression of annexin A10 which led to a significant decrease in cell proliferation, invasion, and migration as well as a reduction in tumor size. In contrast, down-regulation of annexin A10 by siRNA increased the cell proliferation, invasion, and migration in PC-3 cells. Taken together, targeting annexin A10 with statins could be used in preventing or treating prostate cancer [68].

S100 proteins are known to regulate cell functions through interacting with other proteins, particularly with annexins [69]. The interaction between annexin A2 and S100A10 plays an important role in tumor metastasis and neo-angiogenesis [70]. Therefore, inhibiting this interaction could bring therapeutic benefits in cancer treatment. Several inhibitors have been identified using biochemical screening and receptor-guided random docking techniques based on '1,2,4-triazole' structure. One of these compounds was found to be a potent inhibitor: 2-[(5-{[(4,6-dimethylpyrimidin-2-yl)sulfanyl]methyl}-4-(furan-2-ylmcthyl)-4H-1,2,4-triazol-3-yl)sulfanyl] N-[4-(propan-2-yl)phenyl]acetamide [71].

Various chemicals can cause DNA damage and mutagenesis such as As^{3+} or reactive oxygen species, and mutagenesis has an important role in cancer initiation and progression [72]. Annexin A1 is known to participate in signal transduction of growth factors and cell proliferation or differentiation. Nevertheless, in certain types of cancers, the expression of annexin A1 can be reduced such as squamous cell carcinoma, whereas it can be increased in other cancers such as bladder cancer [73]. Moreover, in some cancer cells, the expression of annexin A1 is found higher in nucleus than in cytosol, which indicates that the nuclear presence of annexin A1 could correlate with progression of certain cancers [74]. Annexin A1 requires calcium signaling and tyrosine phosphorylation in order to translocate into the nucleus. This process is triggered by DNA-damaging agents and oxidative stress [75]. Signals of damage in DNA form a mono-ubiquitinated annexin A1, which stimulates translesion DNA synthesis by heavy metals [76]. Since annexin A1 is thought to involve in responses of DNA damage and mutagenesis, the inhibition of binding activity of annexin A1 by several substances including flavonoids has been researched. Results have revealed that Quercetin, Silibinin, and Genistein inhibited the binding activity of annexin A1 in a concentration-dependent manner. Moreover, they inhibited thymidine kinase gene mutation induced by As^{3+} in lymphoma cells through suppressing the translesion DNA synthesis which was mediated by mono-ubiquitinated annexin A1 in the nucleus [77]. These findings indicate that annexin A1 could be a novel target protein in preventing DNA damage induced by gene mutation.

Hepatocarcinoma is one of the most common malignancies with a high mortality rate and no effective treatment. A study has shown that in a mouse hepatocarcinoma cell line (Hca-P), down-regulating the expression of annexin A7 decreases the proliferation and induces apoptosis [78]. To investigate the role of it further, an experiment targeting annexin A7 has been performed. In order to down-regulate the expression of annexin A7, an RNA interference technique (RNAi) was used to demonstrate the changes in cell viability where annexin A7 levels are altered after Cisplatin treatment. According to data obtained, following the down-regulation of annexin A7, treatment with Cisplatin reduced the proliferation of Hca-P cells significantly and induced apoptosis. Additionally, altering the expression of annexin A7 decreased the expression of Bcl2 and increased the expression of caspase-3 and cytochrome-C, which indicates that presence of annexin A7 inhibits apoptosis through the mitochondrial pathway [79] (see **Figure 1**).

Annexin A1 is known to participate in the process of inflammation along with a wide range of cellular activities [2]. It has been revealed that annexin A1 plays a role in the process of apoptosis in inflammatory cells as well [80]. Experiments have shown that elevated annexin A1 levels in U937 cells and bronchoalveolar epithelial cells induce apoptosis through caspase-3 activation [81]. Moreover, it has been shown that in thyroid cancer cells, apoptosis induced by TRAIL is also mediated through annexin A1 expression [82]. Additionally, in

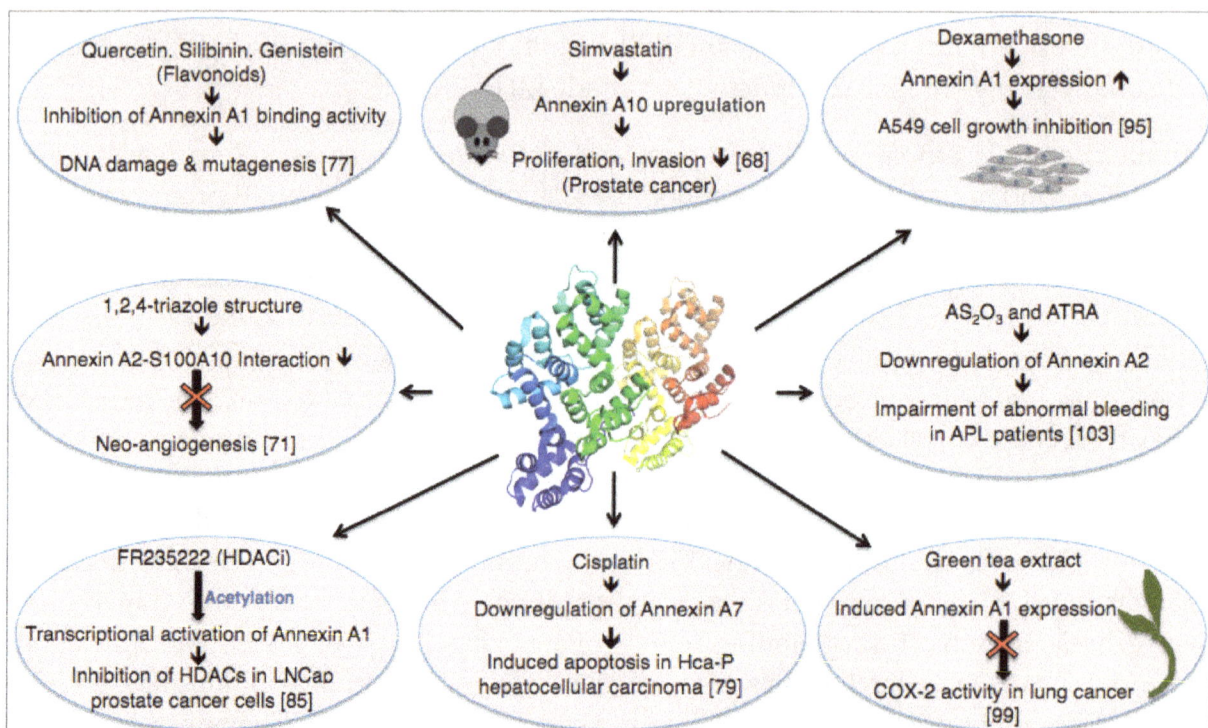

Figure 1. Schematic representation of annexin-targeted novel studies (the centered protein figure was prepared by Pymol Educational Program using annexin IV protein (PDB ID: 2ZOC) from Protein Data Bank).

prostate cancer cells, down-regulation of annexin A1 has been suggested to contribute in cancer initiation and progression [83]. On the other hand, up-regulation of annexin A1 has decreased the cell viability and induced apoptosis through caspase activity [84], which indicates that annexin A1 could be taken as a tumor-suppressor protein in prostate cancer cell line (LNCaP).

Experiments have shown that the expression of annexin A1 decreases in prostate cancer cells. Therefore, the mechanism of this reduction has been investigated. The fact that annexin A1 levels only decrease and are not completely eliminated brings the possibility that dysregulation of annexin A1 occurs at the level of gene transcription [85]. It has been proposed that deacetylation of histone proteins leads to altered gene expressions [86]. The turnover of histone acetylation is mediated by histone acetyltransferases (HATs) and histone deacetylases (HDACs). These enzymes can induce and inhibit transcription [87], and they show dysregulated activities in human cancers leading to neoplastic transformation of tumor cells [88]. Hence, the balance of HAT/HDAC has been a target in cancer therapy. Various compounds have shown antitumor effects through inhibiting HDACs such as valproic acid and some cyclic peptides (FK228) [89].

Recently, a novel compound, FR235222, with inhibitory effect on histone deacetylases has been isolated from a fungus [90]. Experiments have revealed that FR235222 induces apoptosis and regulates annexin A1 expression in leukemia cell lines. The possible mechanism suggested was that reduced levels of annexin A1 could be mediated by deacetylation of histone proteins [85]. To confirm this hypothesis, the effect of FR235222 on apoptosis and annexin A1 expression has been studied in prostate cancer cell lines (LNCaP). Western blotting results have shown that FR235222 induces the expression of annexin A1 in a time-dependent manner with a peak at 48 h. Also, experiments with actinomycin D indicated that the increase of annexin A1 was at transcription level. In contrast, when annexin A1 expression was down-regulated by siRNA transfection protocol, a partial decrease in FR235222-induced apoptosis has been observed by 26% and in caspase-3 activity by 22% in LNCaP cells [91]. These findings suggest that transcriptional activation of annexin A1 is induced by FR235222 through acetylation of histone proteins and inhibition of HDACs in LNCaP cells, and the increased levels of annexin A1 lead to apoptosis through caspase activity.

Lung cancer is one of the most common cancer types with a high rate of mortality [92]. Studies have shown that inflammation participates in the development of lung cancer. One of the components of inflammatory pathways is the COX-2/PGE$_2$ pathway. Increased expression of COX-2 is often seen in human non-small cell lung cancer (NSCLC). This leads to over-expression of PGE$_2$ which involves in various cancer-related activities such as resistance to apoptosis, angiogenesis, invasion, and metastasis [93]. Annexin A1 acts as a phospholipase A2 inhibitor and is associated with several functions such as cell differentiation, cell growth arrest, and anti-inflammation [94]. The effect of annexin A1 in human NSCLC cell line (A549) has been investigated. Studies have concluded that Dexamethasone increased the expression of annexin A1 in A549 cells which inhibited cell growth [95]. In contrast, gene deletion of annexin A1 led to an excessive inflammatory stimuli characterized by increased leukocyte migration and IL-1B generation [17].

Green tea (*Camellia sinensis* leave extract) is known to contain polyphenols which are natural antioxidants. Accumulated data have shown that green tea exhibits a protective role against various cancers including lung cancer [96]. It has been observed that green tea extract (GTE) induced annexin A1 in human urothelial cells and in lung cancer (A549) cells in a dose-dependent manner [97]. Moreover, GTE-induced annexin A1 also mediated cytoskeletal actin remodeling, which led to an increase in cell adhesion and decrease in cell motility. Additionally, inhibition of COX-2 and PGE2 was observed in NSCLC cell lines following GTE-induced annexin A1 expression. In contrast, silencing annexin A1 expression overturned the inhibitory effect of GTE on COX-2. These results suggest that GTE shows its effect through inducing annexin A1 expression, therefore targeting annexin A1 could be a promising mechanism in preventing lung cancer [98].

Annexin A2 is present in various cell types including endothelial cells, neuronal cells, and cancer cells. It acts as a co-receptor for plasminogen and tissue plasminogen activator (tPA) [99]. In acute promyelocytic leukemia (APL) cells, annexin A2 is found to be overexpressed. This causes plasmin to be highly produced leading to hyperfibrinolysis and then abnormal bleeding in patients [100]. A study has been performed to investigate the regulation of annexin A2 expression in APL cells as well as the effect of arsenic trioxide (As_2O_3) and all-trans retinoic acid (ATRA). Results have shown that annexin A2 is expressed abnormally on the surface of APL cells. Additionally, it has been observed that annexin A2 exhibits a unique activity of binding the tPA substrate plasminogen leading to enhanced plasminogen activity in APL cells [101]. Following the administration of As_2O_3 and ATRA in patients with APL, the expression of annexin A2 was significantly down-regulated on the surface of APL cells compared to the control group. Bleeding started to disappear a week after the treatment with ATRA and As_2O_3 as well as parameters of fibrinolysis [102]. These findings suggest that targeting annexin A2 could help treat the abnormal bleeding in patients with APL.

Author details

Filiz Bakar

Address all correspondence to: fbakar@ankara.edu.tr

Department of Biochemistry, Faculty of Pharmacy, Ankara University, Ankara, Turkey

References

[1] Crumpton MJ, Dedman JR. Protein terminology tangle. Nature. 1990;**345**:212. DOI: 10.1038/345212a0

[2] Gerke V, Moss SE. Annexins: From structure to function. Physiological Reviews. 2002;**82**: 331-371. DOI: 10.1152/physrev.00030.2001

[3]   Filipenko NR, Waisman DM. The C-terminus of annexin II mediates binding to F-Actin. Journal of Biological Chemistry. 2001;**276**:5310-5315. DOI: 10.1074/jbc.M009710200

[4]   Rosengarth A, Luecke H. A calcium-driven conformational switch of the N-terminal and core domains of annexin A1. Journal of Molecular Biology. 2003;**326**:1317-1325. DOI: 10.1016/S0022-2836(03)00027- 5

[5]   Janshoff A, Ross M, Gerke V, Steinem C. Visualization of annexin I binding to calcium-induced phosphatidylserine domains. ChemBiochem. 2001;**8**:587-590. DOI: 10.1002/1439-7633(20010803)2:7/8<587::AID-CBIC587>3.0.CO;2-Q

[6]   Babiychuk EB, Draeger A. Annexins in cell membrane dynamics: Ca(2+)-regulated association of lipid microdomains. Journal of Cell Biology. 2000;**150**:1113-1124

[7]   Tomas A, Moss SE. Calcium- and cell cycle-dependent association of annexin 11 with the nuclear envelope. Journal of Biological Chemistry. 2003;**278**:20210-20216. DOI: 10.1074/jbc.M212669200

[8]   Tomas A, Futter C, Moss SE. Annexin 11 is required for midbody formation and completion of the terminal phase of cytokinesis. Journal of Cell Biology. 2004;**165**:813-822. DOI: 10.1083/jcb.200311054

[9]   Solito E, Nuti S, Parente L. Dexamethasone-induced translocation of lipocortin (annexin) 1 to the cell membrane of U-937 cells. British Journal of Pharmacology. 1994;**112**:347-348

[10] Brownstein C, Falcone DJ, Jacovina A, Hajjar KA. A mediator of cell surface-specific plasmin generation. Annals of the New York Academy of Sciences. 2001;**947**:143-155. DOI: 10.1111/j.1749-6632.1997.tb52013.x

[11] Rand JH. Antiphospholipid antibody-mediated disruption of the annexin V antithrombotic shield: A thrombogenetic mechanism for the antiphospholipid syndrome. Journal of Autoimmunity. 2000;**15**:107-111. DOI: 10.1006/jaut.2000.0410

[12] Kim J, Hajjar KA. Annexin II: A plasminogen-plasminogen activator co-receptor. Frontiers in Bioscience. 2002;**7**:341-348. DOI: 10.2741/kim

[13] Menell JS, Cesarman GM, Jacovina AT, McLaughlin MA, Lev EA, Hajjar KA. Annexin II and bleeding in acute promyelocytic leukemia. The New England Journal of Medicine. 1999;**340**:994-1004. DOI: 10.1056/NEJM199904013401303

[14] Romisch J, Schuler E, Bastian B, Burger T, Dunkel FG, Schwinn A, Hartmann AA, Paques EP. Annexins I to VI: Quantitative determination in different human cell types and in plasma after myocardial infarction. Blood Coagulation and Fibrinolysis. 1992;**3**:11-17

[15] Christmas P, Callaway J, Fallon J, Jones J, Haigler HT. Selective secretion of annexin 1, a protein without a signal sequence, by the human prostate gland. Journal of Biological Chemistry. 1991;**266**:2499-2507

[16] Perretti M, Croxtall JD, Wheller SK, Goulding NJ, Hannon R, Flower RJ. Mobilizing lipocortin 1 in adherent human leukocytes downregulates their transmigration. Nature Medicine. 1996;**2**:1259-1262. DOI: 10.1038/nm1196-1259

[17] Hannon R, Croxtall JD, Getting SJ, Roviezzo F, Yona S, Paul-Clark MJ, Gavins FN, Perretti M, Morris JF, Buckingham JC, Flower RJ. Aberrant inflammation and resistance to glucocorticoids in annexin 1-/- mouse. FASEB Journal. 2003;**17**:253-255. DOI: 10.1096/fj.02-0239fje

[18] Pandey S, Ranjan R, Pandey S, Mishra RM, Seth T, Saxena R. Effect of ANXA2 gene single nucleotide polymorphism (SNP) on the development of osteonecrosis in Indian sickle cell patient: A PCR-RFLP approach. Indian Journal of Experimental Biology. 2012;**50**:455-458

[19] Miyamura H, Nishizawa H, Ota S, Suzuki M, Inagaki A, Egusa H, Nishiyama S, Kato T, Pryor-Koishi K, Nakanishi I, Fujita T, Imayoshi Y, Markoff A, Yanagihara I, Udagawa Y, Kurahashi H. Polymorphisms in the annexin A5 gene promoter in Japanese women with recurrent pregnancy loss. Molecular Human Reproduction. 2011;**17**:447-452. DOI: 10.1093/molehr/gar008

[20] Rodriguez-Garcia MI, Fernandez JA, Rodriguez A, Fernandez MP, Gutierrez C, Torre-Alonso JC. Annexin V autoantibodies in rheumatoid arthritis. Annals of the Rheumatic Diseases. 1996;**55**:895-900. DOI: 10.1136/ard.55.12.895

[21] Bakar F, Unlütürk U, Baskal N, Nebioglu S. Annexin V expression and anti-annexin V antibodies in type 1 diabetes. Journal of Clinical Endocrinology and Metabolism. 2014;**99**:932-937. DOI: 10.1210/jc.2013-2592

[22] Hofmann S, Franke A, Fischer A, Jacobs G, Nothnagel M, Gaede KI, Schurmann M, Muller-Quernheim J, Krawczak M, Rosenstiel P, Schreiber S. Genome-wide association study identifies ANXA11 as a new susceptibility locus for sarcoidosis. Nature Genetics. 2008;**40**:1103-1106. DOI: 10.1038/ng.198

[23] Flower RJ, Rothwell NJ. Lipocortin-1: Cellular mechanisms and clinical relevance. Trends in Pharmacological Sciences. 1994;**15**:71-76. DOI: 10.1016/0165-6147(94)90281-X

[24] Cirino G, Flower RJ, Browning JL, Sinclair LK, Pepinsky RB. Recombinant human lipocortin 1 inhibits thromboxane release from guinea-pig isolated perfused lung. Nature. 1987;**328**:270-272. DOI: 10.1038/328270a0

[25] Ahn SH, Sawada H, Ro JY, Nicolson GL. Differential expression of annexin I in human mammary ductal epithelial cells in normal and benign and malignant breast tissues. Clinical and Experimental Metastasis. 1997;**15**:151-156. DOI: 10.1023/A:1018452810915

[26] Shen D, Nooraie F, Elshimali Y, Lonsberry V, He J, Bose S, Chia D, Seligson D, Chang HR, Goodglick L. Decreased expression of annexin A1 is correlated with breast cancer development and progression as determined by a tissue microarray analysis. Human Pathology. 2006;**37**:1583-1591. DOI: 10.1016/j.humpath.2006.06.001

[27] Kang H, Ko J, Jang SW. The role of annexin A1 in expression of matrix metalloproteinase-9 and invasion of breast cancer cells. Biochemical and Biophysical Research Communications. 2012;**423**:188-194. DOI: 10.1016/j.bbrc.2012.05.114

[28] Zhang L, Yang X, Zhong LP, Zhou XJ, Pan HY, Wei KJ, Li J, Chen WT, Zhang ZY. Decreased expression of Annexin A1 correlates with pathologic differentiation grade in oral squamous cell carcinoma. Journal of Oral Pathology and Medicine. 2009;**38**:362-370. DOI: 10.1111/j.1600-0714.2008.00678.x

[29] Liua Y, Liua YS, Wub PF, Lic Q, Daia WM, Yuana S, Xua ZH, Liua TT, Miaoa ZW, Fanga WG, Chena YH, Lia B. Brain microvascular endothelium induced-annexin A1 secretion contributes to small cell lung cancer brain metastasis. The International Journal of Biochemistry and Cell Biology. 2015;**66**:11-19. DOI: 10.1016/j.biocel.2015.06.019

[30] Hajjar KA, Krishnan S. Annexin II: A mediator of the plasmin/plasminogen activator system. Trends in Cardiovascular Medicine. 1999;**9**:128-138. DOI: 10.1016/S1050-1738(99)00020-1

[31] Hajjar KA, Mauri L, Jacovina AT, Zhong F, Mirza UA, Padovan JC, Chait BT. Tissue plasminogen activator binding to the annexin II tail domain: Direct modulation by homocysteine. Journal of Biological Chemistry. 1998;**273**:9987-9993. DOI: 10.1074/jbc.273.16.9987

[32] Johnsson N, Marriott G, Weber K. p36, the major cytoplasmic substrate of src tyrosine protein kinase, binds to its p11 regulatory subunit via a short amino-terminal amphiphatic helix. The EMBO Journal. 1988;**7**:2435-2442

[33] Kassam G, Manro A, Braat CE, Louie P, Fitzpatrick SL, Waisman DM. Characterization of the heparin binding properties of annexin II tetramer. Journal of Biological Chemistry. 1997;**272**:15093-15100. DOI: 10.1074/jbc.272.24.15093

[34] Hajjar KA, Jacovina AT, Chacko J. An endothelial cell receptor for plasminogen/tissue plasminogen activator. I. Identity with annexin II. Journal of Biological Chemistry. 1994;**269**:21191-21197

[35] Chiang Y, Rizzino A, Sibenaller ZA, Wold MS, Vishwanatha JK. Specific down-regulation of annexin II expression in human cells interferes with cell proliferation. Molecular and Cellular Biochemistry. 1999;**199**:139-147. DOI: 10.1023/A:1006942128672

[36] Huang Y, Yan CH, Fu SB. The cloning and expression of apoptosis associated gene ANNEXIN A2 induced by p53 gene. Chinese Journal of Medical Genetics. 2005;**22**:661-664

[37] Madureira PA, Hill R, Miller VA, Giacomantonio C, Lee PW, Waisman DM. Annexin A2 is a novel cellular redox regulatory protein involved in tumorigenesis. Oncotarget. 2011;**2**:1075-1093. DOI: 10.18632/oncotarget.375

[38] Sharma MR, Rothman V, Tuszynski GP, Sharma MC. Antibody-directed targeting of angiostatin's receptor annexin II inhibits Lewis Lung Carcinoma tumor growth via blocking of plasminogen activation: Possible biochemical mechanism of angiostatin's action. Experimental and Molecular Pathology. 2006;**81**:136-145. DOI: 10.1016/j.yexmp.2006.03.002

[39] Spijkers-Hagelstein JA, Mimoso Pinhancos S, Schneider P, Pieters R, Stam RW. Src kinase-induced phosphorylation of annexin A2 mediates glucocorticoid resistance in MLL rearranged infant acute lymphoblastic leukemia. Leukemia. 2013;**27**:1063-1071. DOI: 10.1038/leu.2012.372

[40] Vishwanatha JK, Chiang Y, Kumble KD, Hollingsworth MA, Pour PM. Enhanced expression of annexin II in human pancreatic carcinoma cells and primary pancreatic cancers. Carcinogenesis. 1993;**14**:2575-2579. DOI: 10.1093/carcin/14.12.2575

[41] Brichory FM, Misek DE, Yim AM, Krause MC, Giordano TJ, Beer DG, Hanash SM. An immune response manifested by the common occurrence of annexins I and II autoantibodies and high circulating levels of IL-6 in lung cancer. Proceedings of the National Academy of Sciences of the United States of America. 2001;**98**:9824-9829. DOI: 10.1073/pnas.171320598

[42] Deng S, Jing B, Xing T, Hou L, Yang Z. Overexpression of annexin A2 is associated with abnormal ubiquitination in breast cancer. Genomics Proteomics Bioinformatics. 2012;**10**:153-157. DOI: 10.1016/j.gpb.2011.12.001

[43] Singh P, Wu H, Clark C, Owlia A. Annexin II binds progastrin and gastrin-like peptides, and mediates growth factor effects of autocrine and exogenous gastrins on colon cancer and intestinal epithelial cells. Oncogene. 2007;**26**:425-440. DOI: 10.1038/sj.onc.1209798

[44] Wu N, Liu S, Guo C, Hou Z, Sun MZ. The role of annexin A3 playing in cancers. Clinical and Translational Oncology. 2013;**15**:106-110. DOI: 10.1007/s12094-012-0928-6

[45] Yip KT, Das PK, Suria D, Lim CR, Ng GH, Liew CC. A case-controlledvalidation study of a blood based seven gene biomarker panel for colorectal cancer in Malaysia. Journal of Experimental and Clinical Cancer Research. 2010;**29**:128. DOI: 10.1186/1756-9966-29-128

[46] Mussunoor S, Murray GI. The role of annexins in tumour development and progression. Journal of Pathology. 2008;**216**:131-140. DOI: 10.1002/path.2400

[47] Butsushita K, Fukuoka S, Ida K, Arii Y. Crystal structures of sodium-bound annexin A4. Bioscience Biotechnology and Biochemistry. 2009;**73**:2274-2280. DOI: 10.1271/bbb90366

[48] Kaetzel MA, Chan HC, Dubinsky WP, Dedman JR, Nelson DJ. A role for annexin IV in epithelial cell function. Inhibition of calcium-activated chloride conductance. The Journal of Biological Chemistry. 1994;**269**:5297-5302

[49] Lin L, Huang H, Juan H. Revealing the molecular mechanism of gastric cancer marker annexin A4 in cancer cell proliferation using exon arrays. PLoS One. 2012;**7**:44615. DOI: 10.1371/journal.pone.0044615

[50] Mogami T, Yokota N, Asai-Sato M, Yamada R, Koizume S, Sakuma Y, Yoshihara M, Nakamura Y, Takano Y, Hirahara F, Miyagi Y, Miyagi E. Annexin A4 is involved in proliferation, chemo-resistance and migration and invasion in ovarian clear cell adenocarcinoma cells. PLoS One. 2013;**8**:80359. DOI: 10.1371/journal.pone.0080359

[51] Wang JJ, Liu Y, Zheng Y, Lin F, Cai GF, Yao XQ. Comparative proteomics analysis of colorectal cancer. Asian Pacific Journal of Cancer Prevention. 2012;13:1663-1666. DOI: 10.7314/APJCP.2012.13.4.1663

[52] Saint-Guirons J, Zeqiraj E, Schumacher U, Greenwell P, Dwek M. Proteome analysis of metastatic colorectal cancer cells recognized by the lectin Helix pomatia agglutinin (HPA). Proteomics. 2007;7:4082-4089. DOI: 10.1002/pmic.200700434

[53] Lin LL, Chen CN, Lin WC, Lee PH, Chang KJ, Lai YP, Wang JT, Juan HF. Annexin A4: A novel molecular marker for gastric cancer with Helicobacter pylori infection using proteomics approach. Proteomics Clinical Applications. 2008;2:619-634. DOI: 10.1002/prca.200780088

[54] Yamashita T, Nagano K, Kanasaki S, Maeda Y, Furuya T, Inoue M, Nabeshi H, Yoshikawa T, Yoshioka Y, Itoh N, Abe Y, Kamada H, Tsutsumi Y, Tsunoda S. Annexin A4 is a possible biomarker for cisplatin susceptibility of malignant mesothelioma cells. Biochemical and Biophysical Research Communications. 2012;421:140-144. DOI: 10.1016/j.bbrc.2012.03.144

[55] Zimmermann U, Balabanov S, Giebel J, et al. Increased expression and altered location of annexin IV in renal clear cell carcinoma: A possible role in tumour dissemination. Cancer Letters. 2004;209:111-118. DOI: 10.1016/j.canlet.2003.12.002

[56] Chen W, Chen L, Cai Z, Liang D, Zhao B, Zeng Y, Liu X, Liu J. Overexpression of annexin A4 indicates poor prognosis and promotes tumor metastasis of hepatocellular carcinoma. Tumour Biology. 2016;37(7):9343-9355. DOI: 10.1007/s13277-016-4823-6

[57] Lizarbe MA, Barrasa JI, Olmo N, et al. Annexin–phospholipid interactions. Functional implication. International Journal of Molecular Science. 2013;14:2652-2683. DOI: 10.3390/ijms14022652

[58] van Genderen HO, Kenis H, Hofstra L, et al. Extracellular annexin A5: functions of phosphatidylserine-binding and two-dimensional crystallization. Biochimica et Biophysica Acta. 2008;1783:953-963. DOI: 10.1016/j.bbamcr.2008.01.030

[59] Guo W, Man X, Yuan H, et al. Proteomic analysis on portal vein tumor thrombus associated proteins for hepatocellular carcinoma. Zhonghua yi xue za zhi. 2007;87:2094-2097

[60] Sun MZ, Liu S, Tang J. Proteomics investigation of mouse hepatocarcinoma cell lines with different lymph node metastasis capacities. Chemical Journal of Chinese Universities. 2009;30:517-524

[61] Dooley TP, Reddy SP, Wilborn TW, et al. Biomarkers of human cutaneous squamous cell carcinoma from tissues and cell lines identified by DNA microarrays and qRTPCR. Biochemical and Biophysical Research Communications. 2003;306:1026-1036

[62] Wehder L, Arndt S, Murzik U, et al. Annexin A5 is involved in migration and invasion of oral carcinoma. Cell Cycle. 2009;8:1552-1558. DOI: 10.4161/cc.8.10.8404

[63] Peng B, Guo C, Guanb H, Liuc S, Sun MZ. Annexin A5 as a potential marker in tumors. Clinica Chimica Acta. 2014;**427**:42-48. DOI: 10.1016/j.cca.2013.09.048

[64] Sato H, Ogata H, de Luca LM. Annexin V inhibits the 12-O-tetradecanoylphorbol-13-acetate-induced activation of Ras/extracellular signal-regulated kinase (ERK) signaling pathway upstream of Shc in MCF-7 cells. Oncogene. 2000;**19**:2904-2912. DOI: 10.1038/sj.onc.1203615

[65] Srivastava M, Bubendorf L, Raffeld M, Bucher C, Torhorst J, Sauter G, Olsen C, Kallioniemi OP, Eidelman O, Pollard HB. Prognostic impact of ANX7-GTPase in metastatic and HER2-negative breast cancer patients. Clinical Cancer Research. 2004;**10**(7):2344-2350. DOI: 10.1158/1078-0432.CCR-03-0278

[66] Shirvan A, Srivastava M, Wang MG, Cultraro C, Magendzo K, McBride OW, Pollard HB, Burns AL. Divergent structure of the human synexin (annexin VII) gene and assignment to chromosome 10. Biochemistry. 1994;**33**:6888-6901. DOI: 10.1021/bi00188a019

[67] Fitzpatrick JM, Schulman C, Zlotta AR, Schroder FH. Prostate cancer: A serious disease suitable for prevention. BJU International. 2009;**103**:864-870. DOI: 10.1111/j.1464-410X.2008.08206.x

[68] Miyazawa Y, Sekine Y, Kato H, Furuya Y, Koike H, Suzuki K. Simvastatin up-regulates Annexin A10 that can inhibit the proliferation, migration and invasion of androgen independent human prostate cancer cells. The Prostate. 2016;**77**:337-349. DOI: 10.1002/pros.23273

[69] Santamaria-Kisiel L, Rintala-Dempsey AC, Shaw GS. Calcium-dependent and independent interactions of the S100 protein family. Biochemistry Journal. 2006;**396**:201-214. DOI: 10.1042/BJ20060195

[70] Ling Q, Jacovina AT, Deora A, Febbraio M, Simantov R, Silverstein RL, Hempstead B, Mark WH, Hajjar KA. Annexin II regulates fibrin homeostasis and neoangiogenesis in vivo. Journal of Clinical Investigations. 2004;**113**:38-48. DOI: 10.1172/JCI19684

[71] Reddy TR, Li C, Guo X, Fischer PM, Dekker LV. Design, synthesis and SAR exploration of tri substituted 1,2,4-triazoles as inhibitors of the annexin A2–S100A10 protein interaction. Bioorganic and Medicinal Chemistry. 2014;**22**:5378-5391. DOI: 10.1016/j.bmc.2014.07.043

[72] Wang Z. DNA damage-induced mutagenesis: A novel target for cancer prevention. Molecular Interventions. 2001;**1**:269-281

[73] Lim LHK, Pervaiz S. Annexin 1: The new face of an old molecule. FASEB Journal. 2007;**21**:968-975. DOI: 10.1096/fj.06-7464rev

[74] Liu Y, Wang HX, Lu N, Mao YS, Liu F, Wang Y, Zhang HR, Wang K, Wu M, Zhao XH. Translocation of annexin I from cellular membrane to the nuclear membrane in human esophageal squamous cell carcinoma. World Journal of Gastroenterology. 2003;**9**:645-649. DOI: 10.3748/wjg.v9.i4.645

[75] Mohiti J, Caswell AM, Walker JM. The nuclear location of annexin V in the human osteo-sarcoma cell line MG-63 depends on serum factors and tyrosine kinase signaling path-ways. Experimental Cell Research. 1997;**234**:98-104. DOI: 10.1006/excr.1997.3584

[76] Hirata F, Thibodeau LM, Hirata A. Ubiquitination and SUMOylation of annexin AI and helicase activity. Biochemica et Biophysica Acta. 2010;**1800**:899-905. DOI: 10.1016/j.bbagen.2010.03.020

[77] Hirata F, Harada T, Corcoran GB, Hirata A. Dietary flavonoids bind to mono-ubiq-uitinated annexin A1 in nuclei, and inhibit chemical induced mutagenesis. Mutation Research. 2014;**759**:29-36. DOI: 10.1016/j.mrfmmm.2013.11.002

[78] Huang Y, Wang Q, Du Y, Bai L, Jin F, Zhang J, et al. Inhibition of annexin A7 gene and protein induces the apotosis and decreases the invasion, migration of the hepato-carcinoma cell line. Biomedicine and Pharmacotherapy. 2014;**7**:819-824. DOI: 10.1016/j.biopha.2014.07.001

[79] Huang Y, Dua Y, Zhang X, Bai L, Mibrahim M, Zhang J, Wei Y, Li C, Fan S, Wanga H, Zhao Z, Tang J. Down-regulated expression of Annexin A7 induces apoptosis in mouse hepatocarcinoma cell line by the intrinsic mitochondrial pathway. Biomedicine and Pharmacotherapy. 2015;**70**:146-150. DOI: 10.1016/j.biopha.2015.01.009

[80] Parente L, Solito E. Annexin 1 more than an anti-phospholipase protein. Inflammation Research. 2004;**53**:125-132. DOI: 10.1007/s00011-003-1235-z

[81] Debret R, El Btaouri H, Duca L, Rahman I, Radke S, Haye B, Sallenave JM, Antonicelli F. Annexin A1 processing is associated with caspase-dependent apoptosis in BZR cells. FEBS Letters. 2003;**546**:195-202

[82] Petrella A, Festa M, Ercolino SF, Zerilli M, Stassi G, Solito E, Parente L. Induction of annexin-1 during TRAIL-induced apoptosis in thyroid carcinoma cells. Cell Death and Differentiation. 2005;**12**:1358-1360. DOI: 10.1038/sj.cdd.4401645

[83] Kang JS, Calvo BF, Maygarden SJ, Caskey LS, Mohler JL, Ornstein DK. Dysregulation of annexin I protein expression in highgrade prostatic intraepithelial neoplasia and pros-tate cancer. Clinical Cancer Research. 2002;**8**:117-123

[84] Hsiang CH, Tunoda T, Whang YE, Tyson DR, Ornstein DK. The impact of altered annexin I protein levels on apoptosis and signal transduction pathways in prostate can-cer cells. Prostate. 2006;**66**:1413-1424. DOI: 10.1002/pros.20457

[85] Petrella A, D'Acunto W, Rodriquez M, Festa M, Tosco A, Bruno I, Terracciano S, Taddei M, Gomez Paloma L, Parente L. Effects of FR235222, a novel HDAC inhibitor, in pro-liferation and apoptosis of human leukemia cell lines: Role of annexin A1. European Journal of Cancer. 2008;**44**:740-749. DOI: 10.1016/j.ejca.2008.01.023

[86] Strahl BD, Allis CD. The language of covalent histone modifications. Nature. 2000;**403**: 4041-4045. DOI: 10.1038/47412

[87] Gregory PD, Wagner K, Horz W. Histone acetylation and chromatin remodeling. Experimental and Cellular Research. 2001;**265**:195-202. DOI: 10.1006/excr.2001.5187

[88] Mahlknecht U, Hoelzer D. Histone acetylation modifiers in the pathogenesis of malignant disease. Molecular Medicine. 2000;**6**:623-644

[89] Emanuele S, Lauricella M, Tesoriere G. Histone deacetylase inhibitors: Apoptotic effects and clinical implications. International Journal of Oncology. 2008;**33**:637-646. DOI: 10.3892/ijo_00000049

[90] Mori H, Urano Y, Abe F, Furukawa S, Furukawa S, Tsurumi Y, Sakamoto K, Hashimoto M, Takase S, Hino M, Fujii T. FR235222, a fungal metabolite, is a novel immunosuppressant that inhibits mammalian histone deacetylase (HDAC). I. Taxonomy, fermentation, isolation, and biological activities. The Journal of Antibiotics. (Tokyo). 2003;**56**:72-79

[91] D'Acunto CW, Fontanella B, Rodriquez M, Taddei M, Parente L, Petrella A. Histone deacetylase inhibitor FR235222 sensitizes human prostate adenocarcinoma cells to apoptosis through up-regulation of Annexin A1. Cancer Letters. 2010;**295**:85-91. DOI: 10.1016/j.canlet.2010.02.016

[92] Siegel R, Ma J, Zou Z, Jemal A. Cancer statistics. CA A Cancer Journal for Clinicians. 2014;**64(1)**:9-29. DOI: 10.3322/caac.21208

[93] Lee JM, Yanagawa J, Peebles KA, Sharma S, Mao JT, Dubinett SM. Inflammation in lung carcinogenesis: New targets for lung cancer chemoprevention and treatment. Critical Reviews in Oncology/Hematology. 2008;**66**:208-217. DOI: 10.1016/j.critrevonc.2008.01.004

[94] Solito E, de Coupade C, Parente L, Flower RJ, Russo-Marie F. Human annexin 1 is highly expressed during the differentiation of the epithelial cell line A 549: Involvement of nuclear factor interleukin 6 in phorbol ester induction of Annexin 1. Cell Growth and Differentiation. 1998;**9**:327-336

[95] Croxtall JD, Flower RJ. Lipocortin 1 mediates dexamethasone-induced growth arrest of the A549 lung adenocarcinoma cell line. Proceedings of the National Academy of Sciences of the United States of America. 1992;**89**:3571-3575

[96] Lu G, Liao J, Yang G, Reuhl KR, Hao X, Yang CS. Inhibition of adenoma progression to adenocarcinoma in a 4-(methylnitrosamino)-1-(3-pyridyl)-1- butanone-induced lung tumorigenesis model in A/J mice by tea polyphenols and caffeine. Cancer Research. 2006;**66**:1149-11501. DOI: 10.1158/0008-5472.CAN-06-1497

[97] Xiao GS, Jin YS, Lu QY, Zhang ZF, Belldegrun A, Figlin R, Pantuck A, Yen Y, Li F, Rao J. Annexin-I as a potential target for green tea extract induced actin remodeling. International Journal of Cancer. 2006;**120**:111-120. DOI: 10.1002/ijc.22164

[98] Lu QY, Jin Y, Mao JT, Zhang ZF, Heber D, Dubinett SM, Rao J. Green tea inhibits cycolo-oxygenase-2 in non-small cell lung cancer cells through the induction of Annexin-1. Biochemical and Biophysical Research Communications. 2012;**427**:725-730. DOI: 10.1016/j.bbrc.2012.09.125

[99] Senell JS, Cesarman GM, Jacovina AT, Mclaughlin MA, Lev EA, Hajjar KA. Annexin II and bleeding in acute promyelocytic leukemia. The New England Journal of Medicine. 1999;**340**:994-1004. DOI: 10.1056/NEJM199904013401303

[100] Barbui T, Finazzi G, Falanga A. The impact of all-trans retinoic acid on the coagulopathy of acute promyelocytic leukemia. Blood. 1998;**91**:3093-3102

[101] Hajjar KA, Acharya SS. Annexin II and regulation of cell surface fibrinolysis. Annals of the New York Academy Sciences. 2000;**902**:265-271. DOI: 10.1111/j.1749-6632.2000.tb06321.x

[102] Zhang X, Zhou H, Wang J, Yang L, Hua Y, Shen G, Guo P, Qiao Z, Song S. Arsenic trioxide, retinoic acid and Ara-c regulated the expression of annexin II on the surface of APL cells, a novel co-receptor for plasminogen/tissue plasminogen activator. Thrombosis Research. 2002;**106**:63-70. DOI: 10.1016/S0049-3848(02)00075-0

5

Anticancer Effects of Some Medicinal Thai Plants

Pongtip Sithisarn and Piyanuch Rojsanga

Abstract

Ethanolic extracts from thirty Thai edible plants collected from Sa Keao province, Thailand, were screened for *in vitro* antiproliferative effect on HCT-116 human colon cancer cell line using cell titer 96 aqueous one solution cell proliferation assay. It was found that leaf extract of *Crateva adansnii*, fruit and leaf extracts of *Ardisia elliptica*, shoot extract of *Colocasia esculenta*, leaf extract of *Cratoxylum fomosum*, and leaf extract of *Millettia leucantha* exhibited antiproliferative activities. The fruit extract of *Ardisia elliptica* showed the highest antiproliferative activity. Ethanolic extract of the stems from *C. fenestratum* and its dichloromethane and aqueous fractions showed antiproliferative activity to human colorectal cancer cells (HCT-116) determined by cell growth assay. Berberine, one of the major alkaloid in the stems of *C. fenestratum*, also promoted antiproliferative effect. Extracts from the leaves of three *Azadirachta* species in Thailand, *A. indica*, *A. indica* var. *siamensis*, and *A. excelsa*, were reported to promote *in vitro* antioxidant effects determined by various methods. Ten *Russula* mushroom collected from northeastern part of Thailand were tested for *in vitro* antioxidant activities using photochemiluminescence assay for both lipid-soluble and water-soluble antioxidant capacities. *R. medullata* extract exhibited the highest antioxidant effects in both lipid-soluble and water-soluble models.

Keywords: anticancer, *Coscinium fenestratum*, berberine, *Azadirachta*, *Russula*

1. Introduction

Cancer cells uncontrollably divide to form masses of tissue, which are called tumors. Tumors can grow and interfere with the functions of many bodily systems including the digestive, nervous, and cardiovascular systems. Cancer has been reported to be the first in the rank of causes of the death in the Thai population. Liver, colon, and lung cancers are the most prevalent cancers in Thai males, while breast, cervical, and colon cancers are the most prevalent cancers in Thai females [1].

The development of cancer or carcinogenesis occurs through a multistep process involving the mutation, selection of cells with a progressive increasing capacity for proliferation, survival, invasion, and metastasis [2]. The first step in the process, tumor initiation, relates to the genetic alteration leading to the changes in normal cells. Then, in the promotion or development stage, the cells abnormally proliferate leading to the outgrowth of a population of clonally derived tumor cells [2]. This stage can be stimulated by carcinogens, which are a group of substances such as tobacco, asbestos, arsenic, radiation such as gamma and X-rays, sun light, polycyclic hydrocarbons, nitrosamines, and aflatoxins: these substances do not directly cause cancers but promote or aid the development of cancers [2, 3]. After that, tumor progression continues as additional mutations occur within the cells of the tumor population to further advantage the cancer cells, such as more rapid growth, which will allow them to become dominant within the late tumor population. The process is called clonal selection, since a new clone of tumor cells evolves on the basis of its increased growth rate or other properties such as survival, invasion, or metastasis. Clonal selection continues throughout tumor development, so tumors continuously become more rapid-growing and increasingly malignant [2].

2. Cancer therapy

The modern treatments for cancers mainly are surgery, radiation, and chemotherapy. However, most of chemotherapeutic drugs are not specific to only cancer cells, but also cause damage to normal cells, especially bone marrow, mucous glands, mucous membranes, hair, and nails and can lead to the suppression of the immune system [3]. The success of chemotherapy depends on the number of cancer cells, the proliferation rate, the duration of the drug administration, and the therapeutic interval. To avoid drug resistance, polychemotherapy is always used instead of monochemothearpy [3]. The anticancer drugs can also cause some other side effects including nausea, vomiting, agranulocytosis, inhibition of spermatogenesis and ovulation, alopecia, inflammation of mucous membranes, and terratogenesis [3].

Some compounds separated from natural products are now being developed as modern medicines for the treatments of cancers including paclitaxel, catharanthus alkaloids, and derivatives of podophyllotoxin.

Paclitaxel was separated from the bark of *Taxus brevifolia* Nutt. (Pacific Yew), which is a tree in Taxaceae. Paclitaxel will bind with b-tubulin and stimulate the aggregation of a tubulin subunit to become a nonphysiological microtubule composed of 12 proto-filaments, which cause the inhibition of cell cycles in mitosis and interphase (G_2-phase) and lead to cell apoptosis. This compound is normally used in an injection formulation as the adjuvant chemotherapy for the treatments of ovarian, breast, and bronchial cancers [3].

Some alkaloids are separated from the leaves of *Catharanthus roseus* (L.) G. Don., such as vincristine and vinblastine. Vincristine is used for the treatment of lymphatic leukemia, neuroblastoma, and Wilms tumor, while vinblastine is used to treat lymphogranuloma (Morbus Hodgin), lymphosarcoma, testicular carcinoma, and chorionic carcinoma [3].

Podophyllotoxin was separated from the rhizome of *Podophyllum peltatum* L. or American mandrake. Two derivatives of podophyllotoxin, etoposide and teniposide, are now being developed and used as anticancer drugs. Etoposide is used for the treatment of bronchial cancer, testicular carcinoma, and chorionic carcinoma, while tenoposide is used to treat brain or bladder cancers [3]. The chemical structures of some anticancer compounds from natural products are shown in **Figure 1**.

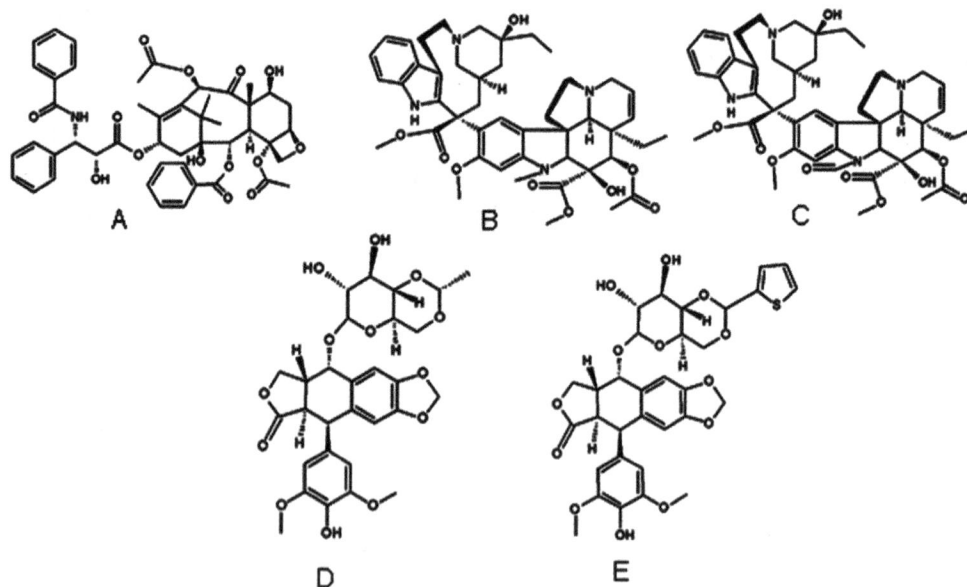

Figure 1. Chemical structures of some anticancer compounds from natural products. A = paclitaxel, B = vinblastine, C = vincristine, D = etoposide, E = teniposide.

3. Anticancer effects of medicinal plants and natural products

Natural products from plants, animals, marine sources, and minerals have been used for the treatments of ailments and diseases for a long time. In Thai traditional medicine, the word "cancer" could refer to the symptom of chronic wound, abscess, emaciation, and weak [4]. Active phytochemicals in plants can be classified into two main groups of primary metabolites, which are the compounds necessary for plant growth and development such as carbohydrates, proteins, and fats. Another group is secondary metabolites, which promote the defense mechanisms or support the lives of the plants; they include polyphenolic compounds, flavonoids, terpenoids, and alkaloids [5]. Ethanolic extracts from thirty Thai local edible plants collected from Wang Nam Yen district, Sa Keao province, Thailand were screened for the *in vitro* anti-proliferative effect on HCT-116 human colon cancer cell lines using a cell titer 96 aqueous one solution cell proliferation assay. It was found that six ethanolic plant extracts, including a leaf extract of *Crateva adansnii*, fruit and leaf extracts of *Ardisia elliptica*, a shoot extract of *Colocasia esculenta*, a leaf extract of *Cratoxylum fomosum*, and a leaf extract of *Millettia leucantha* exhibited antiproliferative activities on the HCT-116 cell line. The fruit extract of *Ardisia elliptica* showed the highest antiproliferative activities with an IC_{50} value of 5.12 ± 0.54 µg/ml [6]. The mechanisms of the action of medicinal plants for anticancer effects have been reported as following [4]:

3.1. Inhibition of cell division in the cancer cell cycle

Alpha-mangostin from mangosteen (*Garcinia mangostana*) fruit rind promoted inhibitory effects to breast cancer cell line (MDA-MB-231) by inhibition of cell division in G1 and S phases [7]. Methanol extract of *Morus alba* L. leaves inhibited liver cancer cell line Hep G2 by inhibition of cell division in G2/M phase [8]. Cucurbitacin B, a triterpenoid from *Trichosanthes cucumerina* L., also inhibited breast cancer cell division in G2/M phase [9].

3.2. Induction of cancer cell apoptosis

This mechanism includes some minor mechanisms which stimulate anticancer genes, induction of caspase enzymes, induction of free radical formation, inhibition or induction of enzymes relating to histone protein, and the formation of spingosine or ceramide [4]. Dehydrocostus lactone from the root of *Saussurea lappa* induced the apoptosis of liver cancer cells Hep G2 and PLC/PRF/5 via p53 protein [10]. Water extract of the seed from *Sapindus rarak* Candolle. induced lung cancer cells A549 apoptosis through the induction of the caspase enzyme [11], while methanol extract of *Derris scandens* Benth. induced apoptosis of colon cancer cells SE480 by increased caspase-3 activity and down-regulated Bcl-2 and up-regulated Bax protein of SW480 cells; it also significantly induced cell necrosis determined by the release of LDH [12]. Alpha-mangostin separated from the fruit rind of mangosteen also upregulated Bax and down-regulated Bcl-2 proteins in rat liver tissue [13]. Methanol extract from stem bark of *Myristica fragrans* Houtt. promoted the apoptosis of lymphoblast Jurkat by controlling the SIRT1 gene [14]. G1 b, a glycospingolipid from *Murdannia loriformis* (Hassk.) R.S.Rao & Kammathy, inhibited breast, lung, colon, and liver cell lines [15].

3.3. Immune stimulation

Methanol extract from the leaves of *Moringa oleifera* Lam. exhibited immune stimulation effect both cell-mediated immunity and humoral immunity by induction of neutrophile production and stimulation of macrophages in animals damaged by the toxicity of anticancer drugs [16].

In Thai traditional medicine, there are some medicinal formulas compose of several plants in different ratios. These formulas are traditionally used for a long time usually for the treatments of cancers in patient with the late stage cancers, patients who cannot improve after treatment with chemotherapy, radiation or surgery, patients with cancers in several organs or patients with incurrent diseases [4]. The sources of anticancer herbal formulas usually come from local traditional doctors or priests in the temples (in Thai, temple is called as "Wat"), with the normal method of preparation being the decoction of plant materials with water [4]. A herbal remedy from Wat Tha-it (Tha-it temple), Ang Thong province, Thailand, composed of several plant materials including *Gelonium multiflorum* A. Juss., *Erycibe ellip-tilimba* Merrill & Chun, *Balanophora abbreviate* Blume, *Smilax china* L., *Smilax glabra* Wall. ex Roxb., and *Millingtonia hortensis* Linn. was reported to significantly promote synergistic effects on doxorubicin in the treatment of A549 cancer cells by the inhibition of cell divisions in the G2/M phase [4, 17]. Another herbal remedy is from a Thai herbal nursing home, Wat Khampramong, Sakon Nakhon province comprises of several plant materials such as *Rhinacanthus nasutus* (L.) Kurz, *Acanthus ebrateatus* Wall., *Smilax glabra* Wall. ex Roxb.,

Artemisia annua L., *Angelica sinensis* (Oliv.) Diels, *Salacia chinensis* L., and *Orthosiphon aristatus* Miq [18]. This herbal remedy can inhibit the growth of some cancer cell lines such as breast adenocarcinoma MDA-MB 231, synovial sarcoma SW982, hepatocellular carcinoma HepG2, cervical adenocarcinoma HeLa, and lung carcinoma A549 [18].

4. Some potential Thai medicinal plants with anticancer effects

4.1. *Coscinium fenestratum* (Gaertn.) Colebr

NAG-1 or nonsteroidal anti-inflammatory drug (NSAID)-activated gene was identified in COX-negative cells by PCR-based subtractive hybridization from an NSAID-induced library as a divergent member of the TGF-β superfamily [19]. The overexpression of NAG-1 in cancer cells results in growth arrest and an increase in apoptosis, suggesting that NAG-1 has antitumorigenic activity [20]. NAG-1 expression is also upregulated by a number of dietary compounds, medicinal plants, and anticancer drugs [21–25]. *Coscinium fenestratum* is one of the medicinal plants that promoted antiproliferative effects on colon cancer cell lines with mechanisms related to NAG-1 [20].

Coscinium fenestratum (Gaertn.) Colebr. is a large climber with yellow wood and sap, known in the Thai language as Hamm or Khamin khruea. The genus *Coscinium* belongs to the tribe Coscinieae of the family Menispermaceae. This genus comprises two species, which are *Coscinium blumeanum* Miers. and *C. fenestratum* (Gaertn.) Colebr. Both of them are stout woody climbers growing in the tropical rain forest regions of Asia [26]. *Coscinium* species are characterized by the axillary flowers, extra-axillary or cauliflorous in racemiform, or peduncled subumbellate aggregate, of 20–50 cm in length. The inflorescences are axillary or cauliflorous with 6–12 florets. Male flowers are sessile or with pedicels, up to 1 mm. Sepals are broadly elliptic to obovate with the inner 3–6 spreading, yellow, and 1.5–2 mm long. Stamens are 6 with 1 mm long. The Sepals of female flower are as in male flowers. Staminodes are 6 and claviform with 1 mm long. Drupes are subglobose, tomentellous, brown to orange or yellowish, 2.8–3 cm diameter. Pericarp is drying woody. Seeds are whitish and subglobose with the enveloping condyle. The leaves are subpeltate or ovate, large, hard-coriaceous, palmately nerved, reticulate, and densely hairy beneath [26]. Physical characteristic of the *Coscinium fenestratum* stem (cross section) is shown in **Figure 2**.

The stem decoction and maceration extracts of *Coscinium fenestratum* have been traditionally used in the Northeastern part of Thailand for the treatment of various diseases such as cancer, diabetes mellitus, and arthritis [27]. The ethanolic extract of the stems from *C. fenestratum* and its dichloromethane and aqueous fractions showed antiproliferative activity on human colorectal cancer cells (HCT-116) determined by a cell growth assay. Berberine, one of the major alkaloids in the stems of *C. fenestratum*, also promoted an antiproliferative effect [20]. The mechanisms of action of the extracts from *C. fenestratum* were reported as the activation of proapoptotic proteins and pparγ [20]. It was also reported that berberine facilitated the apoptosis of cancer cells, and the molecular targets for its activity are NAG-1 and AFT3 [24]. The chemical structure of Berberine is shown in **Figure 3**.

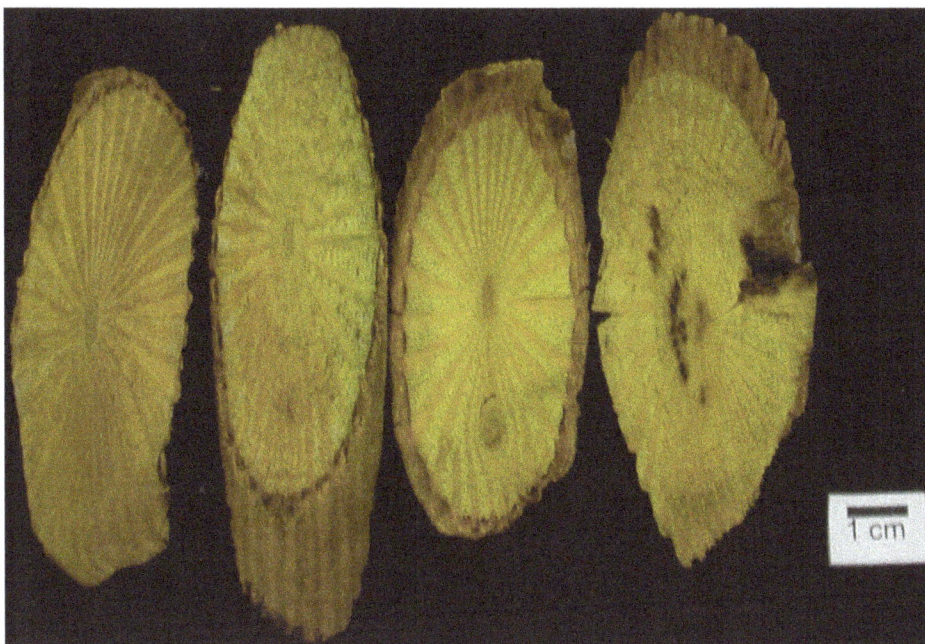

Figure 2. Physical characteristic of *Coscinium fenestratum* stem purchased from Nongkhai province, Thailand (cross section ×1).

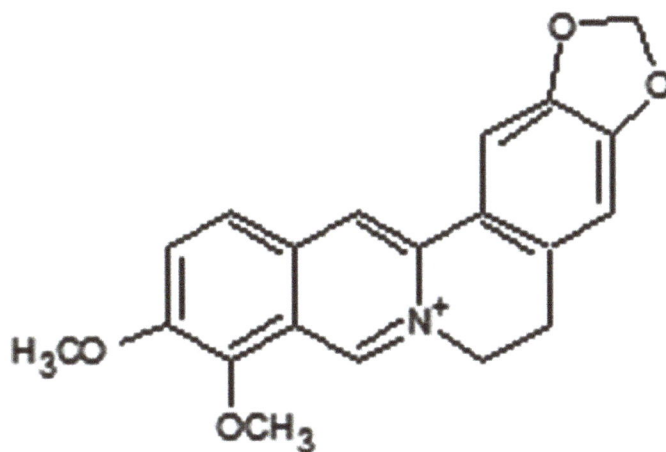

Figure 3. Chemical structure of Berberine.

4.2. *Azadirachta* plants

Oxidative stress is considered to be of some importance for many ailments and pathologies; including cardiovascular diseases, cancers, rheumatoid arthritis, and Alzheimer's disease [28]. Polyphenolic compounds have been reported to have important anticancer and chemo-preventive effects [29]. Phenolic acids such as gallic acid, ellagic acid, and ferulic acid induce apoptosis in cancer cells, activated caspase, prevented cancer formation, and suppress the angiogenesis of cancer [29–32]. Flavonoids such as quercertin and kaempferol also promote apoptosis, inhibit oncogenes, and generated cell cycle arrest [29, 33–35].

Suttajit et al. [36] studied the antioxidant activities of extracts from many Thai medicinal plants using a ABTS-metmyoglobin assay and reported some plants with high antioxidant activities; including *Uncaria gambier* Roxb., *Piper betle* Linn., *Camellia sinensis* (L.) Kuntze., *Azadirachta indica* A. Juss. var. *siamensis* Valeton., *Curcuma zedoaria* Roxb., *Syzygium aromaticum* (L.) Merr. & Perry and *Tamarindus indica* Linn. When focusing on Thai medicinal plants, the Siamese neem tree (*Azadirachta indica* A. Juss. var. *siamensis* Valeton.) is an interesting plant that showed high antioxidant activity in the screening test [36, 37]. Moreover, there are reports about its antioxidant potential based on the antioxidant content as the butylated hydroxyanisole (BHA) equivalent of Thai indigenous vegetable extracts. From this report, the Siamese neem tree leaf extract appeared to be a high potency antioxidant, containing more than 100 mg BHA equivalent in 100 g fresh weight.

Azadirachta plants comprise of three different plant species; *Azadirachta indica* A. Juss or *A. indica* A. Juss var. *indica* (neem), *Azadirachta indica* A. Juss. var. *siamensis* Valeton (Siamese neem tree), and *Azadirachta excela* (Jack) Jacobs. (marrango tree). The Siamese neem tree leaves are wider, longer, and thicker than the leaves of neem, while the marrango tree has the widest, longest, and thickest leaves. The margin of the leaflet of Siamese neem tree is crenate to entire, while the margin of neem is serrate and that of marrango tree is entire to undulate. The colors of the leaflet blade of the Siamese neem tree, neem, and marrango tree are green, light green, and dark shiny green, respectively [38, 39]. The physical characteristics of Siamese neem tree, neem, and marrango tree leaves are shown in **Figure 4**.

The leaves and flowers of Siamese neem tree and neem have been traditionally used as element tonics and antipyretic and gastric secretion stimulating agents, while the stem bark of all *Azadirachta* plants is used to treat amoebic dysentery and diarrhea [40, 41]. There also reports suggesting that polysaccharides and limonoids found in neem bark, leaves, and seed oil reduce tumors and cancers and showed effectiveness against lymphocytic leukemia [42–44]. Moreover, the young leaves and flowers of the Siamese neem tree are popularly consumed as vegetables [39].

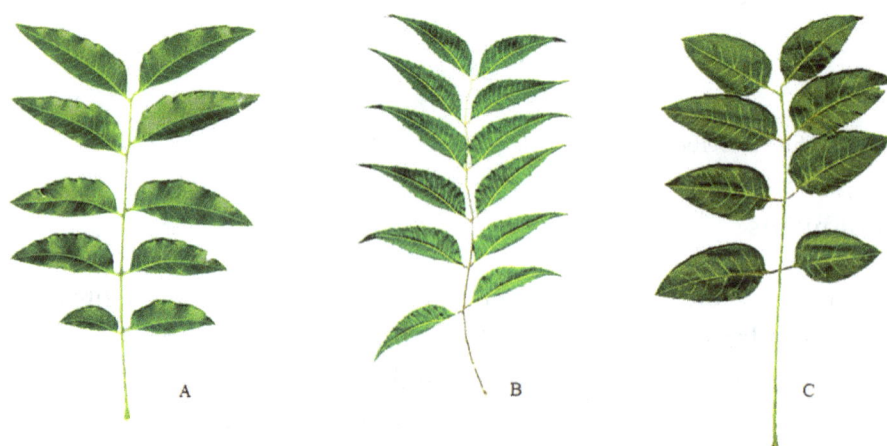

Figure 4. Physical characteristics of *Azadirachta* plants; A = Siamese neem tree (*Azadirachta indica* var. *siamensis*), B = neem (*Azadirachta indica*), C = marrango tree (*Azadirachta excela*).

For the antioxidant effect, *Azadirachta* plants were reported to promote *in vitro* activities tested by various methods. Extracts from the leaves of *A. indica*, *A. indica* var. *siamensis*, and *A. excelsa* were reported to promote *in vitro* antioxidant effects determined by a DPPH scavenging assay, Fremy's salt assay, ESR detection of POBN spin adducts, and an oxygen consumption assay [45, 46]. The leaf's aqueous and flower ethanol extracts from the Siamese neem tree provide antioxidant activity on lipid peroxidation formation induced by UV-irradiation of a Chago K-1 bronchogenic cell culture at a concentration of 100 µg/ml determined by the thiobarbituric acid reactive substances (TBARS) method [47].

Cloning and expression analysis of genes involving flavonoid biosynthesis showed that Siamese neem tree leaves total RNA contained nucleotide sequences related to enzymes F3'H, FLS, DFR, and F3'5'H, which could be responsible for the biosynthesis of the antioxidant flavonoids [48]. Some flavonoids that were separated from Siamese neem tree and neem leaves and flowers are kaempferol, myricetin, quercetin, and rutin [39, 49–51]. The chemical structures of some flavonoids found in *Azadirachta* plants are shown in **Figure 5**.

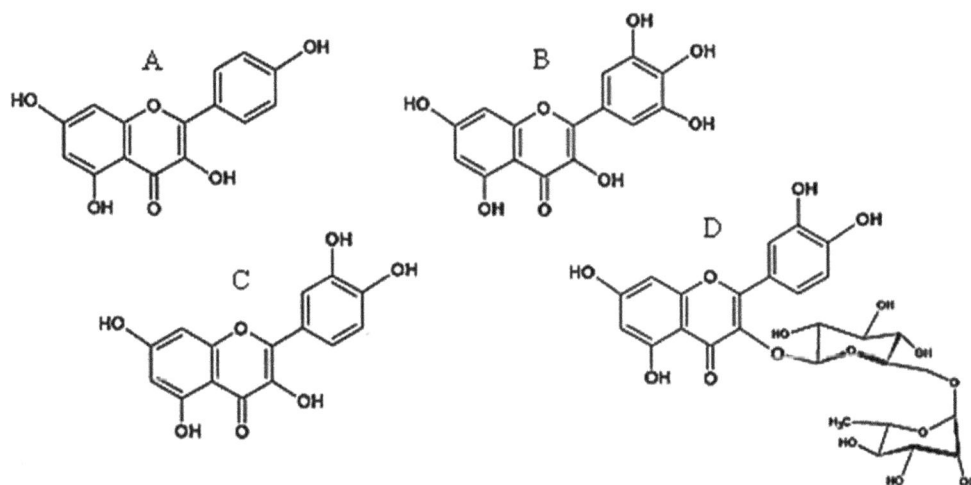

Figure 5. Chemical structures of some flavonoids found in *Azadirachta* plants. A = kaempferol, B = myricetin, C = quercetin, D = rutin.

4.3. *Russula* mushrooms

It is well established that many compounds separated from mushrooms can be used as immuno-modulators or as biological response modifiers [52]. Several mushroom species in Basidiomycetes have been reported to possess anti-tumor activity [53, 54].

Many phytochemical compounds have been reported in various mushrooms, and they can be classified into two main groups: high molecular weight compounds such as beta-glucan and other polysaccharides [55] and low molecular weight compounds including polyphenolics, flavonoids, and terpenoids [52]. Polyphenolics such as caffeic acid, chlorogenic acid, ferulic acid, and gallic acid and flavonoids such as myricetin and catechin were found in *Agaricusbisporus*, *Boletus edulis*, *Calocybe gambosa*, and *Cantharellus cibarius* [56]. Triterpeniods were found in *Agaricus bisporus*, *Ganoderma lucidum*, and *Russula lepida*. Moreover, aristolane sesquiterpenoids were also found in *Russula lepida* [57]. Polysaccharides were found in *Agaricus bisporus*, *Agaricus brasiliensis, Ganoderma lucidum*, and *Phellinus linteus* [58]. Some polysaccharides such as beta-glucan are reported to promote immunomodulatory effects via CR3, the leukocytemembrane receptor for β-glucans [59]. The mechanisms of the action of the mushrooms to promote anticancer effects have been reported as NF-κB inhibitors, protein kinase inhibitors, protein and DNA alkylating agents, modulators of G1/S and G2/M phases, inhibitors of MAPK protein kinase signaling pathways, aromatase and sulfatase inhibitors, matrix metalloproteinases inhibitors, cyclooxygenase inhibitors, DNA topoisomerases, and DNA polymerase inhibitors and anti-angiogenic substances [52].

A previous study reported the presence of 1147 mushroom species in the Northeast part of Thailand. They are composed of 647 consumed mushroom species, 222 trade mushroom species, and 400 poisonous mushroom species [60]. Thirty-seven species of these mushrooms are used in traditional medicine [60]. However, there are still some mushrooms in Thailand, especially in the Northeastern part of the country, that have never been studied for their biological properties and phytochemical compounds.

The Russula mushroom's shape resembles an umbrella. There have a clear cap and stem, with the gills underneath the cap. The cap is thin and has an underlying radius arranged around the center. The mushroom has no ring and no latex in the cap. The mushroom is fresh, soft, fragile, and perishable [61]. There are around 750 worldwide species of *Russula* [62, 63]. The distribution of the *Russula* species shows that they are present in several countries, including the United States of America, Sweden, France, Norway, Madagascar, Italy, Belgium, Taiwan, China, Japan, and Thailand [64]. In Thailand, *Russula* mushrooms have been found in 17 provinces in the Northeastern region of Thailand [65]. Numerous *Russula* mushrooms have been consumed as food such as *R. monspeliensis*, *R. virescens*, *R. alboareolata*, *R. medullata*, and *R. helios* [65, 66]. Various *Russula* mushrooms have been traditionally used for the treatments of various diseases such as *R. cyanoantha* and *R. nobilis*, which are used for the treatment of fever; *R. luteotacta*, which is used for wound healing; and *R. delica* and *R. parazurea*, which are used for the treatment of gastritis and high blood pressure, while *R. acrifolia* is used for treatments of skin cancer [36]. Moreover, some *Russula* mushrooms have also been traditionally used for tonic purposes such as *R. cyanoxantha, R. nobilis, R. delica, R. parazurea, R. acrifolia*, and *R. luteotacta* [67]. In addition, *Russula luteotacta* has been used as a sleep promoting agent [67]. Physical characteristics of some *Russula* mushrooms found in Thailand are shown in **Figure 6**.

Ten *Russula* mushroom collected from northeastern part of Thailand: *R. crustosa, R. delica, R. monspeliensis, R. velenovskyi, R. virescens, R. lepida, R. alboareolata, R. paludosa, R. medullata*, and *R. helios* were tested for their *in vitro* antioxidant activities using a photochemiluminescence assay for both lipid-soluble and water-soluble antioxidant capacities. *R. medullata* extract exhibited the highest antioxidant effects in both lipid-soluble and water-soluble models with antioxidant capacities of 1.1658 nmol of trolox equivalence and 1.323 nmol of ascorbic acid equivalence, respectively [68].

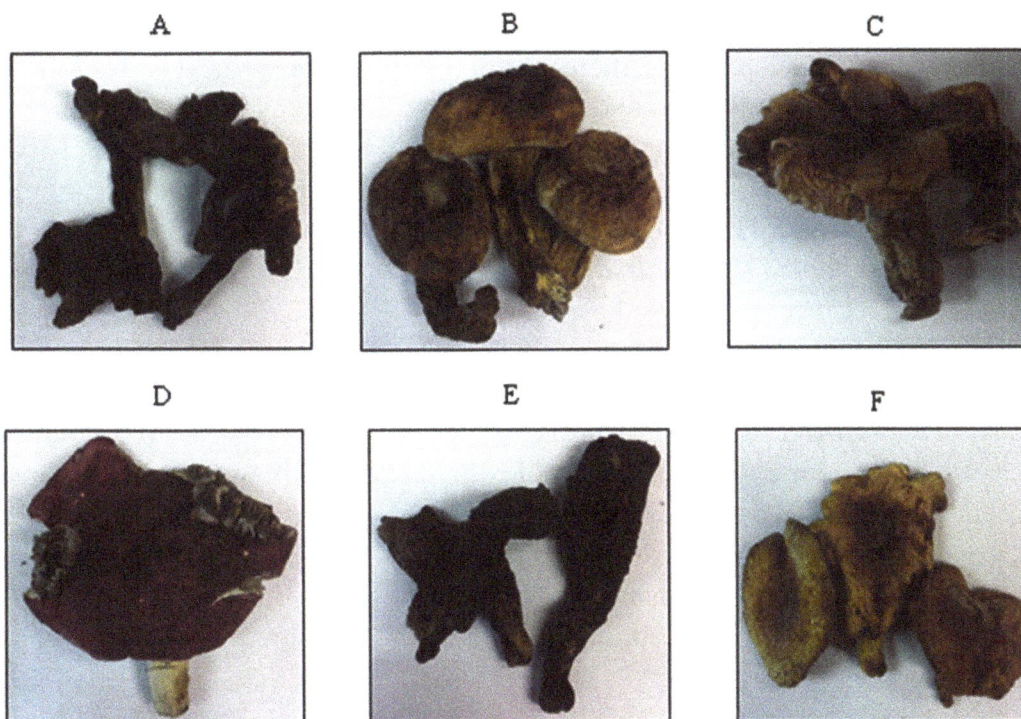

Figure 6. Physical characteristics of some Russula mushrooms found in Thailand; A = *Russula crustosa* Peck, B = *Russula delica* Fries, C = *Russula monspeliensis* Sarnari, D = *Russula velenovskyi* Melzer & Zvára, E = *Russula virescens* (Schaeff) Fries, F = *Russula alboareolata* Hongo.

Some chemical constituents have been reported from *Russula* mushrooms including phenolic acids such as ρ-hydroxy-benzoic acid, chlorogenic acid, ferulic acid, caffeic acid, protocate-chuic acid, and coumaric acid and flavonoids such as quercetin, chrysin, and catechin [69–71]. Some terpeniods were also found in *Russula* mushrooms including aristolane and marasmane [57, 72]. The chemical structures of the constituents found in *Russula* mushrooms are shown in **Figure 7**.

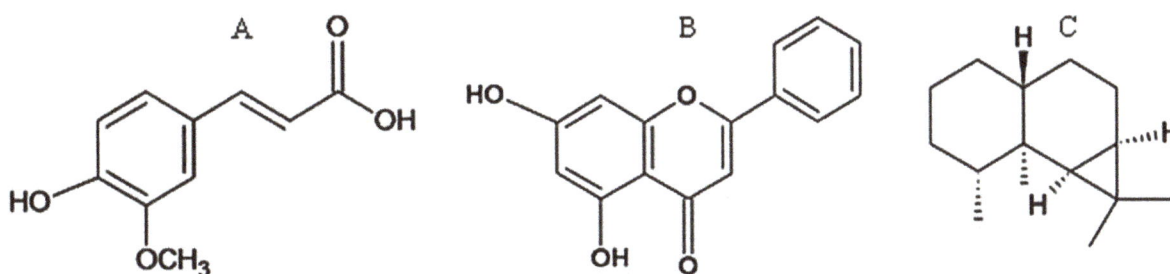

Figure 7. Chemical structures of some flavonoids found in *Russula* mushrooms. A = ferulic acid, B = chrysin, C = aristolane.

5. Conclusion

Natural products have been main sources of drug discoveries including the development of active compounds or formulas for the treatment of cancers. Even though it has become difficult to discover or synthesize new active components, with the knowledge and intelligence regarding traditional medicine, there are still several ethnomedical herbal formulas and regional plants that could be studied and developed for further medicinal utilizations. Herbal remedies from Wat Tha-it and Wat Khampramong, Thailand, are examples of the efforts to develop anticancer therapies from traditional knowledge. Both remedies can inhibit the growth of various cancer cell lines. The stem extract and active compound, Berberine from the Thai medicinal plant *Coscinium fenestratum*, significantly promoted anti-proliferative activity on human colorectal cancer cells with the mechanism of action via NAG-1 and AFT3. Plants in the genus *Azadirachta* have been traditionally used as a tonic. They promote significant antioxidant activities, which could support the body's systems and prevent oxidative stress, which is one of the causes of carcinogenesis. *Russula* is the local mushroom species in the Northeastern part of Thailand. They promote significant antioxidant effects in both lipid-soluble and water-soluble models. These plants and natural products have the potential to be sources of anticancer compounds or active extracts for the treatments of cancer. However, standardization and quality control of the extract or active compounds should be performed before studying the toxicity, *in vivo* biological activity tests, and further clinical studies in the future.

Acknowledgements

The authors acknowledge the Thailand Institute of Scientific and Technological Research for the support in supplying the photos of *Russula* mushrooms. The authors would like to thank Dr. Prapaipat Klungsupya for her valuable guidance and support about photochemiluminescence assays. The authors also thank Ms. Charinan Jaengklang for her assistance in the *Russula* mushrooms work.

Author details

Pongtip Sithisarn[1]* and Piyanuch Rojsanga[2]

*Address all correspondence to: pongtip.sit@mahidol.ac.th

1 Department of Pharmacognosy, Faculty of Pharmacy, Mahidol University, Bangkok, Thailand

2 Department of Pharmaceutical Chemistry, Faculty of Pharmacy, Mahidol University, Bangkok, Thailand

References

[1] Attasara P, Buasom R (2009). Hospital-based cancer registry. National Cancer Institute. Department of Medical Services. Ministry of Public Health. [Access on January 10, 2017] http://www.nci.go.th/th/File_download/Nci%20Cancer%20Registry/hospital%20based%20cancer%20registry.pdf

[2]   Cooper GM, Sunderland MA (2000). The development and causes of cancer. The cell: a molecular approach. 2nd edition. Sinauer Associates.

[3]   Jiratchariyakul W (2015). Anticancer substances in medicinal plants. M and M Laser Printing Co. Ltd. Bangkok (book in Thai).

[4]   Kummalue T (2012). Anticancer mechanisms of medicinal plants, a medical research. Faculty of Medicine Siriraj Hospital, Mahidol University. Bangkok (book in Thai).

[5]   Evans WC (2009). Trease and Evans Pharmacognosy. 16th edition. Elsevier. London.

[6]   Ondee S, Sithisarn P, Ruangwises N, Rojsanga P (2015). Anti-proliferative activity on colorectal cancer cells of thirty Thai edible plants. Proceeding in the 1st international conference on pharmacy education and research network of ASEAN, Bangkok, Thailand, December, 2-4.

[7]   Shibata MA, Iinuma M, Morimoto J, Kurose H, Akamatsu K, Okuno Y, Akao Y, Otsuki Y (2011). α-Mangostin extracted from the pericarp of the mangosteen (*Garcinia mangostana* Linn) reduces tumor growth and lymph node metastasis in an immunocompetent xenograft model of metastatic mammary cancer carrying a p53 mutation. BMC Med. 9(69):1-18.

[8]   Naowaratwattana W, De-eknamkul W, De Mejia EG (2010). Phenolic containing organic extracts of mulberry (Morusalba L.) leaves inhibit Hep G2 hepatoma cell through G2/M phase arrest, induction of apoptosis, and inhibition of topoisomerase II alpha activity. J Med Food. 13(5):1045-56.

[9]   Dakeng S, Duangmano S, Jiratchariyakul W, U-pratya Y, Bogler O, Patmasiriwat P (2012). Inhibition of Wnt signaling by cucurbitacin B in breast cancer cells: reduction of Wnt-associated proteins and reduced translocation of galectin-3-mediated β-catenin to the nucleus. J Cell Biochem. 113(1):49-60.

[10] Hsu YL, Wu LY, Kuo PL (2009). Dehydrocostus lactone, a medicinal plant-derived sesquiterpene lactone, induces apoptosis coupled to endoplasmic reticulum stress in liver cancer cells. J Pharmacol Exp Ther. 329(2):808-19.

[11] Kummalue T, Sujiwattanarat P, Jiratchariyakul W (2011). Apoptosis inducibility of Sapindusrorak water extract on A549 human lung cancer cell line. J Med Plant Res. 5(7):1087-94.

[12] Kaewkon W, Khamprasert N, Limpeanchob N (2011). Derris scandens Benth extract induced necrosis rather than apoptosis of SW480 colon cancer cell. Thai J Pharmacol. 33(2):118-21.

[13] Moongkarndi P, Jaisupa N, Kosem N, Konlata J, Samer J, Pattanapanyasat K, Rodpai E (2015). Effect of purified α-mangostin from mangosteen pericarp on cytotoxicity, cell cycle arrest and apoptotic gene expression in human cancer cells. World J Pharm Sci. 3(8):1473-84.

[14] Chirathaworn C, Kongcharoensuntorn W, Dechdoungchan T, Lowanitchapat A, Sa-nguanmoo P, Poovorawan Y (2007). Myristica fragrans Houtt. methanolic extract

induces apoptosis in a human leukemia cell line through SIRT1 mRNA downregulation. J Med Assoc Thai. 90(11):2422-8.

[15] Jiratcgariyakul W, Okabe H, Moongkarndi P, Frahm AW (1998). Cytotoxic glycosphingo-lipid from Murdannia loriformis (Hassk.) Rolla Rao et Kammathy. Thai J Phytopharm. 5(1):10-20.

[16] Sudha P, Syed M, Sunil D, Gowda C (2010). Immunomodulatory activity of methanolic leaf extract of Moringa oleifera in animals. Indian J Physiol Pharmacol. 54(2):133-40.

[17] Srisapoomi T, Jiratchariyakul W, O-partkiattikul N, Kummalue T (2008). Effects of two Thai herbal remedies on the sensitivity of chemotherapeutic agents in human cancer cells. Asian J Trad Med. 3(4):144-52.

[18] Soonthornchareonnon N, Sireeratawong S, Wiwat C, Ruangwises N, Wongnopphavich A, Jaijoy K (2011). Research and development of anti-cancer formula from Wat Khampramong. National Research Council of Thailand. Faculty of Pharmacy, Mahidol University, Bangkok.

[19] Baek SJ, Kim KS, Nixon JB, Wilson LC, Eling TE (2001). Cyclooxygenase inhibitors regu-late the expression of a TGF-beta superfamily member that has proapoptotic and antitu-morigenic activities. Mol Pharmacol 59:901-8.

[20] Rojsanga P, Sukhthankar M, Krisanapan C, Gritsanapun W, Lawson DB, Baek SJ (2010). In vitro anti-proliferative activity of alcoholic stem extract of Coscinium fenestratum in human colorectal cancer cells. Exp Ther Med. 1:181-6.

[21] Baek SJ, Kim JS, Jackson FR, Eling TE, McEntee MF, Lee SH (2004). Epicatechin gallate induced expression of NA G-1 is associated with growth inhibition and apoptosis in colon cancer cells. Carcinogenesis. 25:2425-32.

[22] Baek SJ, Wilson LC, Eling TE (2002). Resveratrol enhances the expression of non-steroi-dal anti-inflammatory drug-activated gene (NA G-1) by increasing the expression of p53. Carcinogenesis. 23: 425-34.

[23] Martinez JM, Sali T, Okazaki R, Anna C, Hollingshead M, Hose C, Monks A, Walker NJ, Baek SJ, Eling TE (2006). Drug-induced expression of nonsteroidal anti-inflam-matory drug-activated gene/macrophage inhibitory cytokine-1/prostate-derived factor, a putative tumor suppressor, inhibits tumor growth. J Pharmacol Exp Ther. 318:899-906.

[24] Rojsanga P, Sukhthankar M, Baek SJ (2007). Berberine, a natural isoquinoline alkaloid, induces NAG-1 and AFT3 expression in human colorectal cancer cells. Cancer Lett. 258(2): 230-40.

[25] Lee SH, Cekanova M, Baek SJ (2008). Multiple mechanisms are involved in 6-gingerol-induced cell growth arrest and apoptosis in human colorectal cancer cells. Mol Carcinog. 47:197-208.

[26] Forman LL (1991). Menispermaceae. Bangkok: The Forest Herbarium.300-65.

[27] Wattanathorn J, Uabundit N, Itarat W, Mucimapura S, Laopatarakasem P, Sripanidkulchai B (2006). Neurotoxicity of Coscinium fenestratum stem, a medicinal plant used in traditional medicine. Food Chem Toxicol. 44:1327-33.

[28] Cross EC (1987). Oxygen radicals and human disease. Ann Intern Med. 107: 526-45.

[29] Carocho M, Ferreira ICFR (2013). The role of phenolic compounds in the fight against cancer-a review. Anticancer Agents Medicinal Chem. 13:1236-58.

[30] Ji B, Hsu W, Yang J, Hsia T, Lu C, Chiang J, Yang J, Lin C, Lin J, Suen L, Wood WG, Chung J (2009). Gallic acid inducesapoptosisviacaspase-3 and mitochondrion-dependent pathways in vitro and suppresses lung xenograft tumor growth in vivo. J Agric Food Chem. 57:7596-7604.

[31] Kim S, Gaber MW, Zawaski JA, Zhang F, Richardson M, Zhang XA, Yang Y (2009). The inhibition of glioma growth in vitro and in vivo by a chitosan/ellagic acid composite biomaterial. Biomaterials. 30:4743-51.

[32] Baskaran N, Manoharan S, BalakrishnanS, Pugalendhi P (2010). Chemopreventive potential of ferulic acid in 7,12-dimethylbenz[a]anthracene-induced mammary carcinogenesis in Sprague-Dawley rats. Eur J Pharmacol. 637:22-9.

[33] Nair H, Rao KVK, Aalinkeel R, Mahajan S, Chawda R, Schwartz SA (2004). Inhibition of prostate cancer cell colony formation by the flavonoid quercetin correlates with modulation of specific regulatory genes. Clin Diagn Lab Immunol. 11:63-9.

[34] Yuan Z, Chen L, Fan L, Tang M, Yang G, Yang H, Du X, Wang G, Yao W, Zhao Q, Ye B, Wang R, Diao P, Zhang W, Wu H, Zhao X, Wei Y (2006). Liposomal quercetin efficiently suppresses growth of solid tumors in murine models. Clin Cancer Res. 12:3193-9.

[35] Zhang H, Zhang M, Yu L, Zhao Y, HeN, Yang, X (2012).Antitumor activitiesofquercetin and quercetin-50,8-disulfonate in human colon and breast cancer cell lines. Food Chem Toxicol. 50:1589-99.

[36] Suttajit S, Khansuwan U, Suttajit M (2002). Antioxidative activity of Thai medicinal herbs. Thai J Pharm Sci. 26(suppl.):32.

[37] Trakoontivakorn G, Saksitpitak J (2000). Antioxidative potential of Thai indigenous vegetable extracts. Journal of Food Research and Product Development. Kasetsart University. 30(3):164-76.

[38] Sombatsiri K, Ermel K, Schmutterer H (1995). Other Meliaceous plants containing ingredients for integrated pest management and further purpose. In: Schmutter H. The neem tree Azadirachtaindica A. Juss. and other meliaceous plants. Germany: VCH.

[39] Sithisarn P, Gritsanapan W (2008). Siamese neem tree: A plant from kitchen to antioxidative health supplement. Advances in Phytotherapy Research. Research Signpost. Kerala. India.

[40] Clayton T, Soralump P, Chaukul W, Temsiririrkkul R (1996). Medicinal plants in Thailand volume 1. Bangkok: Amarin Printing.

[41] Te-Chato S, Rungnoi O (2000). Induction of somatic embryogenesis from leaves of Sadao Chang (Azadirachta excelsa (Jack) Jacobs). Sci Horticult. 86:311-21.

[42] Arivazhagan S, Balasenthil S, Nagini S (2000). Garlic and neem extracts enhance hepatic glutathione-dependent enzymes during N-methyl-N-nitro-N-nitrosoguanidine (MNNG)-induced gastric carcinogenesis in rats. Phytother Res. 14:291-3.

[43] Akudugu J, Gade G, Bohm L (2001). Cytotoxicity of axadirachtin A in human glioblastoma cell lines. Life Sci. 68:1153-60.

[44] Subapriya R, Nagini S (2003). Ethanolicneem leaf extracts protects againstN-methyl-N-nitro-N-nitrosoguanidine-induced gastric carcinogenesis inWistar rats. Asian Pac J Cancer Prev. 4:215-23.

[45] Sithisarn P, Gritsanapan W, Supabphol R (2004). Free radical scavenging activity of three Azadirachta plants. Proceeding in the 21st Annual Research meeting in Pharmaceutical Sciences, Bangkok, Thailand, December, 23-24, 2004.

[46] Sithisarn P, Carlsen CU, Andersen ML, Gritsanapan W, Skibsted LH (2007). Antioxidative effects of leaves from Azadirachta species of different provenience. Food Chem. 104: 1539-49.

[47] Sithisarn P, Supabphol R, Gritsanapan W (2005). Antioxidant activity of Siamese neem tree. J Ethophamacol. 99: 109-12.

[48] Sithisarn P, Suksangpanomrung M, Gritsanapan W (2007). Gene expression of enzymes related to biosynthesis of antioxidative flavonoids in Siamese neem tree leaves. Planta Med. 73: 222.

[49] Pankadamani KS, Seshadri TR (1952). Survey of anthoxanthins. Proc Indian Acad Sci Ser A 36: 157-69.

[50] Nakov N, Labode O, Akahtaedzhiev K (1982). Study of the flavonoid composition of *Azadirachta indica*. Farmatsiya (Sofia). 32:24-8.

[51] Siddiqui S, Mahmood T, Siddiqui BS, Faizi S (1985). Studies in the nonterpenoial constituents of Azadirachtaindica. Pak J Sci Ind Res. 28(1):1-4.

[52] Zaidman BZ, Yassin M, Mahajna J, Wasser SP (2005). Medicinal mushroom modulators of molecular targets as cancer therapeutics. Appl Microbiol Biotechnol. 67: 453-68.

[53] Mizuno T (1995). Bioactive biomolecules of mushrooms: food function and medicinal effect of mushroom fungi. Food Rev Int. 11:7-21.

[54] Wasser SP (2002). Medicinal mushrooms as a source of antitumor and immunomodulating polysaccharides. Appl Microbiol Biotechnol. 60:258-274.

[55] Jaruntorn B, Chanida H (2010). Spatial distribution of Beta glucan containing wild mushroom communities in subtropical dry forest, Thailand. Fungal Divers. 46(1): 29-42.

[56] Palacios I, Lozano M, Moro C, D'Arrigo M, Rostagno MA, Martínez JA, García-Lafuente A, Guillamón E, Villares A (2011). Antioxidant properties of phenolic compounds occurring in edible mushrooms. Food Chem. 128:674-8.

[57] Jian-Wen T, Ze-Jun D, Ji-Kai L (2000). New terpenoids from Basidiomycetes Russula lepida. Helv Chim Acta. 83:3191-7.

[58] Kozarski M, Klaus A, Niksic M, Jakovljevic D, Helsper JPFG, Van Griensven LJLD (2011). Antioxidative and immunomodulating activities of polysaccharide extracts of the medicinal mushrooms Agaricusbisporus, Agaricusbrasiliensis, Ganodermalucidum and Phellinuslinteus. Food Chem. 129(4):1667-75.

[59] Xia Y, Vetvicka V, Yan J, Hanikyrova M, Mayadas T, Ross GD (1999). The beta-glucan-binding lectin site of mouse CR3 (CD11b/CD18) and its function in generating a primed state of the receptor that mediates cytotoxic activation in response to iC3b-opsonized target cells. J Immunol. 162:2281-90.

[60] The Bureau of Thai Indigenous Medicine, Department for Development of Thai Traditional and Alternative Medicine. Ministry of Public Health (2011). Mushrooms are health food from folk medicine. The Bureau of Thai Indigenous Medicine, Department for Development of Thai Traditional and Alternative Medicine. Ministry of Public Health. Nonthaburi. (book in Thai).

[61] Sonoamuang N (2010). Wild mushrooms of Thailand: biodiversity and utilization. Department of Plant Science and Natural Resources. Faculty of Agriculture, Khon Kaen University.

[62] Joshi S, Bhatt RP, Stephenson SL (2012). The current status of the family Russulaceae in the Uttarakhand Himalaya, India. Mycosphere. 3(4):486-501.

[63] Jain N, Pande V (2013). Diversity analysis of ectomycorrhizal genus Russula using RAPD markers. Octa Jour Env Res. 1(4):332-5.

[64] Buyck B, Hofstetter V, Eberhardt U, Verbeken A, Kauff F (2008). Walking the thin line between *Russula* and *Lactarius*: the dilemma of Russula subsect. Ochricompactae. Fungal Divers. 28:15-40.

[65] Manassila M, Sooksa-Nguan T, Boonkerd N, Rodtongb S, Teaumroonga N (2005). Phylogenetic diversity of wild edible Russula from Northeastern Thailand on the basis of internal transcribed spacer sequence. Science Asia. 31:323-8.

[66] Quiñónez-Martínez M, Ruan-Soto F, AguilarMoreno IE, Garza-Ocañas F, LebgueKeleng T, Lavín-Murcio PA, Enríquez-Anchondo ID (2014). Knowledge and use of edible mushrooms in two municipalities of the Sierra Tarahumara, Chihuahua, Mexico. J Ethnobiol Ethnomed. 10(67):1-13.

[67] Sanmeea R, Dellb B, Lumyongc P, Izumorid K, Lumyong S (2003). Nutritive value of popular wild edible mushrooms from northern Thailand. Food Chem. 82: 527-32.

[68] Jaengklang C, Jarikasem S, Sithisarn P, Klungsupya P (2015). Determination on antioxidant capacity and TLC analysis of ten Thai Russula mushroom extracts. Isan J Pharm Sci. 10:241-50.

[69] Yaltirak T, Aslim B, Ozturk S, Alli H (2009). Antimicrobial and antioxidant activities of Russula delica Fr. Food Chem Toxicol. 47:2052-6.

[70] Chen XH, Xia LX, Zhou HB, Qiu GZ (2010). Chemical composition and antioxidant activities of Russula griseocarnosa sp. nov. J Agric Food Chem. 58:6966-71.

[71] Kalogeropoulos N, Yanni AE, Koutrotsios G, Aloupi M (2013). Bioactive microconstituents and antioxidant properties of wild edible mushrooms from the island of Lesvos, Greece. Food Chem Toxicol. 55:378-85.

[72] Clericuzio M, Cassino C, Corana F, Vidari G (2012). Terpenoids from Russula lepida and Russula amarissima (Basidiomycota, Russulaceae). Phytochemistry. 84:154-9.

6

Lupan-Skeleton Pentacyclic Triterpenes with Activity against Skin Cancer: Preclinical Trials Evolution

Codruţa Şoica, Diana Antal, Florina Andrica,

Roxana Băbuţa, Alina Moacă, Florina Ardelean,

Roxana Ghiulai, Stefana Avram, Corina Danciu,

Dorina Coricovac, Cristina Dehelean and

Virgil Păunescu

Abstract

Skin cancer is an increasingly frequent pathology, with a dangerous high percentage of malignant melanoma. The use of synthetic chemotherapy raises the problem of severe adverse effects and the development of resistance to treatment. Therefore, the use of natural therapies became the focus of numerous research groups due to their high efficacy and lower systemic adverse effects. Among natural products evaluated as therapeutical agents against skin cancer, betulinic acid was emphasized as a highly selective anti-melanoma agent and is currently undergoing phase II clinical trials as topical application. Several other pentacyclic triterpenes exhibit antiproliferative activities. This chapter aims to present the latest main discoveries in the class of pentacyclic triterenes with antitumor effect and the evolution of their preclinical trials. Furthermore, it includes reports on plant sources containing pentacyclic triterpenes, as well as the main possibilities of their water solubilization and cancer cell targeting. A review on recent data regarding mechanisms of action at cellular and molecular levels complements information on the outstanding medicinal potential of these compounds.

Keywords: pentacyclic triterpenes, betulinic acid, lupane, preclinic, mechanism of action

1. Introduction

Skin cancer represents one of the most frequent cancers with an increasing incidence over the past decades [1]. Malignant melanoma, squamous cell carcinoma and basal cell carcinoma represent 98% of all skin cancers [2]. Malignant melanoma determines a higher mortality compared to nonmelanoma skin cancers, being responsible of 75% of skin cancer deaths [2, 3]. Sun exposure is one of the major risk factors, but it influences differently the types of skin cancer. Squamous cell carcinoma is more often related to chronic sun exposure, while malignant melanoma is caused by intermittent sun exposure and overexposure in childhood [4].

Nonmelanoma skin cancer is considered to have the highest incidence of all cancers and occurs more frequently in people with white skin [5]. However, 232,000 new cases of malignant melanoma were diagnosed in 2012, with the highest incidence in Australia. The number of deaths due to this type of skin cancer was 55,000 worldwide in the same year [6]. Malignant melanoma cases tripled in the last 30 years in the United States and Europe [1]. According to World Health Organization [7], each year occur 132,000 cases of melanoma skin cancers worldwide. The increasing incidence is associated with an increase of treatment costs. This aspect underscores the important role of prevention and early detection efforts for this type of cancer [8].

Even though numerous efforts were made for finding effective treatments in melanoma, prognosis for these patients remains unsatisfactory. The standard treatment in early stages is represented by surgical excision, followed by an adjuvant therapy or enrollment in a clinical trial [9]. An early detection of melanoma and a proper treatment increase the chances for cure. Surgery, chemotherapy, immunotherapy or radiation therapy can be used for the treatment [10]. Interferon-α (IFN-α) is used as an adjuvant therapy in patients with high-risk cutaneous melanoma, improving mainly disease-free survival but also overall survival, though not without side effects [11]. An improvement of survival in patients with stage III melanoma has been noticed for ipilimumab therapy. This monoclonal antibody increases the immune response and is approved for treatment in advanced melanoma, but also causes gastrointestinal, endocrine and hepatic adverse effects [12]. New drugs have also been used in the treatment of patients with inoperable or stage IV cutaneous malignant melanoma. The BRAF inhibitors vemurafenib and dabrafenib, the anti-PD1 (programmed death 1) antibodies pembrolizumab and nivolumab or the MEK (mitogen-activated protein kinase) inhibitors trametinib and cobimetinib are new agents proposed in melanoma therapy [13]. Associations of BRAF inhibitors (dabrafenib) and MEK inhibitors (trametinib) have also been evaluated in order to improve overall survival and to delay the appearance of drug resistance in patients with metastatic melanoma with BRAF mutations [14].

In nonmelanoma skin cancer, the therapy is different depending on the severity of the tumor. Standard excision or Mohs micrographic surgery (MMS), radiotherapy, photodynamic therapy (PDT), cryosurgery and topical treatment with imiquimod or 5-fluorouracil are employed in the management of this type of skin cancer [15].

Despite the numerous studies and the advances in targeted therapy and immunotherapy, the treatment options in melanoma are limited [9]. The main inconveniences of chemotherapeutic agents currently used in skin cancer are the severe side effects and the multi-drug resistance [16].

Due to these disadvantages of conventional therapies, new alternatives have been investigated in order to find compounds that can serve for the synthesis of new drugs [16]. Plant-derived compounds are intensively studied as anticancer agents, many studies being performed to evaluate their properties in different types of cancer, including skin cancer [17].

2. Plant sources of pentacyclic triterpenes with lupane scaffold

Plants have gained over the time an important place in the prevention and treatment of various medical conditions. Extracts from plants were obtained since ancient times following simple procedures and used as teas, potions and ointments in an attempt to alleviate pain and to cure diseases. Natural sources of drugs remain an important branch in pharmaceutical drug discovery and therapeutic implementation. Combinatorial chemistry as an initial source of information was unable to offer the expected amount of final products, but is considered a tool for preliminary analysis of new drugs even on cancer treatment. Several groups of researchers provided routes to refine and improve the skeleton of natural compound and to prepare novel active agents [18]. Links between natural sources, synthetic chemistry and knowledge about genetic analysis of microbes are new trends in preclinical evaluations [18, 19]. Drugs derived from nature may be fall in one of the following categories: natural product botanical, derived from natural product or made by total synthesis but with the specification that the pharmacophore is in relation with a natural product [18].

During the last decades, natural remedies are engaged in an unprecedented evolution aimed at an increased efficacy. The development of sophisticated technologies in the fields of phytochemistry, drug formulation and pharmacology, as well as the focus on the mechanism of action on a cellular and molecular level, enables the obtainment of highly efficient drugs from plants.

One of the numerous categories of plant phytochemicals are triterpenes (**Figures 1–3**). So far, over 20,000 triterpenes have been isolated from the plant kingdom. They include a variety of structural subtypes: squalene, lanostane, dammarane, tetranortriterpenoids, lupane, oleanane, ursane, hopane and other [20, 21]. Pentacyclic triterpenes, their natural sources and biological effects are presented in **Table 1**.

Among plant sources containing lupan-skeleton pentacyclic triterpenes (**Figure 2**), birch bark has received particular attention due to its high content in these substances, its well-proven application and uses over the time [41]. Currently, it is acknowledged that the outer birch bark is a rich source of pentacyclic triterpenes, which include: betulin (B lup-20 (29)-ene-3β, 28-diol), betulinic acid (BA, 3β acid, hydroxy-lup-20 (29)-en-28-oic) and lupeol

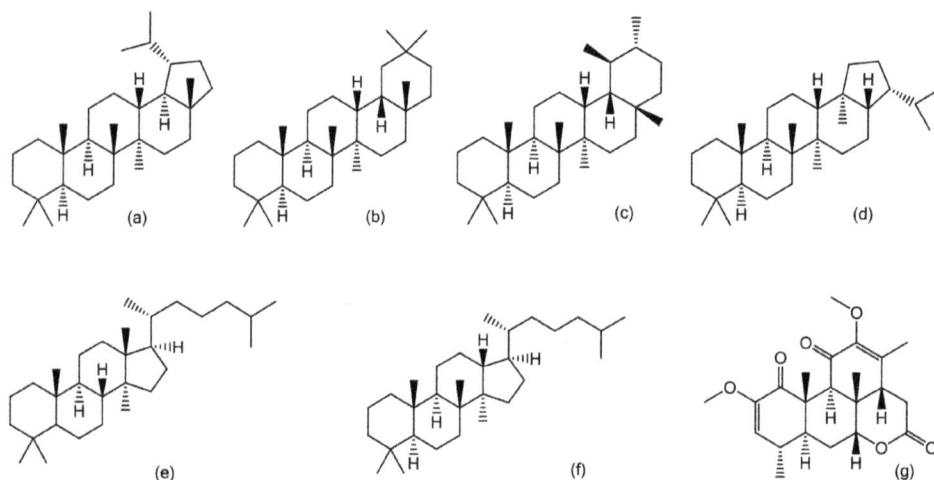

Figure 1. Triterpene structures (a) lupane; (b) oleanane; (c) ursane; (d) hopane; (e) lanostane; (f) dammarane and (g) quassin.

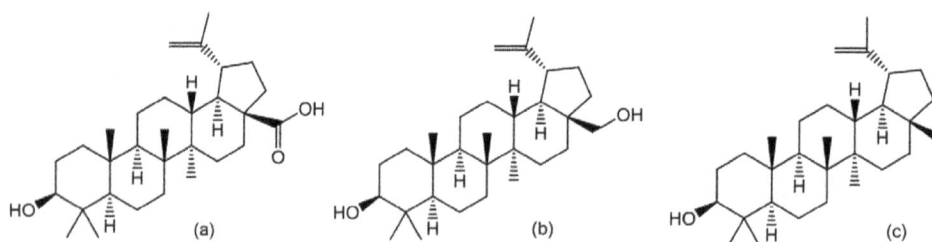

Figure 2. Lupan skeleton triterpenes (a) betulinic acid; (b) betulin and (c) lupeol.

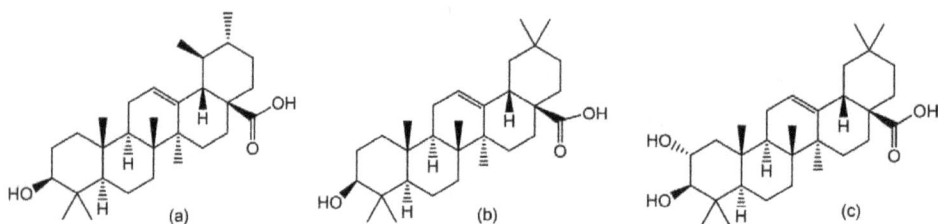

Figure 3. Other triterpenes (a) ursolic acid; (b) oleanolic acid and (c) maslinic acid.

(L, Lup-20 (29)-en-3-ol). The development of birch bark extracts, their applications and bioactivity has comprehensively been reviewed [42]. By analyzing birch bark extract, it was shown that betulin is present in the highest amount, while betulinic acid content is lower. However, it is possible that plants from different geographical regions present a variable content in pentacyclic triterpene, which requires a rigorous analysis of the content [43]. Differences between barks of birch species regard the content in: betulin, betulinic acid, betulinic aldehyde, lupeol, oleanolic acid, oleanolic acid 3-acetate, betulin 3-caffeate, erythrodiol and other.

Substance	Plant (family)	Plant part	Study/effect	Reference
BA	*Ziziphus mauritiana* Lam. (Rhamnaceae)	Stem bark	*In vitro*—inhibitory effect on (MEL-1, -2, -3, -4) cells; apoptotic effect on MEL-2 cells *In vivo*—antitumor effect on athymic mice injected with MEL-2 cells	[22]
BE, LU	*Betula x caerulea* Blanch., *Betula cordifolia* Regel, *Betula papyrifera* Marsh., *Betula populvolia* Marsh. (Betulaceae)	Bark	N/A	[23]
BA, LU, BE, UA, OA	*Syzygium formosanum* Hay. Mori (Myrtaceae)	Leaves	N/A	[24]
BE, BA, UA	*Diospyros leucomelas* Poir. (Ebenaceae)	Leaves	*In vivo*—anti-inflammatory activity on Swiss mice, for induced ear edema and induced paw edema	[25]
OA	*Rosa canina* L. (Rosaceae)	Rose hip, powder	*In vitro*—immunomodulatory activity on Mono Mac 6, obtained when a mixture of OA, BA and UA was used	[26]
BA	*Rosmarinus officinalis* L. (Labiatae)	Stems and leaves	*In vivo*—antidepressant-like effect in the TST, for Swiss mice; anti-immobility effect	[27]
BE, BA	*Betula pendula* Roth, syn. *Betula verrucosa* (Betulaceae)	Bark	*In vitro*—cytotoxic effect in EPG85-257 and EPP85-181 cells line	[28]
A, BA, BE, LU, UA, OA	*Ligustrum pricei* Hayata, *Ligustrum sinense* Lour., *Ligustrum lucidum* W.T.Aiton (Oleaceae)	Leaves	*In vivo*—analgesic and anti-inflammatory effect on Sprague Dawley rats	[29]
OA, BA	*Viscum album* L. (Santalaceae) – harvested from *Malus domestica* Borkh.	Sprout	*In vitro*—cytotoxic and apoptotic effect on B16.F10 cells	[30]
OA, BA	*Viscum album* L. (Santalaceae) – harvested from *Malus domestica* Borkh.	Sprout	*In vivo*—antiapoptotic, antiproliferative effect on C57BL/6NCrL mice injected with B16.F10	[31]
BE, UA	*Myrica cerifera* L. (Myricaceae)	Bark	*In vitro*—cytotoxic activity against HL60, A549 and SK-BR-3 cell lines	[32]
LU	*Taraxacum* sp. Dandelion (Asteraceae)	Root	*In vitro*—cytostatic, not cytotoxic effect on B16 2F2 cells; inhibition of cells proliferation by differentiation	[33]
LU	*Lactuca indica* L. (Asteraceae)	N/A	*In vivo*—prevents local tumor progression, distant metastasis in dogs with COMM Dogs: two miniature Dachshunds, two Beagles, two miniature Schnauzers, one Golden Retriever, one Labrador Retriever, one American Cocker Spaniel, one Cavalier King Charles Spaniel and 1 mixed-breed dog	[34]
LU	*Lactuca indica* L. (Asteraceae)	N/A	*In vivo*—tumor growth suppression and induced cell cycle arrest in C57BL/6 mice injected with B16 2F2 cells	[35]

Substance	Plant (family)	Plant part	Study/effect	Reference
LU	*Bombax ceiba* L. (Malvaceae)	Stem Bark	*In vitro*—antiangiogenic effect on SK-MEL-2, A549 and B16-F10 cell lines	[36]
BA, OA	*Paeonia rockii* ssp. rockii T.Hong & J.J.Li (Paeoniaceae)	Root	*In vitro*—antiapoptotic effect induced selectively in the M-14 cell line	[37]
UA	*Salvia officinalis* L. (Lamiaceae)	N/A	*In vivo*—antiprotease and antimetastatic effects on C57BL/6N mice injected with B16 cells	[38]
BA	*Avicennia officinalis* L. (Acanthaceae)	Leaves	*In vivo*—anti-inflammatory effect on rats	[39]
BA, UA, MA	*Bridelia cambodiana* Gagnep. (Phyllanthaceae)	Whole plant	*In vitro*—cytotoxic effect against HL60 and LCC cell lines	[40]

BA (betulinic acid); BE (betulin); LU (lupeol); UA (ursolic acid); OA (oleanolic acid); MA (maslinic acid); N/A (not applicable); MEL-1, -2, -3, -4 (human melanoma cell line); Mono Mac 6 (human monocytic cell line); TST (tail suspension test); EPG85-257 (human gastric carcinoma cell line); EPP85-181 (human pancreatic carcinoma cell line); B16.F10 (murine melanoma cell line); HL60 (human promyelocytic leukemia cell line); A549 (human lung carcinoma cell line); SK-BR-3 (human breast cancer cell line); B16 2F2 (mouse melanoma derived subclone with high differentiation capability); COMM (canine oral malignant melanoma); SK-MEL-2 (human melanoma cell line); M-14 (human melanoma cell line); B16 (mouse melanoma cell line derived from spontaneous skin tumor); LLC (mouse lewis lung carcinoma).

Table 1. Bioactivity of various plant products containing pentacyclic triterpenes.

3. Obtainment of lupane-skeleton triterpenes with efficacy in skin cancer

Pentacyclic triterpenes from plants are secondary metabolites with high lipophilicity. Therefore, they are mainly located in hydrophobic histological structures. In the cork of trees, which represents the outer tissue of the secondary bark, triterpenes are associated with suberin; a well-known example is birch bark [44]. Triterpenes are as well components of cuticular and epicuticular waxes covering leaves [45] and fruits [46].

Betulin was isolated for the first time in the 1788 by Lowitz [47] from birch cork. The elucidation of its structure was performed by only in 1953 by Guider et al. [48]. Additional plant sources for betulin include hornbeam (*Carpinus betulus* L) and hazel (*Corylus avellana* L.), plants which are phylogenetically closely related to birch [49]. Betulinic acid, a triterpene of major therapeutic relevance, was isolated under the name of "graciolon" from *Gratiola officinalis* [50] and recognized as such only 40 years later [51]. "Platanolic acid," isolated from *Platanus acerifolia* bark [52], proved later to be betulinic acid as well [53]. Furthermore, betulinic acid could be obtained from an alcoholic extract of *Cornus florida* L. bark [54]. Ko and co-workers [55] used mistletoe (*Viscum album*) to obtain an ethanol extract enriched in triterpenes, including betulinic acid and botulin.

The obtainment of triterpenes from the plant matrices employs as a first step extraction with organic solvents such as methanol or ethanol [56]. Other solvents are chloroform, dichloromethane, ethyl acetate, petroleum ether or various mixtures thereof, in accordance with the low polarity of these phytocompounds. Recovery procedures may include Soxhlet extraction, maceration and ultrasound-assisted processes [57]. In order to progressively enrich/isolate triterpenes, the usual phytochemical approaches are employed: partition among solvents of increasing polarity, column chromatography on silica gel, countercurrent chromatography and preparative chromatography. Triterpene acids are extracted after alkalinization with sodium hydroxide [57] or calcium hydroxyde [58]. Pure betulin was prepared from a crude mixture using a chromatographic column with silica gel as a stationary phase and a mixture of hexane and ethyl acetate as eluent, followed by recrystallization from 75% ethyl alcohol [59]. An effective preparation of crystalline betulin (99% purity) from birch bark is clearly described in a recent work, following the steps to remove betulinic acid and lupeol. Additionally, the authors demonstrate the obvious relationship between the cytotoxic activity of betulin and its purity [58]. The analytic determination of triterpenes in samples is performed by reverse-phase HPTLC and gas chromatography, coupled with the detection using mass spectrometry detection, is a widely used method for analysis of betulin and other triterpenes in samples. High-performance thin-layer chromatography (HPTLC) is a valuable straightforward tool for the visualization of impurities [60].

Betulinic acid received high attention due to its properties to inhibit the growth of cancer cell lines, without being cytotoxic to normal cells. In plant materials used as sources of triterpenes such as birch, the content in betulinic acid is much lower than that in betulin. For this reason, various attempts have been made to obtain betulinic acid, using betulin as a starting point. In the study of Melnikova and co-workers [61], the most intense catalytic activity was noticed for aluminum salts, which also have a selective activity. The reaction proceeds via the intermediate betulonic acid, purified by recrystallization. Betulonic acid is reduced with $NaBH_4$ (THF or isopropanol) at room temperature to obtain a mixture of 3α-betulinic acid and betulinic acid-3β [61].

Enzymatic transformations, privileged for their simplicity, eco-friendliness and safety, are currently a mainstay in the obtainment of drugs. In an enzymatic approach, the fungus *Armillaria luteo-virens* Sacc ZJUQH100-6 was employed in the biotransformation of betulin into betulinic acid [62]. Optimization of the obtainment was monitored by variation of parameters like pH, glucose, betulin content, addition of tween 80 and stage of inoculation; the presence of the surfactant had a significant impact on the yield of the biotransformation.

While betulin is readily available from birch and other plants, its anticancer activity is only moderate. Being an accessible starting point for derivatizations, betulin has been the subject of many researches, aiming to obtain compounds with enhanced anticancer activities [63]. The acetylated derivates were tested for antiproliferative effect on several cell lines: colorectal adenocarcinoma, leukemia and breast cancer. By esterificating betulin with propionic acid in dichloromethane solution in the presence of dicyclohexylcarbodiimide and 4-dimethyl-aminopyridine, derivatives: 28-O-propynoylbetulin and 3.28-A, IB, dipropynoylbetulin were obtained. Column chromatography was employed in order to obtain the pure components with a yield of 60% in the case of the first derivative and 12% in the second. The reaction of betulin with propargyl chloroformate and 3-butyl-1-yl chloroformate in benzene, in the presence of pyridine, resulted in the formation of a mixture of 28-O-propargyloxycarbonylbetulin mono-esters and 28-O- (3-butynyloxycarbonyl) toxin and di-3,28-A sheep-di (pro-pargyloxycarbonyl)

3.28-A toxin and sheep-di (3-butyn-yloxycarbonyl) toxin. The resulting mixture was separated by column chromatography; thus, pure components were obtained in a 64–69% yield for mono-esters and 23–27% in the case of diesters [64].

4. Advanced formulation of lupane triterpenes

The most challenging aspect of the biomedical use of lupane triterpenes is their low water solubility which subsequently causes poor bioavailability [65]; so far, several delivery systems have been developed in order to achieve superior pharmacokinetic outcomes. The current subchapter aims to review the most recent and promising delivery options for betulin, betulinic acid and lupeol.

The first step in the attempt to modulate the aqueous solubility of an insoluble compound relies in its convenient derivatization with water-soluble partners; such an attempt was conducted by Drag-Zalesinska and co-workers [66], who prepared mono- and diesters of betulin and betulinic acid with amino acids. All esters revealed higher water solubilities and significant cytotoxic activity via apoptosis induction; the type of ester as well as the type of the amino acid side chain strongly influences the biological effect of the respective compounds [66]. C(2)-propargyl-substituted pentacyclic triterpenoids conjugated with 1,2,3-triazole glucopyrano-sides were synthesized via "click" chemistry in order to achieve optimized water solubility as well as pharmacokinetic and pharmacological properties [67].

Cyclodextrin (CD) complexation represents an attractive solution to increase the aqueous solubility of numerous compounds; through their hydrophobic interior and hydrophilic surface, cyclodextrins are able to accommodate various lipophilic guest molecules which can thus be water-solubilized. According to molecular studies [68], the bulky structures of betulinic acid and betulin fit best inside the cavity of γ-CD and its semisynthetic derivatives, such as hydroxypropyl-γ-CD (HPGCD). As a result of HPGCD complexation, a 14-fold increased water solubility was reported for BA accompanied by superior biological activity [69], i.e., strong antiangiogenic and antitumor effect [70, 71]. Similar outcomes were achieved in terms of anti-melanoma activity tested on B16 cell line (murine melanoma) [72]. Fontanay et al. conducted a study on the inclusion of hydroxy pentacyclic triterpenoid acids, including BA, inside native γ-CD [73]; the physicochemical analysis revealed the formation of a 1:1 complex with a significantly improved aqueous solubility.

β-CD derivatives also served as complexation partners for BA, and its inclusion in the cyclo-dextrin hydrophilic matrix led to significantly improved dissolution rate and, subsequently, antiproliferative in vitro activity against MCF7 (breast cancer) cell line [74]. The same tumor cell line was involved in the study of the biological activity of betulinic acid accommodated inside native β-CD [75]; a dose-dependent antiproliferative activity was reported, through mitochondria-mediated apoptosis induction and G2/M cell cycle arrest.

An important parameter in the cyclodextrin inclusion process is the stability constant of the final complex, its value giving the measure of the potential use of the complex as biologically active agent; significantly high stability constants were achieved for both betulin and betulinic acid in complex with newly synthesized hydrophilic γ-CD derivatives [76]. Such a high stability constant characterizes a strong interaction between the host- and the guest molecule, thus enabling the delivery of the active drug at the target site in the absence of systemic adverse effects. Both complexes, with betulin and betulinic acid, respectively, were *in vitro* and *in vivo* tested, revealing moderate *in vitro* antiproliferative activity; however, *in vivo* results on murine models showed a significant decline in tumor size and volume [77, 78].

The inclusion of betulin inside HPGCD led to optimized outcomes in terms of bioavailability and antiproliferative activity [79, 80]; similar results were reported for betulin complexation with hydrophilic β-CD derivatives that caused stronger inhibitory activity against MCF7 (breast cancer) cell line than pure betulin [74].

Lupeol was also subjected to inclusion inside γ-CD by kneading in a 1:2 molar ratio; the complex revealed optimized antiproliferative and antiangiogenic activities compared to the pure drug [81].

The use of triterpenes as mixtures such as total extract of birch outer bark may trigger simultaneously various mechanisms of apoptosis induction and therefore result in an additive or synergistic effect. Hertrampf et al. [82] used HPBCD as solubilizer for birch total extract; a series of dilutions were prepared using the main ingredient, betulin, as a reference to calculate concentrations. The study reported the multivalent cytotoxic activity of the birch bark at lower concentrations than previously used presumably due to a higher bioavailability of triterpenes provided by cyclodextrin solubilization; moreover, a synergistic effect was suggested. Triterpene-rich mistletoe extract (6.9% BA) was solubilized by Strüh et al. [30] by using HPBCD and tested against B16F10 melanoma cell line; a dose-dependent reduction of cellular ATP was reported accompanied by high cytotoxicity due to DNA fragmentation. The research was continued by in vivo studies on C57BL/6 mice bearing B16F10 subcutaneous melanoma, revealing an increased antitumor effect and a prolonged mice survival [31].

An alternative research direction was the preparation of cyclodextrin conjugates instead of inclusion complexes; "click chemistry" was involved in the synthesis of triazole-bridged conjugates between β-CD and pentacyclic triterpenes [83]. All bioconjugates showed higher hydrophilicity than the parent compound, and several conjugates displayed significant cytotoxicity on various cancer cell lines; in addition, the cyclodextrin conjugation led to the disappearance of haemolytic toxicity. The authors continued their research by synthesizing α-CD conjugates with several pentacyclic triterpenes including BA [84]; all conjugates exhibited lower hydrophobicity than the parent molecules accompanied by significant anti-HCV (hepatitis C virus) entry activity.

An excellent review was published in 2016 by Lima et al. [85], describing the main attempts to use cyclodextrins as nanocarriers for various terpenes; the authors concluded that cyclodextrins are feasible tools in improving the pharmacological profile of terpenes, limited mainly by the scarce pharmacokinetic and clinical studies.

Liposomes are small vesicles displaying one or more phospholipidic layers and an aqueous core [86] that may incorporate both lipophilic and hydrophilic compounds [87, 88]. Betulinic acid was trapped inside large liposomes by Mullauer et al. [89] and administered to mice bearing experimental models of colon (SW480) and lung (A549) cancer; no systemic adverse effects were reported following parenteral (i.v.) and oral administration. Similar studies reported liposomal and proliposomal formulations with BA with 95% yield of the incorporation process [90]. Phospholipidic nanosomes prepared by means of supercritical fluids were used to entrap BA in order to increase its efficacy as antiviral agent [91, 92]. Several betulin derivatives such as 28-acetylenic derivatives [93] and pyrazoles and 1,2,3-triazole derivatives [94] were synthesized and formulated as liposomes; the nanoformulations exhibited strong apoptotic activity due to both higher biological effect of the active compound and optimized delivery. PEG-ylated BA liposomes were obtained by Liu et al. in 2016, entrapping BA in the lipid bilayer of the liposomes by the ethanol injection technique [95]; the hydrophilic outer PEG layer ensured improved sustained release and antitumor effect compared to free BA or BA liposomes.

Another attractive option in drug delivery is the use of micro- and nanoemulsions; a nanoemulsion containing BA was prepared using flax-seed oil as lipophilic phase and the high-pressure homogenization method [96]; the *in vivo* testing on the chorioallantoic membrane (CAM assay) revealed a significant antiangiogenic activity. The same procedure was applied for betulin nanoemulsion, followed by *in vivo* testing by CAM assay and experimental murine cancer model; the study reported strong anti-inflammatory, antiproliferative and antiangiogenic activities of the incorporated betulin as well as its potential benefits in inhibiting metastasis [97]. An oil-in-water nanoemulsion with BA was prepared through the use of phospholipase-catalyzed modified phosphatidylcholine as emulsifier in an ultrasound device; various factors such as composition, ultrasound amplitude, temperature and pH significantly influenced nanoparticle size and stability [98].

A different approach consists in the administration of betulin via the nasal route; in order to avoid mouth sedimentation of betulin particles, the solvent exchange method was used to limit particle sizes to nanoscale, thus leading to higher bioavailability of betulin in the lower respiratory tract [99].

Water solubility may be increased through grinding with hydrophilic polymers (i.e., polyvinylpyrrolidone, polyethylene glycol, arabinogalactan) [100, 101]; solid dispersions of BA with various hydrophilic polymers (*i.e.*, Soluplus, HPMCAS-HF, Kollidon VA64, Kollidon K90, Eudragit RLPO) in 1:4 (w/w) ratio were prepared and analyzed by Yu et al. [102] in 2014, revealing a great potential to increase BA water solubility. Moreover, hydrophilic bioconjugates can be synthesized between active drugs and hydrophilic polymers. BA-monomethoxy polyethylene glycol (mPEG) conjugate was synthesized by covalent bonding of the carboxyl moiety of BA and the amine groups of mPEG [103]; the conjugate exhibited cytotoxicity through cell apoptosis on hepatic cancer cells (Hep3B, Huh7) as well as *in vivo* antitumor efficacy in Ehrlich ascites tumor (EAT) model while lacking any sign of biochemical and histological toxicity. A step further was represented by the use of multiarm-PEGs as conjugation partner which offer a high density of functional groups; through the formation of an ester bond, BA was linked to eight-arm PEG (8arm-PEG) and then to a targeting molecule (folate) followed by the self-assembly into nanoparticles [104]. A second anticancer drug, hydroxycamptothecin, was added by nanoprecipitation; the ensemble achieved a dramatically increased cytotoxicity, prolonged blood circulation, enhanced tumor targeting and lower systemic toxicity than the free drugs; in addition, a synergistic antitumor efficacy was reported [104]. BA also shows the ability to self-assemble into nano- and microfibers with antileukemic efficacy and cytoprotective activity as well [105].

Biodegradable polymeric nanospheres based on poly(lactide-co-glycolide)-poly(ethylene glycol) (PLGA-PEG) were prepared by nanoprecipitation to incorporate 40% BA [106]; the study reported an increased cytotoxicity and lower IC50 value compared to the pure drug. PLGA was used as building material by interfacial deposition for nanocapsules that efficiently entrapped lupeol [107]. Polymer matrixes can be involved in regional chemotherapy, an approach that avoids systemic adverse effects [108] and allows the controlled release of the pure drug; betulin was incorporated as model compound in such a matrix (poly(3,4-ethylenedioxythiophene), its release being conducted by passive or active mode. The novel formulation exhibited efficient cytotoxic activity against KB and MCF7 cancer cell lines.

BA conjugates with carboxyl-functionalized single-walled carbon nanotubes were synthesized via π–π stacking interaction, leading to a 20% loading of the active drug [109]; following physicochemical and biological analysis, the authors reported the controlled, prolonged release of the drug, with no sign of toxicity on normal fibroblasts and significant cytotoxicity against A549 (lung cancer) cell line. The research continued by coating the nanotubes with four biopolymers: tween 20, tween 80, polyethylene glycol and chitosan in order to further improve biocompatibility [110]; the procedure induced sustained and prolonged release compared to the uncoated nanotubes, while cytotoxicity depended on the chosen biopolymer.

Metallic nanoparticles were also used as nanocarriers for pentacyclic triterpenes; as an example, magnetic nanoparticles coated with chitosan were loaded with BA and exhibited a pseudo-second-order kinetic model release of the active drug [111]; the nanoparticles were cytotoxic on MCF7 cells in a dose-dependent manner while lacking toxicity against normal mouse fibroblast cells. Silver nanoparticles coated with BA were involved in the in vitro testing on a panel of cancer cell lines, including A375 (murine melanoma) [112]; the new formulation revealed strong antiproliferative and antimigratory activity, in particular against melanoma cells.

5. Innovative approaches in preclinical evaluations of pentacyclic triterpenes of the lupane series in skin cancer

Preclinical trials are important in the initial evaluation of new drugs, formulations or specific new design of pathology. They are complex processes with an uncertain ending, as just a reduced percent of evaluations lead to a market product. It is estimated that around 90% of tested drugs are not launched to the market [113]. Despite intense of basic research, the actual delivery of accepted drugs is scarce.

The classical route of a tested compound in preclinical trials includes *in vitro* tests followed by *in vivo* tests on animals [113]. These tests may be conceived in a variety of ways and are constantly improved and diversified. The mainstay of preclinical tests regarding a potential efficacy against skin cancer types is *in vitro* tests using different types of cell lines. In this regard, lupane triterpenes were tested on human melanoma (G361, SK-MEL-28, MEL-2, SK-MEL2, A375), mouse melanoma (B16-F1, B16 2F2) and human skin epidermoid carcinoma A431. In case of betulin, the latter showed a particularly high sensitivity (with a IC50 value below 10µM), while various types of human melanoma cell lines may display a high variation range of the sensitivity to betulin, with differences in IC50 values of one order of magnitude, from 12.4 to over 250 µM [114]. For betulinic acid, IC50 was 154 µM when tested on A375 melanoma [115], and 70 µM when tested on B16-F10 murine melanoma [116]. Information of particular relevance for the actual clinical utilization as anticancer agent comes from comparative data on the cytotoxicity against normal cells and cancer cell lines. Betulin, for example, is more cytotoxic against cancerous cells than nontumoral ones [114]. Further steps in preclinical evaluation are the investigation of the mechanism of action; lupeol, betulin, betulinic acid and their semi-synthetic derivatives have so far shown significant effects on apoptosis and cell cycle regulation [117, 118]. As inflammation is an important player in the pathogenesis of cancer, the anti-inflammatory effects and mechanisms are as well explored to give a correct picture of the antitumoral potential [117]. Furthermore, it is important to explore the antimigratory potential of natural products, as it has a seminal importance for malignant melanoma—a cancer type with a high invasiveness [119]. A global approach to relevant preclinical tests regarding triterpenes should thus be multi-component. In this regard, our workgroup has established an efficient battery of tests for aimed at establishing the potential of natural triterpenes with anticancer/anti-inflammatory activity as agents against skin cancer. The module of preclinical evaluations includes as follows:

- **Step 1**: *in vitro* tests on normal cells (e.g., HaCat) comparing with specific pathological tests; evaluation of cytotoxic activity;

- **Step 2:** *in vitro* evaluations concerning the impact on apoptosis, and observations of specific markers via DAPI/HOPI staining, and evaluation of Annexin V, caspases and other cellular markers [120];

- **Step 3:** *in vivo* embryonated egg membrane assay for toxicological evaluation (HET CAM assay) and investigations of the potential to affect angiogenesis; future aspects include cultivation of cancer cells on embryonated eggs and direct research of the therapeutic potential;

- **Step 4:** *in vivo* tests including a large number of experimental protocols: photochemical model, inoculation of murine cells, xenograft of human pathological cells on adequate mouse hosts and correlations with therapeutical surveillance. Furthermore, histopathological evaluations and immuno-histochemical assays are correlated with innovative approaches like RAMAN skin evaluation, noninvasive methods for skin quality and surface damage characterization.

Additional determinations could require selection of cells from a primary experimental tumor, cultivation of cells and evaluation of compounds, PET animal observations and other methods applied for a detailed pathologic surveillance of drugs.

6. Pentacyclic triterpenes: mechanism of action at cellular and molecular level

Apoptosis is a programmed cell death consisting in morphological changes including cell shrinkage, nuclear condensation, chromosomal DNA fragmentation, plasma membrane blebbing and caspase activation [121]. In this regard, apoptosis is considered a crucial physiological process in tumor clearance, being a major target for anticancer drugs [122]. The molecular mechanisms of apoptosis can include extrinsic and intrinsic pathways. The extrinsic pathway of apoptosis is initiated by external signals, which can activate TNF/Fas-receptor, which in turn activates procaspase-8 [123]. The activated caspase-8 is involved into the caspase-3, -6 and -7 cascade activation [124]. Caspases are important cellular enzymes synthesized as inactive zymogens, which can be activated into their active tetrameric forms by various apoptotic signals [124]. The activation of caspase-3, -6 and -7 leads to cell death not only by breaking down the cytoskeleton, but also the nucleus.

The intrinsic pathway of apoptosis, known as the mitochondrial pathway, is initiated by internal stimuli which can activate the proapoptotic genes from the outer membrane of mitochondria. Bcl-2 family proteins (Bax, Bak, Bcl-xs) are important proapoptotic genes involved in permeabilization of the mitochondrial membrane in order to release cytochrome c in cytosol, where it binds to the caspase-activating protein apoptotic protease activating factor-1 (APAF-1) and with the procaspase-9, transforming into an apoptosome [124]. The apoptosome releases the activated form of caspase-9, which is also involved into the caspase-3, -6 and -7 activations, which lead to cell death [123].

Previous evidences showed that the pentacyclic triterpens, especially betulin, betulinic acid, lupeol and ursolic acid, have induced apoptosis in different types of cancer cells via activation of the mitochondrial pathway and not to the death receptor pathway (extrinsic way) [125, 126]. These data have been supported by Drag-Zalesinska et al. [118] study in which betulin and betulinic acid proved to induce apoptosis in human metastatic melanoma cells (Me-45) by releasing cytochrome c or the apoptosis inducing factor (AIF) through the mitochondrial membrane. Liu et al. [122] have also demonstrated that betulinic acid, as well as betulin, could kill CNE2 cells through the mitochondrial pathway. Betulinic acid induced the DNA fragmentation, caspase activation and cytochrome c release but independent of Bax proteins [115, 122]. Moreover, betulinic acid has been also involved in activation of nuclear factor kappa B (NF-κB) responsible for apoptosis in various types of cancer cells [127].

The increased production of reactive oxygen species (ROS) caused by betulin and betulinic acid stimulation [128, 129] has been considered a stress factor involved in the depolarization of mitochondrial membrane [130]. Furthermore, both calcium overload and ATP depletion were additional stress factors responsible for increasing the permeability of the inner mitochondrial membrane through formation of nonspecific pores [116]. For instance, the dimethylaminopyridine triterpenoid derivatives have also caused the depolarization of the mitochondrial membrane in situ, in order to increase the permeability transition pore [131].

Unlike the previous data, the study of Şoica et al. [77] on B164A5 murine melanoma cells and on a mouse melanoma model showed that BE and its derivatives had no effect on caspase-2 regulation, the apoptotic mechanism of betulin being suggested to be probably through the transformation of BE into betulinic acid inside the cells.

According to the study of Muceniece et al. [132] *in vitro*, betulin had a mimetic effect on melanocortin (MC) receptor, especially on MC-1 subtype. This observation has been also supported by Şoica et al. [77] study in which botulin had revealed strong inhibitory effects on B64A5 murine melanoma cells, by binding to the melanocortin receptors. Betulin has been not involved by itself in stimulation of cAMP generation, but it acted as a weak antagonist on alpha-melanocyte-stimulating hormone (alpha-MSH)-induced cAMP accumulation in B16-F1 mouse melanoma cells [132].

In vitro and *in vivo* studies have also revealed that the birch bark extract and betulin have significantly increased the expression of PARP-1 in melanoma cells [118], exhibiting interferon-inducing activity [133].

According to Zhang et al. [126] study, betulinic acid induced apoptosis by suppressing the cyclic AMP-dependent transcription factor ATF-3 and NF-κB pathways and decreasing the expression of topoisomerase I, p53 and lamin B1. On one hand, earlier studies indicated that betulinic acid had induced apoptosis of cells due to the p53 pathways [134]. This conclusion has been also supported by Tiwari et al. [135] study, in which BA proved a dose-dependent apoptotic effect on both p53 mutant and wild-type cells probably because of its involvement in p53-independent apoptotic pathway. On the other hand, a recent study has shown that the apoptotic effect of betulinic acid in human metastatic melanoma cells (Me-45) had been independent of p53-apoptotic pathway [118]. The presumable mechanisms of action of betulinic acid and betulin in skin cancer are depicted in **Figure 4**.

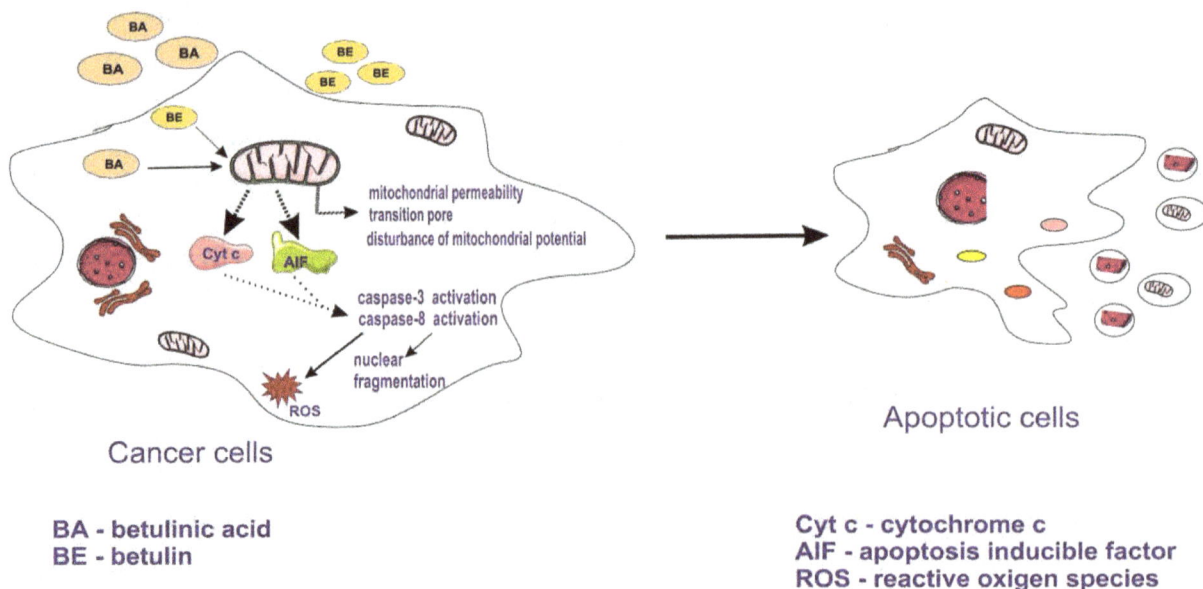

Figure 4. The mechanism of action of betulinic acid and betulin in skin cancer.

Lupeol is a complex multitarget phytochemical, being involved in controlling IL-1 receptor-associated kinase-mediated toll-like receptor 4 (IRAK-TLR4), Bcl-2 family, nuclear factor kappa B (NF-κB), phosphatidylinositol-3-kinase (PI3-K)/Akt and Wnt/β-catenin signaling pathways [136]. According to the Tarapore et al. study, the anticarcinogenic effect of lupeol has been related to the Wnt/β-catenin signaling pathway. That study has revealed that lupeol caused a dose-dependent decrease in Wnt target genes in Mel 1011 cells. Moreover, there has been also observed a decrease of nuclear β-catenin expression, associated with an enhancement of plasmatic β-catenin expression in melanoma cells (Mel 928 and Mel 1241). Consequently, lupeol has been involved in blocking the movement of β-catenin between cytoplasm and nucleus [137].

An *in vivo* study on Swiss Albino mice showed that lupeol exerted apoptotic effects through the enhancement of bax and caspase-3 genes expression and downregulation of bcl-2 anti-apoptotic genes [138].

Unlike botulin and betulinic acid, lupeol has also induced apoptosis via extrinsic pathway by enhancing the expression of FADD protein and Fas receptors [127].

Ursolic acid has strongly increased the IR-induced apoptotic effect in various types of cancer cells, likely DU145, CT26 and B16F10, playing a major role in DNA fragmentation, mitochondrial dysfunction and apoptotic marker modulation [139]. Moreover, ursolic acid has induced apoptosis in M4Beu cells human melanoma through intrinsic pathway by enhancing the caspase-3 activity in a dose-dependent manner, correlated with a low caspase-9 activity [140]. Ursolic acid has also proved to act as an inhibitor of the endogenous reverse transcriptase (RT) activity in the following tumor cells: melanoma (A375), glioblastoma (U87) and thyroid anaplastic carcinoma (ARO), as well as on nontransformed human fibroblast cell line (WI-38), exhibiting strong antiproliferative effects [141].

The mechanism of apoptosis induced by pentacyclic triterpens is not fully understood, although, according to the previous studies, we can conclude that these triterpens exhibited strong apoptotic effects, especially via intrinsic pathway, being involved in increasing the permeability of inner mitochondrial membrane, activation of caspase-9 and 3, as well as cell death.

7. Conclusion

Pentacyclic triterpenes represent an important issue in the field of antiskin cancer formulations; nowadays, the researches focus on the development of nanoformulations that provide multiple advantages over the classical pharmaceutical formulations, including the possibility of being decorated with targeting moieties that significantly improve the antiproliferative activity of the loaded active drug. Different mechanisms of action have been identified so far at cellular and molecular level, in particular for betulinic acid; however, future studies are needed in order to fully comprehend the intimate details of the anticancer treatment with pentacyclic triterpenes and formulations thereof.

Acknowledgements

This work was supported by a grant financed by the University of Medicine and Pharmacy "Victor Babes" Timisoara (Grant PIII-C4-PCFI-2016/2017-03, acronym NANOCEL to C.S. and V.P.).

Author details

Codruţa Şoica[1†*], Diana Antal[1†], Florina Andrica[1], Roxana Băbuţa[1], Alina Moacă[1], Florina Ardelean[1], Roxana Ghiulai[1], Stefana Avram[1], Corina Danciu[1], Dorina Coricovac[1], Cristina Dehelean[1] and Virgil Păunescu[2]

*Address all correspondence to: codrutasoica@umft.ro

1 Faculty of Pharmacy, "Victor Babeş" University of Medicine and Pharmacy, Timişoara, Romania

2 Faculty of Medicine, "Victor Babeş" University of Medicine and Pharmacy, Timişoara, Romania

† These authors are equally conributed

References

[1] Katalinic A, Waldmann A, Weinstock MA, Geller AC, Eisemann N, Greinert R, Volkmer B, Breitbart E. Does skin cancer screening save lives? An observational study comparing trends in melanoma mortality in regions with and without screening. Cancer. 2012;**118**(21):5395-5402. DOI: 10.1002/cncr.27566

[2] de Vries E, Trakatelli M, Kalabalikis D, Ferrandiz L, Ruiz-de-Casas A, Moreno-Ramirez D, Sotiriadis D, Ioannides D, Aquilina S, Apap C, Micallef R, Scerri L, Ulrich M, Pitkänen S, Saksela O, Altsitsiadis E, Hinrichs B, Magnoni C, Fiorentini C, Majewski S, Ranki A, Stockfleth E, Proby C, EPIDERM Group. Known and potential new risk factors for skin cancer in European populations: A multicentre case-control study. British Journal of Dermatology. 2012;**167**(Suppl 2):1-13. DOI: 10.1111/j.1365-2133.2012.11081.x

[3] Guy GP Jr, Thomas CC, Thompson T, Watson M, Massetti GM, Richardson LC, Centers for Disease Control and Prevention (CDC). Vital signs: Melanoma incidence and mortality trends and projections—United States, 1982-2030. MMWR: Morbidity and Mortality Weekly Report. 2015;**64**(21):591-596

[4] Brøndum-Jacobsen P, Nordestgaard BG, Nielsen SF, Benn M. Skin cancer as a marker of sun exposure associates with myocardial infarction, hip fracture and death from any cause. International Journal of Epidemiology. 2013;**42**(5):1486-1496. DOI: 10.1093/ije/dyt168

[5] Lomas A, Leonardi-Bee J, Bath-Hextall F. A systematic review of worldwide incidence of nonmelanoma skin cancer. British Journal of Dermatology. 2012;**166**(5):1069-1080. DOI: 10.1111/j.1365-2133.2012.10830.x

[6]   Ferlay J, Soerjomataram I, Dikshit R, Eser S, Mathers C, Rebelo M, Parkin DM, Forman D, Bray F. Cancer incidence and mortality worldwide: Sources, methods and major patterns in GLOBOCAN 2012. International Journal of Cancer. 2015;**136**(5):E359-E386. DOI: 10.1002/ijc.29210

[7]   World Health Organization. Available from: http://www.who.int/uv/faq/skincancer/en/ [Accessed: February 16, 2017]

[8]   Guy GP Jr, Machlin SR, Ekwueme DU, Yabroff KR. Prevalence and costs of skin cancer treatment in the U.S., 2002-2006 and 2007-2011. American Journal of Preventive Medicine. 2015;**48**(2):183-187. DOI: 10.1016/j.amepre.2014.08.036

[9]   Garbe C, Eigentler TK, Keilholz U, Hauschild A, Kirkwood JM. Systematic review of medical treatment in melanoma: Current status and future prospects. Oncologist. 2011;**16**(1):5-24. DOI: 10.1634/theoncologist.2010-0190

[10] Aris M, Barrio MM. Combining immunotherapy with oncogene-targeted therapy: A new road for melanoma treatment. Frontiers in Immunology. 2015;**6**:46. DOI: 10.3389/fimmu.2015.00046

[11] Mocellin S, Lens MB, Pasquali S, Pilati P, Chiarion Sileni V. Interferon alpha for the adjuvant treatment of cutaneous melanoma. Cochrane Database of Systematic Reviews. 2013;(6):CD008955. DOI: 10.1002/14651858.CD008955.pub2

[12] Eggermont AM, Chiarion-Sileni V, Grob JJ, Dummer R, Wolchok JD, Schmidt H, Hamid O, Robert C, Ascierto PA, Richards JM, Lebbé C, Ferraresi V, Smylie M, Weber JS, Maio M, Konto C, Hoos A, de Pril V, Gurunath RK, de Schaetzen G, Suciu S, Testori A. Adjuvant ipilimumab versus placebo after complete resection of high-risk stage III melanoma (EORTC 18071): A randomised, double-blind, phase 3 trial. Lancet Oncology. 2015;**16**(5):522-530. DOI: 10.1016/S1470-2045(15)70122-1

[13] Svedman FC, Pillas D, Taylor A, Kaur M, Linder R, Hansson J. Stage-specific survival and recurrence in patients with cutaneous malignant melanoma in Europe—A systematic review of the literature. Clinical Epidemiology. 2016;**8**:109-122. DOI: 10.2147/CLEP.S99021

[14] Robert C, Karaszewska B, Schachter J, Rutkowski P, Mackiewicz A, Stroiakovski D, Lichinitser M, Dummer R, Grange F, Mortier L, Chiarion-Sileni V, Drucis K, Krajsova I, Hauschild A, Lorigan P, Wolter P, Long GV, Flaherty K, Nathan P, Ribas A, Martin AM, Sun P, Crist W, Legos J, Rubin SD, Little SM, Schadendorf D. Improved overall survival in melanoma with combined dabrafenib and trametinib. New England Journal of Medicine. 2015;**372**(1):30-39. DOI: 10.1056/NEJMoa1412690

[15] Samarasinghe V, Madan V. Nonmelanoma skin cancer. Journal of Cutaneous and Aesthetic Surgery. 2012;**5**(1):3-10. DOI: 10.4103/0974-2077.94323

[16] Chinembiri TN, du Plessis LH, Gerber M, Hamman JH, du Plessis J. Review of natural compounds for potential skin cancer treatment. Molecules. 2014;**19**(8):11679-11721. DOI: 10.3390/molecules190811679

[17] Wang H, Khor TO, Shu L, Su ZY, Fuentes F, Lee JH, Kong AN. Plants against cancer: A review on natural phytochemicals in preventing and treating cancers and their druggability. Anti-Cancer Agents in Medicinal Chemistry. 2012;**12**(10):1281-1305

[18] Newman DJ, Cragg GM. Natural products as sources of new drugs over the 30 years from 1981 to 2010. Journal of Natural Products. 2012;**75**(3):311-335. DOI: 10.1021/np200906s

[19] Mobegi FM, van Hijum SA, Burghout P, Bootsma HJ, de Vries SP, van der Gaast-de Jongh CE, Simonetti E, Langereis JD, Hermans PW, de Jonge MI, Zomer A. From microbial gene essentiality to novel antimicrobial drug targets. BMC Genomics. 2014;**15**:958. DOI: 10.1186/1471-2164-15-958

[20] Hill RA, Connolly JD. Triterpenoids. Natural Product Reports. 2013;**30**(7):1028-1065. DOI: 10.1039/c3np70032a

[21] Thimmappa R, Geisler K, Louveau T, O'Maille P, Osbourn A. Triterpene biosynthesis in plants. Annual Review of Plant Biology. 2014;**65**:225-257. DOI: 10.1146/annurev-arplant-050312-120229

[22] Pisha E, Chai H, Lee IS, Chagwedera TE, Farnsworth NR, Cordell GA, Beecher CW, Fong HH, Kinghorn AD, Brown DM, Wani MC, Wall ME, Hieken TJ, Das Gupta TK, Pezzuto JM. Discovery of betulinic acid as a selective inhibitor of human melanoma that functions by induction of apoptosis. Nature Medicine. 1995;**1**(10):1046-1051. DOI: 10.1038/nm1095-1046

[23] O'Connell MM, Bentley MD, Campbell CS, Cole BJW. Betulin and lupeol in bark from four white-barked birches. Phytochemistry. 1988;**27**(7):2175-2176. DOI: 10.1016/0031-9422(88)80120-1

[24] Chang CW, Wu TS, Hsieh YS, Kuo SC, Lee Chao PD. Terpenoids of *Syzygium formosanum*. Journal of Natural Products. 1999;**62**(2):327-328

[25] Del Carmen Recio M, Giner RM, Manez S, Gueho J, Julien HR, Hostettmann K, Rios JL. Investigations on the steroidal anti-inflammatory activity of triterpenoids from Diospyros leucomelas. Planta Medica. 1995;**61**(1):9-12. DOI: 10.1055/s-2006-957988

[26] Saaby L, Moesby L, Hansen EW, Christensen SB. Isolation of immunomodulatory triterpene acids from a standardized rose hip powder (*Rosa canina* L.). Phytotherapy Research. 2011;**25**(2):195-201. DOI: 10.1002/ptr.3241

[27] Machado DG, Cunha MP, Neis VB, Balen GO, Colla A, Bettio LEB, Oliveira A, Pazini FL, Dalmarco JB, Simionatto EL, Pizzolatti MG, Rodrigues AL. Antidepressant-like effects of fractions, essential oil, carnosol and betulinic acid isolated from *Rosmarinus officinalis* L. Food Chemistry. 2013;**136**(2):999-1005. DOI: 10.1016/j.foodchem.2012.09.028

[28] Drag M, Surowiak P, Malgorzata DZ, Dietel M, Lage H, Oleksyszyn J. Comparision of the cytotoxic effects of birch bark extract, betulin and betulinic acid towards human gastric carcinoma and pancreatic carcinoma drug-sensitive and drug-resistant cell lines. Molecules. 2009;**14**(4):1639-1651. DOI: 10.3390/molecules14041639

[29] Wu CR, Hseu YC, Lien JC, Lin LW, Lin YT, Ching H. Triterpenoid contents and anti-inflammatory properties of the methanol extracts of Ligustrum species leaves. Molecules. 2011;16(1):1-15. DOI: 10.3390/molecules16010001

[30] Strüh CM, Jäger S, Schempp CM, Scheffler A, Martin SF. A novel triterpene extract from mistletoe induces rapid apoptosis in murine B16.F10 melanoma cells. Phytotherapy Research. 2012;26(10):1507-1512. DOI: 10.1002/ptr.4604

[31] Strüh CM, Jäger S, Kersten A, Schempp CM, Scheffler A, Martin SF. Triterpenoids amplify anti-tumoral effects of mistletoe extracts on murine B16.F10 melanoma in vivo. PLoS One. 2013;8(4):e62168. DOI: 10.1371/journal.pone.0062168

[32] Zhang J, Yamada S, Ogihara E, Kurita M, Banno N, Qu W, Feng F, Akihisa T. Biological activities of triterpenoids and phenolic compounds from *Myrica cerifera* bark. Chemistry & Biodiversity. 2016;13(11):1601-1609. DOI: 10.1002/cbdv.201600247

[33] Hata K, Ishikawa K, Hori K, Konishi T. Differentiation-inducing activity of lupeol, a lupane-type triterpene from Chinese dandelion root (Hokouei-kon), on a mouse melanoma cell line. Biological and Pharmaceutical Bulletin. 2000;23(8):962-967. DOI: 10.1248/bpb.23.962

[34] Yokoe I, Azuma K, Hata K, Mukaiyama T, Goto T, Tsuka T, Imagawa T, Itoh N, Murahata Y, Osaki Y, Minami S, Okamoto Y. Clinical systemic lupeol administration for canine oral malignant melanoma. Molecular and Clinical Oncology. 2015;3(1):89-92. DOI: 10.3892/mco.2014.450

[35] Nitta M, Azuma K, Hata K, Takahashi S, Ogiwara K, Tsuka T, Imagawa T, Yokoe I, Osaki T, Minami S, Okamoto, Y. Systemic and local injections of lupeol inhibit tumor growth in a melanoma-bearing mouse model. Biomedical Reports. 2013;1(4):641-645. DOI: 10.3892/br.2013.116

[36] You YJ, Nam NH, Kim Y, Bae KH, Ahn BZ. Antiangiogenic activity of lupeol from Bombax ceiba. Phytotherapy Research. 2003;17(4):341-344. DOI: 10.1002/ptr.1140

[37] Mencherini T, Picerno P, Festa M, Russo P, Capasso A, Aquino R. Triterpenoid constituents from the roots of *Paeonia rockii* ssp. *rockii*. Journal of Natural Products. 2011;74(10):2116-2121. DOI: 10.1021/np200359v

[38] Jedinák A, Mučková M, Košťálová D, Maliar T, Mašterová I. Antiprotease and antimetastatic activity of ursolic acid isolated from *Salvia officinalis*. Zeitschrift für Naturforschung. 2006;61:777-782

[39] Sumithra M, Kumar JV, Kancharana VS. Influence of methanolic extract of *Avicennia officinalis* leaves on acute, subacute and chronic inflammatory models. International Journal of PharmTech Research. 2011;3(2):763-768

[40] Khiev P, Cai XF, Chin Y, Ahn KS, Lee HK, Oh SR. Cytotoxic terpenoids from the methanolic extract of *Bridelia cambodiana*. Journal of the Korean Society for Applied Biological Chemistry. 2009;52(6):626-631. DOI: 10.3839/jksabc.2009.104

[41] Peyton JL. The Birch: Bright Tree of Life and Legend. Granville, OH, USA: McDonald Woodward Publishing Company; 1994

[42] Krasutsky PA. Birch bark research and development. Natural Product Reports. 2006;23(6):919-942. DOI: 10.1039/b606816b

[43] Cîntă-Pînzaru S, Dehelean CA, Soica C, Culea M, Borcan F. Evaluation and differentiation of the Betulaceae birch bark species and their bioactive triterpene content using analytical FT-vibrational spectroscopy and GC-MS. Chemistry Central Journal. 2012;6(1):67. DOI: 10.1186/1752-153X-6-67

[44] Ekman R. The suberin monomers and triterpenoids from the outer bark of Betula verrucosa. Ehrh. Holzforschung. 1983;37:205-211

[45] Heredia-Guerrero JA, Benítez JJ, Domínguez E, Bayer IS, Cingolani R, Athanassiou A, Heredia A. Infrared and Raman spectroscopic features of plant cuticles: A review. Frontiers in Plant Science. 2014;5:305. DOI: 10.3389/fpls.2014.00305

[46] Szakiel A, Paczkowski C, Pensec F, Bertsch C. Fruit cuticular waxes as a source of biologically active triterpenoids. Phytochemistry Reviews. 2012;11(2-3):263-284

[47] Lowitz JT. Uber eine neue, fast benzoeartige Substanz der Birken [On a novel, nearly benzoin resin like substance of the silver birches]. Chemische Annalen Fur Freunde Der Naturlehre, Arzneygelahrtheit, Haushaltungskunst Und Manufakturen. 1788;2:312-316

[48] Guider JM, Halsall TG, Jones ERH. The chemistry of the triterpenes and related compounds. Part XX. The stereochemistry of ring E of betulin and related compounds. Journal of the Chemical Society (Resumed). 1953:3024-3028. DOI: 10.1039/JR9530003024

[49] Hayek EWH, Jordis U, Moche W, Sauter F. A bicentennial of betulin. Phytochemistry. 1989;28(9):2229-2242. DOI: 10.1016/S0031-9422(00)97961-5

[50] Retzlaff F. Ueber Herba Gratiolae. Archiv der Pharmazie. 1902;240(8):561-568. DOI: 10.1002/ardp.19022400802

[51] Barton DHR, Jones ERH. Optical rotatory power and structure in triterpenoid compounds. Application of the method of molecular rotation differences. Journal of the Chemical Society (Resumed). 1944:659. DOI: 10.1039/jr9440000659

[52] Zellner J, Ziffer D. "Plantanolsaure" aus der Rinde von Platanus orientalis L. Monatshefte für Chemie. 1925;46:323-325

[53] Bruckner V, Kovács J, Koczka I. Occurrence of betulinic acid in the bark of the plane tree. Journal of the Chemical Society. 1948:948-951. DOI: 10.1039/JR9480000948

[54] Robertson A, Soliman G, Owen EC. Polyterpenoid compund. Part I. Betulic acid from Cornus florida, L. Journal of the Chemical Society. 1939:1267-1273. DOI: 10.1039/JR9390001267

[55] Ko BS, Kang S, Moon BR, Ryuk JA, Park S. A 70% ethanol extract of mistletoe rich in betulin, betulinic acid, and oleanolic acid potentiated β-cell function and mass and

enhanced hepatic insulin sensitivity. Evidence-Based Complementary and Alternative Medicine. 2016;**2016**:7836823. DOI: 10.1155/2016/7836823

[56] Goulas V, Manganaris GA. Towards an efficient protocol for the determination of triterpenic acids in olive fruit: A comparative study of drying and extraction methods. Phytochemical Analysis. 2012;**23**(5):444-449

[57] Belem Lima AM, Siani AC, Nakamura MJ, D'Avila LA. Selective and cost-effective protocol to separate bioactive triterpene acids from plant matrices using alkalinized ethanol: Application to leaves of Myrtaceae species. Pharmacognosy Magazine. 2015,**11**(43):470-476. DOI: 10.4103/0973-1296.160453

[58] Šiman P, Filipová A, Tichá A, Niang M, Bezrouk A, Havelek R. Effective method of purification of betulin from birch bark: The importance of its purity for scientific and medicinal use. PLoS One. 2016;**11**(5):e0154933. DOI: 10.1371/journal.pone.0154933

[59] Lugemwa FN. Extraction of betulin, trimyristin, eugenol and carnosic acid using water-organic solvent mixtures. Molecules. 2012;**17**:9274-9282

[60] Joshi H, Saxena GK, Singh V, Arya E, Singh RP. Phytochemical investigation, isolation and characterization of betulin from bark of *Betula utilis*. Journal of Pharmacognosy and Phytochemistry. 2013;**2**:145-151

[61] Melnikova N, Burlova I, Kiseleva T, Klabukova I, Gulenova M, Kislitsin A, Vasin V, Tanaseichuk B. A practical synthesis of betulonic acid using selective oxidation of betulin on aluminium solid support. Molecules. 2012;**17**:11849-11863

[62] Liu J, Fu ML, Chen QH. Biotransformation optimization of betulin into betulinic acid production catalysed by cultured Armillaria luteo-virens Sacc ZJUQH100-6 cells. Journal of Applied Microbiology. 2011;**110**(1):90-97

[63] Pettit GR, Melody N, Hempenstall F, Chapuis JC, Groy TL, Williams L. Antineoplastic agents. 595. Structural modifications of betulin and the X-ray crystal structure of an unusual betulin amine dimer. Journal of Natural Products. 2014;**77**(4):863-872

[64] Boryczka S, Bębenek E, Wietrzyk J, Kempińska K, Jastrzębska M, Kusz J, Nowak M. Synthesis, structure and cytotoxic activity of new acetylenic derivatives of betulin. Molecules. 2013;**18**:4526-4543

[65] Jäger S, Laszczyk MN, Scheffler A. A preliminary pharmacokinetic study of betulin, the main pentacyclic triterpene from extract of outer bark of birch (Betulae alba cortex). Molecules. 2008;**13**:3224-3235

[66] Drag-Zalesinska M, Kulbacka J, Saczko J, Wysocka T, Zabel M, Surowiak P, Drag M. Esters of betulin and betulinic acid with amino acids have improved water solubility and are selectively cytotoxic toward cancer cells. Bioorganic & Medicinal Chemistry Letters. 2009;**19**:4814-4817. DOI: 10.1016/j.bmcl.2009.06.046

[67] Spivak AY, Gubaidullin RR, Galimshina ZR, Nedopekina DA, Odinokov VN. Effective synthesis of novel C(2)-propargyl derivatives of betulinic and ursolic acids and their

conjugation with β-d-glucopyranoside azides via click chemistry. Tetrahedron. 2016;**72**: 1249-1256. DOI: 10.1016/j.tet.2016.01.024

[68] Dehelean C, Şoica C, Peev C, Gruia AT, Şeclaman E. Physico-chemical and molecular analysis of antitumoral pentacyclic triterpenes in complexation with gamma-cyclodextrin. Revista de Chimie. 2008;**59**:887-890

[69] Şoica C, Dehelean C, Peev C, Coneac G, Gruia AT. Complexation with hydroxipropil-gamma cyclodextrin of some pentacyclic triterpenes. Characterisation of their binary products. Farmacia. 2008;**56**:182-190

[70] Dehelean CA, Soica C, Peev C, Ciurlea S, Feflea S, Kasa P Jr. A pharmaco-toxicological evaluation for betulinic acid mixed with hydroxipropilgamma cyclodextrin on in vitro and in vivo models. Farmacia. 2011;**59**:51-59

[71] Dehelean C, Zupko I, Rethy B, Şoica C, Coneac G, Peev C, Bumbacila B. In vitro analysis of betulinic acid in lower concentrations and its anticancer activity/toxicity by changing the hydrosolubility with hydroxipropilgamma cyclodextrin. Toxicology Letters. 2008;**180**:S100

[72] Dehelean CA, Soica C, Muresan A, Tatu C, Aigner Z. Toxicological evaluations for betulinic acid in cyclodextrins complexes on in vitro and in vivo melanoma models. Planta Medica. 2009;**75**:PE3

[73] Fontanay S, Kedzierewicz F, Duval RE, Clarot I. Physicochemical and thermodynamic characterization of hydroxy pentacyclic triterpenoic acid/γ-cyclodextrin inclusion complexes. Journal of Inclusion Phenomena and Macrocyclic Chemistry. 2012;**73**:341-347

[74] Şoica CM, Peev CI, Ciurlea S, Ambrus R, Dehelean C. Physico-chemical and toxicological evaluations of betulin and betulinic acid interactions with hydrophilic cyclodextrins. Farmacia. 2010;**58**:611-619

[75] Sun YF, Song CK, Viernstein H, Unger F, Liang ZS. Apoptosis of human breast cancer cells induced by microencapsulated betulinic acid from sour jujube fruits through the mitochondria transduction pathway. Food Chemistry. 2013;**138**:1998-2007. DOI: 10.1016/j.foodchem.2012.10.079

[76] Wang HM, Soica C, Wenz G. A comparison investigation on the solubilization of betulin and betulinic acid in cyclodextrin derivatives. Natural Product Communications. 2012;**7**:289-291

[77] Şoica C, Dehelean C, Danciu C, Wang HM, Wenz G, Ambrus R, Bojin F, Anghel M. Betulin complex in γ-cyclodextrin derivatives: Properties and antineoplasic activities in in vitro and in vivo tumor models. International Journal of Molecular Sciences. 2012;**13**(11):14992-15011. DOI: 10.3390/ijms131114992

[78] Soica C, Danciu C, Savoiu-Balint G, Borcan F, Ambrus R, Zupko I, Bojin F, Coricovac D, Ciurlea S, Avram S, Dehelean CA, Olariu T, Matusz P. Betulinic acid in complex with a gamma-cyclodextrin derivative decreases proliferation and in vivo tumor development of

non-metastatic and metastatic B164A5 cells. International Journal of Molecular Sciences. 2014;**15**:8235-8255

[79] Dehelean C, Şoica C, Peev C, Ordodi V, Tatu C. Betulinic acid dissolved with PVP dose/effect relationship and its intervention on skin pathology and melanoma. A pharmaco-toxicological evaluation. Timişoara Medical Journal. 2008;**58**(Suppl. 2):345-349

[80] Dehelean C, Şoica C, Ciurlea S, Urşica L, Peev C, Aigner Z. Consequences of increasing betulin hydrosolubility with hydroxipropilgamma cyclodextrin, in vitro analysis of its efficacy/noxious activity. Timişoara Medical Journal. 2008;**58**(Suppl. 2):341-345

[81] Dehelean C, Soica C, Peev C, Ciurlea S, Coneac G, Cinta-Pinzaru S. Pentacyclic triter-penes interventions in skin pathology/toxicity and treatment: In vitro and in vivo cor-relations. Bulletin of the University of Agricultural Sciences and Veterinary Medicine. 2008;**65**:370-375

[82] Hertrampf A, Gründemann C, Jäger S, Laszczyk M, Giesemann T, Huber R. In vitro cytotoxicity of cyclodextrin-bonded birch bark extract. Planta Medica. 2012;**78**(9):881-889. DOI: 10.1055/s-0031-1298473

[83] Xiao S, Wang Q, Si L, Shi Y, Wang H, Yu F, Zhang Y, Li Y, Zheng Y, Zhang C, Wang C, Zhang L, Zhou D. Synthesis and anti-HCV entry activity studies of β-cyclodextrin-pentacyclic triterpene conjugates. ChemMedChem. 2014;**9**:1060-1070. DOI: 10.1002/cmdc.201300545

[84] Xiao S, Wang Q, Si L, Zhou X, Zhang Y, Zhang L, Zhou D. Synthesis and biological evaluation of novel pentacyclic triterpene α-cyclodextrin conjugates as HCV entry inhibitors. European Journal of Medicinal Chemistry. 2016;**124**:1-9. DOI: 10.1016/j.ejmech.2016.08.020

[85] Lima PS, Lucchese AM, Araújo-Filho HG, Menezes PP, Araújo AA, Quintans-Júnior LJ, Quintans JS. Inclusion of terpenes in cyclodextrins: Preparation, characterization and pharmacological approaches. Carbohydrate Polymers. 2016;**151**:965-987. DOI: 10.1016/j.carbpol.2016.06.040

[86] Chang HI, Cheng MY, Yeh MK. Clinically proven liposome-based drug delivery: Formulation, characterization and therapeutic efficacy. Open Access Scientific Reports. 2012;**1**:195. DOI: 10.4172/scientific reports.195

[87] Immordino ML, Dosio F, Cattel L. Stealth liposomes: Review of the basic science, rationale, and clinical applications, existing and potential. International Journal of Nanomedicine. 2006;**1**:297-315

[88] Torchilin VP. Recent advances with liposomes as pharmaceutical carriers. Nature Reviews Drug Discovery. 2005;**4**:145-160

[89] Mullauer FB, van Bloois L, Daalhuisen JB, Ten Brink MS, Storm G, Medema JP, Schiffelers RM, Kessler JH. Betulinic acid delivered in liposomes reduces growth of human lung and colon cancers in mice without causing systemic toxicity. Anticancer Drugs. 2011;**22**:223-233

[90] Khattar D, Kumar M, Mukherjee R, Burman AC, Garg M, Jaggi M, Singh AT, Awasthi A. Proliposomal And Liposomal Compositions Of Poorly Water Soluble Drugs; US Patent 2009/0017105 A1, January 15, 2009, http://www.freepatentsonline.com/y2009/0017105.html

[91] Castor TP. Phospholipid nanosomes. Current Drug Delivery. 2005;2:329-340

[92] Son LB, Kaplun AP, Spilevskiĭ AA, Andiia-Pravdivyĭ IuE, Alekseeva SG, Gribor'ev VB, Shvets VI. Synthesis of betulinic acid from betulin and study of its solubilization using liposomes. Bioorganicheskaia Khimiia. 1998;24:787-793

[93] Csuk R, Barthel A, Kluge R, Ströhl D. Synthesis, cytotoxicity and liposome preparation of 28-acetylenic betulin derivatives. Bioorganic & Medicinal Chemistry. 2010;18:7252-7259

[94] Csuk R, Barthel A, Sczepek R, Siewert B, Schwarz S. Synthesis, encapsulation and anti-tumor activity of new betulin derivatives. Archiv der Pharmazie. 2011;344:37-49

[95] Liu Y, Gao D, Zhang X, Liu Z, Dai K, Ji B, Wang Q, Luo L. Antitumor drug effect of betu-linic acid mediated by polyethylene glycol modified liposomes. Materials Science and Engineering C: Materials for Biological Applications. 2016;64:124-132. DOI: 10.1016/j.msec.2016.03.080

[96] Dehelean CA, Feflea S, Ganta S, Amiji M. Anti-angiogenic effects of betulinic acid administered in nanoemulsion formulation using chorioallantoic membrane assay. Journal of Biomedical Nanotechnology. 2011;7:317-324

[97] Dehelean CA, Feflea S, Gheorgheosu D, Ganta S, Cimpean AM, Muntean D, Amiji MM. Anti-angiogenic and anti-cancer evaluation of betulin nanoemulsion in chicken chorioallantoic membrane and skin carcinoma in Balb/c mice. Journal of Biomedical Nanotechnology. 2013;9:577-589

[98] Cavazos-Garduño A, Ochoa Flores AA, Serrano-Niño JC, Martínez-Sanchez CE, Beristain CI, García HS. Preparation of betulinic acid nanoemulsions stabilized by ω-3 enriched phosphatidylcholine. Ultrasonics Sonochemistry. 2015;24:204-213. DOI: 10.1016/j.ultsonch.2014.12.007

[99] Karlina MV, Pozharitskaya ON, Shikov A, Makarov VG, Mirza S, Miroshnyk I, Hiltunen R. Biopharmaceutical study of nanosystems containing betulin for inhalation adminis-tration. Pharmaceutical Chemistry Journal. 2010;44:501-503

[100] Shakhtshneider TP, Kuznetsova SA, Mikhailenko MA, Malyar YN, Skvortsova G, Boldyrev VV. Obtaining of nontoxic betulin composites with polyvinylpyrrolidone and polyethylene glycole. Journal of Siberian Federal University. Chemistry. 2012;1:52-60

[101] Shakhtshneider TP, Kuznetsova SA, Mikhailenko MA, Zamai AS, Malyar YN, Zamai TN, Boldyrev VV. Effect of mechanochemical treatment on physicochemical and anti-tumor properties of betulin diacetate mixtures with arabinogalactan. Chemistry of Natural Compounds. 2013;49:470-474

[102] Yu M, Ocando JE, Trombetta L, Chatterjee P. Molecular interaction studies of amor-phous solid dispersions of the antimelanoma agent betulinic acid. AAPS PharmSciTech. 2015;16:384-397. DOI: 10.1208/s12249-014-0220-x

[103] Saneja A, Sharma L, Dubey RD, Mintoo MJ, Singh A, Kumar A, Sangwan PL, Tasaduq SA, Singh G, Mondhe DM, Gupta PN. Synthesis, characterization and augmented anticancer potential of PEG-betulinic acid conjugate. Materials Science and Engineering: C. 2017;**73**:616-626

[104] Dai L, Cao X, Liu K-F, Li CX, Zhang GF, Deng LH, Si CL, He J, Lei JD. Self-assembled targeted folate-conjugated eight-arm-polyethylene glycol–betulinic acid nanoparticles for co-delivery of anticancer drugs. Journal of Materials Chemistry B. 2015;**3**:3754-3766

[105] Dash SK, Chattopadhyay S, Karmakar P, Roy S. Anti-leukemic activity of betulinic acid from bulk to self-assembled structure. BLDE University Journal of Health Sciences. 2016;**1**:14-19

[106] Li J. Development, characterization and in vivo evaluation of biodegradable nanospheres and nanocapsules [thesis]. Halle: Martin-Luther University Halle-Wittenberg, Germany; 2012

[107] Silva MAA, Naves LN, Lima EM, Bozinis MCV, Diniz DGA. Development and characterization of lupeol-loaded nanocapsules. In: SINPOSPq: 4th International Symposium of Post-Graduation and Research; 4-6 November 2010; Sao Paulo, Brazil

[108] Krukiewicz K, Cichy M, Ruszkowski P, Turczyn R, Jarosz T, Zak JK, Lapkowski M, Bednarczyk-Cwynar B. Betulin-loaded PEDOT films for regional chemotherapy. Materials Science and Engineering: C. 2017;**73**:611-615

[109] Tan JM, Karthivashan G, Arulselvan P, Fakurazi S, Hussein MZ. Sustained release and cytotoxicity evaluation of carbon nanotube-mediated drug delivery system for betulinic acid. Journal of Nanomaterials. 2014;**2014**:862148. DOI: 10.1155/2014/862148

[110] Tan JM, Karthivashan G, Abd Gani S, Fakurazi S, Hussein MZ. Biocompatible polymers coated on carboxylated nanotubes functionalized with betulinic acid for effective drug delivery. Journal of Materials Science: Materials in Medicine. 2016;**27**:26. DOI: 10.1007/s10856-015-5635-8

[111] Hussein-Al-Ali SH, Arulselvan P, Fakurazi S, Hussein MZ. The in vitro therapeutic activity of betulinic acid nanocomposite on breast cancer cells (MCF-7) and normal fibroblast cell (3T3). Journal of Materials Science. 2014;**49**:8171-8182. DOI: 10.1007/s10853-014-8526-3

[112] Soica C, Coricovac D, Dehelean C, Pinzaru I, Mioc M, Danciu C, Fulias A, Puiu M, Sitaru C. Nanocarriers as tools in delivering active compounds for immune system related pathologies. Recent Patents on Nanotechnology. 2016;**10**(2):128-145

[113] Brodniewicz T, Grynkiewicz G. Preclinical drug development. Acta Poloniae Pharmaceutica. 2010;**67**(6):578-585

[114] Krol SK, Kielbus M, Rivero-Müller AR, Stepulak A. Comprehensive review on betulin as a potential anticancer agent. BioMed Research International. 2015:584189. DOI: 10.1155/2015/58418

[115] Suresh C, Zhao H, Gumbs A, Chetty CS, Bose HS. New ionic derivatives of betulinic acid as highly potent anti-cancer agents. Bioorganic & Medicinal Chemistry Letters. 2012;**22**(4):1734-1738. DOI: 10.1016/j.bmcl.2011.12.102

[116] Saha S, Ghosh M, Dutta SK. A potent tumoricidal co-drug 'Bet-CA' — An ester derivative of betulinic acid and dichloroacetate selectively and synergistically kills cancer cells. Scientific Reports. 2015;**5**:7762. DOI: 10.1038/srep07762

[117] Yadav VR, Prasad S, Sung B, Kannappan R, Aggarwal BB. Targeting inflammatory pathways by triterpenoids for prevention and treatment of cancer. Toxins. 2010;**2**:2428-2466. DOI: 10.3390/toxins2102428

[118] Drąg-Zalesinska M, Drąg M, Poreba M, Borska S, Kulbacka J, Saczko J. Anticancer properties of ester derivatives of betulin in human metastatic melanoma cells (Me-45). Cancer Cell International. 2017;**17**:4. DOI: 10.1186/s12935-016-0369-3

[119] AlQathama A, Prieto JM. Natural products with therapeutic potential in melanoma metastasis. Natural Product Reports. 2015;**32**(8):1170-1182

[120] McIlwain DR, Berger T, Mak TW. Caspase functions in cell death and disease. Cold Spring Harbor Perspectives in Biology. 2013;**5**(4):a008656. DOI: 10.1101/cshperspect.a008656

[121] Alakurtti S, Makela T, Koskimies S, Yli-Kauhaluoma J. Pharmacological properties of the ubiquitous natural product betulin. European Journal of Pharmaceutical Sciences. 2006;**29**(1):1-13. DOI: 10.1016/j.ejps.2006.04.006

[122] Liu Y, Luo W. Betulinic acid induces Bax/Bak-independent cytochrome c release in human nasopharyngeal carcinoma cells. Molecules and Cells. 2012;**33**(5):517-524. DOI: 10.1007/s10059-012-0022-5

[123] Oh SH, Choi JE, Lim SC. Protection of betulin against cadmium-induced apoptosis in hepatoma cells. Toxicology. 2006;**220**(1):1-12. DOI: 10.1016/j.tox.2005.08.025

[124] Li Y, He K, Huang Y, Zheng D, Gao C, Cui L, Jin YH. Betulin induces mitochondrial cytochrome c release associated apoptosis in human cancer cells. Molecular Carcinogenesis. 2010;**49**(7):630-640. DOI: 10.1002/mc.20638

[125] Mullauer FB, Kessler JH, Medema JP. Betulin is a potent anti-tumor agent that is enhanced by cholesterol. PLoS One. 2009;**4**(4):e1. DOI: 10.1371/journal.pone.0005361

[126] Zhang X, Hu J, Chen Y. Betulinic acid and the pharmacological effects of tumor suppression (Review). Molecular Medicine Reports. 2016;**14**(5):4489-4495. DOI: 10.3892/mmr.2016.5792

[127] Laszczyk MN. Pentacyclic triterpenes of the lupane, oleanane and ursane group as tools in cancer therapy. Planta Medica. 2009;**75**(15):1549-1560. DOI: 10.1055/s-0029-1186102

[128] Csuk R, Barthel A, Kluge R, Strohl D, Kommera H, Paschke R. Synthesis and biological evaluation of antitumour-active betulin derivatives. Bioorganic & Medicinal Chemistry. 2010;**18**(3):1344-1355. DOI: 10.1016/j.bmc.2009.12.024

[129] Csuk R, Barthel A, Schwarz S, Kommera H, Paschke R. Synthesis and biological evaluation of antitumor-active gamma-butyrolactone substituted betulin derivatives. Bioorganic & Medicinal Chemistry. 2010;18(7):2549-2558. DOI: 10.1016/j.bmc. 2010.02.042

[130] Saudagar P, Dubey VK. Molecular mechanisms of in vitro betulin-induced apoptosis of Leishmania donovani. American Journal of Tropical Medicine and Hygiene. 2014;90(2):354-360. DOI: 10.4269/ajtmh.13-0320

[131] Bernardo TC, Cunha-Oliveira T, Serafim TL, Holy J, Krasutsky D, Kolomitsyna O, Krasutsky P, Moreno AM, Oliveira PJ. Dimethylaminopyridine derivatives of lupane triterpenoids cause mitochondrial disruption and induce the permeability transition. Bioorganic & Medicinal Chemistry. 2013;21(23):7239-7249. DOI: 10.1016/j.bmc. 2013.09.066

[132] Muceniece R, Saleniece K, Riekstina U, Krigere L, Tirzitis G, Ancans J. Betulin binds to melanocortin receptors and antagonizes alpha-melanocyte stimulating hormone induced cAMP generation in mouse melanoma cells. Cell Biochemistry & Function. 2007;25(5):591-596. DOI: 10.1002/cbf.1427

[133] Dehelean CA, Soica C, Ledeti I, Aluas M, Zupko I, Galuscan A, Cinta-Pinzaru S, Munteanu M. Study of the betulin enriched birch bark extracts effects on human carcinoma cells and ear inflammation. Chemistry Central Journal. 2012;6(1):137. DOI: 10.1186/1752-153X-6-137

[134] Rosas LV, Cordeiro MS, Campos FR, Nascimento SK, Januario AH, Franca SC, Nomizo A, Toldo MP, Albuquerque S, Pereira PS. In vitro evaluation of the cytotoxic and trypanocidal activities of Ampelozizyphus amazonicus (Rhamnaceae). Brazilian Journal of Medical and Biological Research. 2007;40(5):663-670

[135] Tiwari R, Puthli A, Balakrishnan S, Sapra BK, Mishra KP. Betulinic acid-induced cytotoxicity in human breast tumor cell lines MCF-7 and T47D and its modification by tocopherol. Cancer Investigation. 2014;2(8):402-408. DOI: 10.3109/07357907.2014.933234

[136] Tsai FS, Lin LW, Wu CR. Lupeol and its role in chronic diseases. Advances in Experimental Medicine and Biology. 2016;929:145-175. DOI: 10.1007/978-3-319-41342-6_7

[137] Tarapore RS, Siddiqui IA, Saleem M, Adhami VM, Spiegelman VS, Mukhtar H. Specific targeting of Wnt/beta-catenin signaling in human melanoma cells by a dietary triterpene lupeol. Carcinogenesis. 2010;31(10):1844-1853. DOI: 10.1093/carcin/bgq169

[138] Nigam N, Prasad S, George J, Shukla Y. Lupeol induces p53 and cyclin-B-mediated G2/M arrest and targets apoptosis through activation of caspase in mouse skin. Biochemical and Biophysical Research Communications. 2009;381(2):253-258. DOI: 10.1016/j.bbrc.2009.02.033

[139] Koh SJ, Tak JK, Kim ST, Nam WS, Kim SY, Park KM, Park JW. Sensitization of ionizing radiation-induced apoptosis by ursolic acid. Free Radical Research. 2012;46(3):339-345. DOI: 10.3109/10715762.2012.656101

[140] Duval RE, Harmand PO, Jayat-Vignoles C, Cook-Moreau J, Pinon A, Delage C, Simon A. Differential involvement of mitochondria during ursolic acid-induced apoptotic process in HaCaT and M4Beu cells. Oncology Reports. 2008;**19**(1):145-149

[141] Bonaccorsi I, Altieri F, Sciamanna I, Oricchio E, Grillo C, Contartese G, Galati EM. Endogenous reverse transcriptase as a mediator of ursolic acid's anti-proliferative and differentiating effects in human cancer cell lines. Cancer Letters. 2008;**263**(1):130-139. DOI: 10.1016/j.canlet.2007.12.026

7

Lycopene: Multitargeted Applications in Cancer Therapy

Kazim Sahin, Shakir Ali, Nurhan Sahin,
Cemal Orhan and Omer Kucuk

Abstract

Cancer is an uncontrolled growth and division of cells, leading to significant morbidity and mortality and economic burden to the society. Natural products as anticancer molecules have drawn the attention of researchers and have resulted in the development of many successful anticancer drugs, which include camptothecins, epipodophyllotoxins, vinca alkaloids, and taxanes. Another group of compounds with anti-cancer effects include botanicals (phytochemicals) found in the diet. In recent years, a tomato carotenoid lycopene (LYC) has gained attention for its potential health benefits, especially in prevention and treatment of cancer. The studies suggest that the consumption LYC in food or by itself may reduce cancer risk. However, there are insufficient clinical trial data to support the hypothesis. LYC may play a preventive role in a variety of cancers, especially in prostate cancer. It acts by multiple mechanisms including the regulation of growth factor signalling, cell cycle arrest and/or apoptosis induction, metastasis and angiogenesis, as well as by modulating the anti-inflammatory and phase II detoxification enzymes activities. The effects can be attributed to the unique chemical structure of the carotenoid which confers it a strong antioxidant property. In this chapter, we discuss the chemopreventive and anti-cancer properties of LYC, a dietary carotenoid."

Keywords: phytochemicals, lycopene, cancer, molecular, signaling pathway

1. Introduction

Natural products, which can be defined as simple or complex molecules (primary and secondary metabolites) produced naturally by any organism, constitute a diverse group of substances some of which are part of our food, and others have medicinal properties. Over the past few decades, there has been a tremendous increase in research on isolation and purification of compounds of botanical origin and establishing the efficacy of these compounds as potential therapeutic and preventive agents. The natural products have received considerable attention as potential drugs, and a large number of medicinal plants and their formulations have been investigated and found useful in cancer chemotherapy [1]. According to an estimate, more than half of potent anticancer drugs have natural product origin [2]. Some of the plant species that have been used for medicinal purpose and suggested for their beneficial effect in cancer are listed in **Table 1**.

Plant species	Preparation	Effect
Acacia nilotica	Aqueous extracts of bark, gum, flower, and leaves	Effective in chemically-induced hepatocellular carcinoma (HCC) [3] and skin papillomagenesis [4]
Aegle marmelos	Hydro-alcoholic extract of leaf	Remission in Ehlirch ascites carcinoma (EAC) [5]
Aloe vera	Extract	Skin carcinoma [6]
Alstonia scholaris	Alkaloid fraction from bark	UV-induced carcinogenesis [7], DMBA-induced skin carcinogenesis [8] and UV-induced hematological disorder [9]
Azadirchata indica	Ethyl acetate and methanolic fractions of the leaves	DMBA-induced mammary carcinogenesis [10] and prostate cancer [11]
Biophytum sensitivum	Alcoholic extract	Dalton's lymphoma ascites (DLA) and EAC [12]
Boswellia serrata	Triterpenediol preparation	Caspase-8 activation and apoptosis [13]
Butea monosperma	Flower extract	Liver cancer [14]
Cassia auriculata	leaf extract	Decrease Bcl-2/Bax ratio [15]
Cassia occidentalis	Aqueous extracts	Inhibit growth of HCT-15, SW-620, PC-3, MCF-7, SiHa and OVCAR-5 cancer cells [16]
Cassia tora	Methanolic extract	Enhance caspase-3 activity of HeLa cells [17]
Cedrus deodara	Lignan mixture	Effect on leukemia cells [18]
Cheilanthes farinose	Fern	HCC [19]
Cinnamomum cassia		Cervical cancer cells (SiHa) [20]
Garcinia indica	Methanolic extract	Colon, breast and liver cancer [21]
Inula racemosa	Ethanolic extract of roots	Colon, ovary, prostate, lung, CNS and leukemia cells [22]
Lygodium flexuosum	Extract	Induce apoptosis in hepatoma cells [23]
Ocimum viride	Essential oils	Colorectal adenocarcinoma [24]
Oryza sativa	Methanolic extracts	C6 glioma cells [25]
Phyllanthus niruri	Hydro-alcoholic extract	Skin carcinoma [26]
Piper longum	Methanolic extract	Colon cancer [27]

Plant species	Preparation	Effect
Polyalthia longifolia	Ethanolic stem, bark and leave extracts	EAC and DLA [28]
Rhodiola imbricate	Aqueous extract	Increase ROS and arrest cell cycle progression at G2/M phase in K562 cells [29]
Semecarpus anacardium	Nut milk extract	Effect on leukemic cells from the bone marrow [30], induce apoptosis in breast cancer cells through mitochondria mediated apoptosis [31]
Sesbania grandiflora	Sesbania fraction 2, extracted from the flower	Down-regulate NF-kB, Bcl-2, p-Akt, cyclooxygenase-2, inhibits proliferation and induced apoptosis in DLA and SW-480 cells [32]
Terminalia arjuna	Ethanolic extract	Liver cancer [33]
Tinospora cordifolia	Extract	Antitumor and chemopreventive [34]
Trachyspermum ammi	Seed extract	Skin and forestomach tumor multiplicity [35]
Withania somnifera	Hydro-alcoholic extract	Colon cancer model [36], cell cycle disruption and antiangiogenic, property [37]
Zingiber officinale	Extract	Suppressed cell proliferation [38]

Table 1. List of some medicinal plants suggested for beneficial effects in cancer.

2. Natural compounds as lead molecules for cancer therapy and their mechanisms of action

Natural substances such as paclitaxel [39], alkaloids and other substances [1] have demonstrated encouraging antitumor activity in human cancer cells in vivo and in vitro. These molecules act by a variety of mechanisms. For example, paclitaxel, a complex diterpene having a taxane ring with a four-membered oxetane ring and an ester side chain at position C-13, enhances the polymerization of tubulin to stable microtubules and also interacts directly with the microtubules [39]. Other mechanisms of action of antitumor agents include the inhibition of S phase-specific topoisomerase-I (camptothecin) and S and G2 phase-specific topoisomerase-II (etoposide), blockade of G2/M and M/G1 check points (paclitaxel), and prevention of microtubule depolymerization (vinblastine). A new class, commonly known as the vascular disrupting agents (VDA) (e.g., combretastatin A4 phosphate), targets tumor blood vessels. Combretastatin A4 phosphate is a VAD isolated from Combretum caffrum and has been reported to be antimitotic and antiangiogenic, along with the microtubule-depolymerizing property [40]. Substances like berberine, a protoberberine alkaloid found in the roots, rhizomes, stems and bark of berberis, goldenseal (*Hydrastis canadensis*) and *Coptis chinensis*, have also been reported to inhibit different types of cancer [41–49]. They act by inhibiting angiogenesis and by other mechanisms in different cancer models. Mahanine, a purified lead molecule derived from the leaves of Murraya koenigii, which showed antiproliferative activity in leukemic cells, primary cells of leukemic and myeloid patients and inhibited K562 xenograft growth, activates reactive oxygen species (ROS)-mediated mitochondrial apoptotic pathway, death receptor-mediated signaling differentially in MOLT-3 and K562 cells. Piper betle, reported to decrease the mitochondrial membrane potential and induce apoptosis in primary leukemia cells from CML patients in vitro and K562 xenografts in vivo, can also augment the early ROS production [50]. Withaferin A, which induces apoptosis in HL-60 cells through multiple pathways, also enhances early ROS accumulation leading to loss of mitochondrial membrane potential and cytochrome c release, Bax translocation, caspase activation, and PARP cleavage [51]. It enhanced caspase-8 activity, caspase 3-mediated nuclear cleavage of p65/Rel, which was inhibited by N-acetylcysteine, an antioxidant, suggesting the role of early ROS production in withaferin A-mediated apoptotic signaling. The anticancer molecules, such as betulinic acid, a pentacyclic triterpene, have also been reported to directly activate mitochondria-mediated intrinsic pathway and exhibit antitumor activity [50, 52]. Resveratrol, a phytoalexin found in various food products, induces human promyelocytic leukemia cell differentiation, inhibits cyclooxygenase and hydroperoxidase functions and the development of pre-neoplastic lesions in carcinogen-treated mouse mammary glands as well as tumorigenesis in a mouse skin cancer model [53]. Various other substances isolated from plant material and found to be effective in cancer include: 2-deacetoxytaxinine (from the bark of Himalayan yew, *Taxus wallichiana*) [54], curcumin (from *Curcuma longa*) [55], quercetin 3-O-rutinoside (from the fruits of *Barringtonia racemosa*) [56], 13-epi-sclareol (from the roots of *Coleus forskohlii*) [57], corchorusin-D (from *Corchorus acutangulus*) [58], tetranortriterpenoid methyl angolensate (from the root callus extract *Soymida febrifuga*) [59], oleanonic acid (from *Lantana camara*) [60], longitriol and longimide (from the leaves of *Polyalthia longifolia*) [61], 1-hydroxytectoquinone (from *Rubia cordifolia*) [62], 3-(8′(Z),11′(Z)-pentadecadienyl catechol (from *Semecarpus anacardium* nut) [63], β-sitosterol (from *Asclepias curassavica*) [64], sulfonoquinovosyl diacylglyceride (isolated from leaves of *Azadirachta indica*) and nimbolide (from the leaves and flowers of *A. indica*) [65], diallyl disulfide (from *Allium sativum*) [66], arjunic acid (from *Terminalia arjuna*) [67], L-asparaginase, withaferin A, and ashwagandhanolide from (from *Withania somnifera*) [68–70]. Organosulfur from *Allium sativum* (diallyl disulfide and S-allylcysteine) also exhibits good antiproliferative activity [71]. S-allylcysteine is reported to inhibit N-methyl-N′-nitro-N-nitrosoguanidine-induced gastric cancer in rats when administered with tomato carotenoid LYC in a combinatorial approach [72]. A glycoprotein isolated from the bulbs of *Urginea indica* has also been reported to show antitumor activity against an ascites tumor and mouse mammary carcinoma. It inhibited NF-kB, VEGF-induced DNA fragmentation and caspase-3 activation [73].

3. Lycopene

Diets high in fruits and vegetables may reduce the risk of cancers [74–78]. Tomato and tomato-based products have been found to be effective in the stomach, lung and pleural, colorectal, oral/laryngeal/pharyngeal, esophageal, pancreatic, prostate, bladder, breast, cervical and ovarian cancers [79]. Lycopene (LYC) (C40H56; Molar mass, 536.873 g/mol) is a bright red-colored carotenoid pigment found in red fruits and vegetables particularly tomato, carrot, watermelon, guava, etc., (but not in all red fruits, like strawberries, or cherries) and also in some vegetables that are not red, such as parsley and asparagus. The beneficial effects of tomato on health have been attributed to the presence of LYC. LYC is a highly unsaturated, straight-chain hydrocarbon containing 11 conjugated and two non-conjugated double bonds (**Figure 1**).

It is a non-provitamin A carotenoid. The biological significance of carotenoids has been well established and documented. The β-carotene, for example, is converted into retinal, retinoic acid, and apocarotenoids, which plays a very important role in human/animal

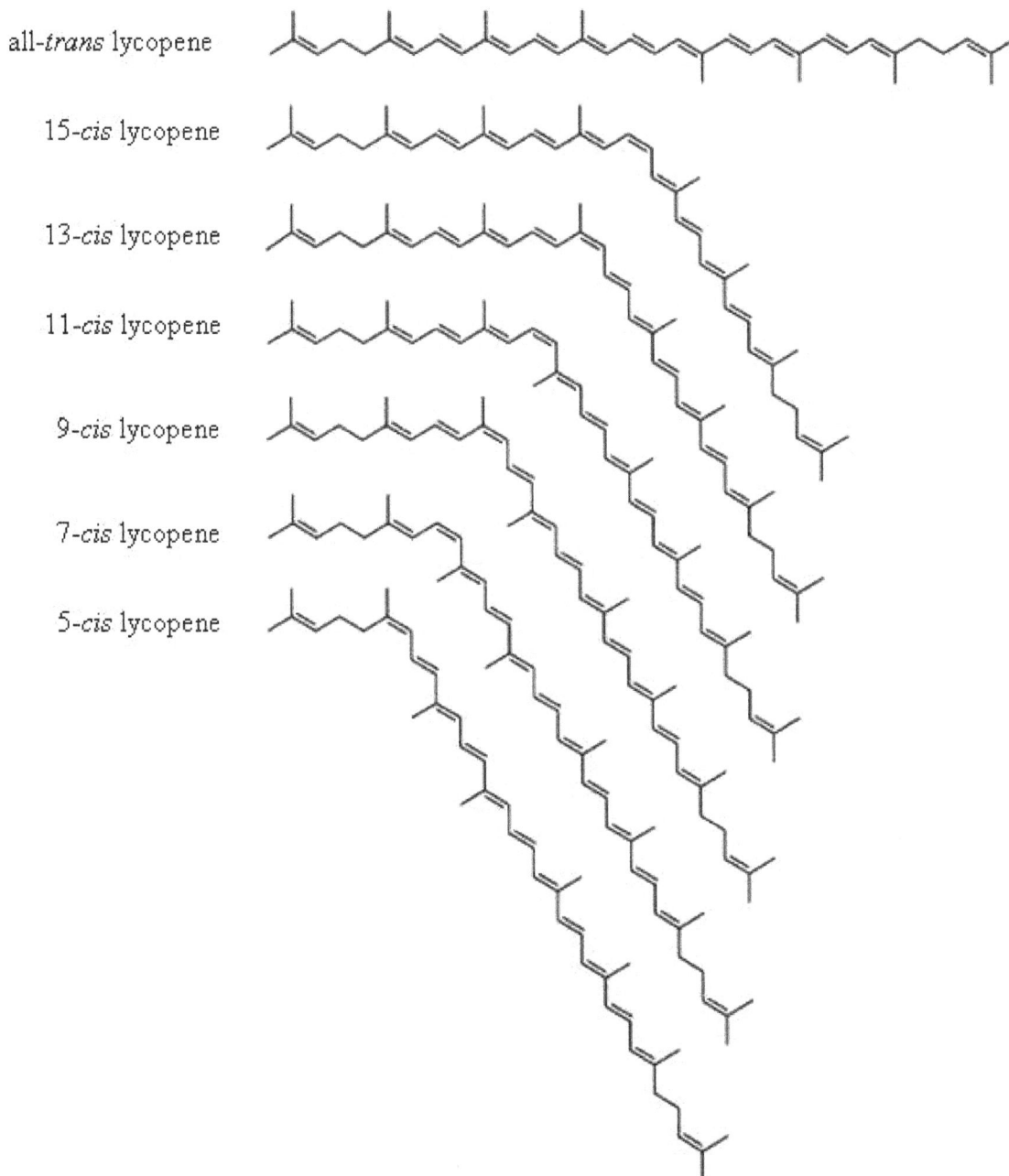

Figure 1. Chemical structures of lycopene isomers.

physiology [80]. LYC is non-provitamin A carotenoid which is not converted to vitamin A. It is a major component found in the serum and other tissues and has been inversely related to cancer and cardiovascular diseases [81]. The molecule acts as an antioxidant and has been reported to have beneficial effects, which can be attributed to its unique chemical structure [82]. LYC can modulate the intercellular gap junction communication, hormonal and immune system, and metabolic pathways.

LYC exists predominantly in trans-configuration, the most thermodynamically stable form, and as a polyene, it undergoes cis-trans isomerization induced by light, thermal energy or chemical reactions. In human plasma, LYC is an isomeric mixture containing 50% of total LYC as cis isomers. All-trans, 5-cis, 9-cis, 13-cis, and 15-cis are most commonly identified isomeric forms of LYC. LYC is poorly absorbed when ingested in its natural trans-form found in tomatoes. Heat processing of tomatoes and tomato products increases the bioavailability of LYC by inducing isomerization of LYC to the cis form [83]. LYC, which when oxidized with potassium permanganate and by atmospheric oxygen catalyzed by a metalloporphyrin, is converted into apo-lycopenals and apo-lycopenones [84]. In addition, a number of other apo-lycopenals have been suggested in fruits, vegetables, and human plasma [85–87].

4. Lycopene: its role and mechanisms of action in cancer

Carotenoid-rich foods have been associated with reduced risk of cancer, such as the prostate and other cancers by various mechanisms [81, 88–95]. The enhanced cytotoxic and apoptosis inducing the activity of LYC has been recorded in different cancer cell lines [96]. The influence of LYC and its oxidation products on the levels of intracellular ROS in three different cell lines has been studied, and in all the cases, the oxidation products increased the ROS levels than the LYC- and control-treated cells. In MCF-7 cells, ROS in control- and LYC-treated groups was lower by 16.3 and 15.5% than in oxidation product treated cells [96].

A number of mechanisms of action have been proposed to explain the anticarcinogenic action of LYC. These include: (i) the inhibition of cancer cell proliferation and induction of differentiation (of cancer cells) by modulating the expression of cell cycle regulatory proteins, (ii) modulation of the IGF-1/IGFBP-3 system, (iii) inhibition of oxidative DNA damage, (iv) modulation of redox signaling, (v) upregulation of gap-junctional gene connexin 43 (Cx43) and increased gap junctional intercellular communication, (vi) inhibition of 5-lipoxygenase, (vii) modulation of carcinogenic metabolizing enzymes, (viii) modulation of immune function, (ix) modulation of IL-6 and androgen, (x) inhibition of IL-6 and androgen, (xi) inhibition of 5-lipoxygenase, (xii) modulation of carcinogen metabolizing enzymes and (xiii) modulation of immune function [97], (xiv) reduction of oxidative stress by modulating ROS-producing enzymes (CYP-P450 enzymes, NADPH oxidase, iNOS, COX-2 and 5-LOX), (xv) inducing antioxidant/detoxifying phase II enzymes (also chemical interaction with radioactive materials), NQO1 and GST [98], (xvi) regulation of nuclear factor E2-related factor 2-antioxidant response element (Nrf2-ARE) system [99], and (xvii) inactivation of growth factor (PDGF, VEGF and IGF)-induced PI3K/AKT/PKB and Ras/RAF/MAPK signaling pathways [100] (**Figure 2**)

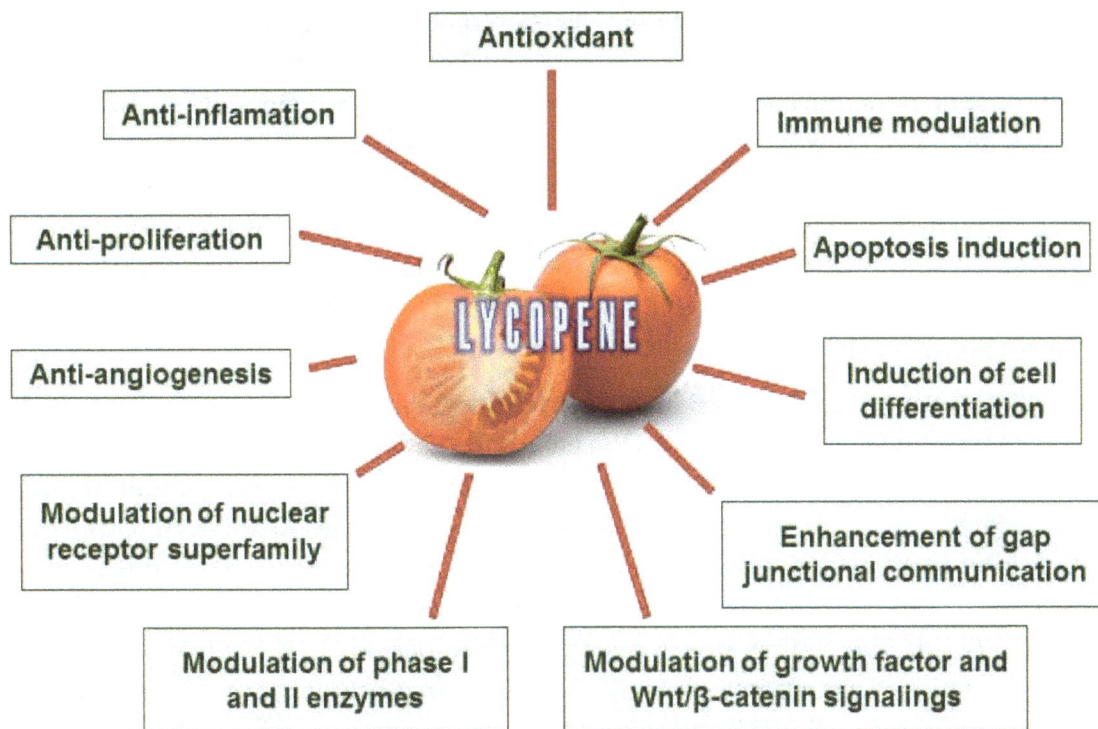

Figure 2. Mechanisms of cancer chemoprevention by lycopene.

4.1. Prostate cancer

The beneficial effects of LYC in prostate cancer (PC) have been extensively reported. A significant inverse correlation between PC and plasma LYC concentration [odds ratio (OR) = 0.17, P-trend = 0.005] has been found between the highest and lowest quintiles of intake [101]. In several experimental studies, LYC has been suggested to suppress PC in vitro and in vivo [102, 103]. It was found to down-regulate the expression of protein kinase B (AKT2) and up-regulate miR-let-7f-1 expression in PC3 cells. Reintroduction of miR-let-7f-1 into PC3 cells was able to inhibit cell proliferation and induce apoptosis. Further research has shown that up-regulation of miR-let-7f-1-targeted AKT2 and AKT2 in PC3 cells can alleviate the effects induced by miR-let-7f-1 [104]. In a recent study published by Tan et al. [105], mice fed semi-purified diets containing 10% tomato powder or 0.25% LYC beadlets up to 18 weeks had higher serum concentrations of total, 5-cis, other cis and all-trans as compared with control in β-carotene 9′,10′-oxygenase (BCO2) +/+ mice. The incidence of PC was lower in animals fed with tomato and LYC when compared with control group. The ability of LYC and tomato to inhibit prostate carcinogenesis was significantly attenuated by loss of BCO2 (P-interaction = 0.0004 and 0.0383, respectively), although the BCO2 genotype did not significantly alter the PC outcome in mice fed with the control AIN-93G diet alone. In another study, the treatment with LYC or metabolite with apo-10-lycopenal increased the BCO2 expression and decreased cell proliferation in androgen-sensitive cell lines, but did not alter BCO2 expression or cell growth in LYC androgen-resistant cells. In particular, restoration of BCO2 expression in PC cells prevented cell proliferation and colony formation independent of LYC exposure [106]. Yang et al. [107] reported that a low or high dose of LYC (4 and 16 mg/kg) and a single β-carotene (16 mg/kg) twice weekly for 7 weeks strongly inhibited the tumor growth, as evidenced by the decrease in tumor volume and tumor weight in thimeric nude mice implanted subcutaneously with human androgen-independent prostate carcinoma PC-3 cells. At high dose level, LYC and β-carotene significantly reduced the expression of PCNA (proliferating cellular nuclear antigen) in tumor tissues and increased insulin-like growth factor-binding protein-3 levels in the plasma. In addition, LYC supplementation at high dose level significantly reduced vascular endothelial growth factor (VEGF) in the plasma. Tang et al. [94] also showed that supplemental LYC inhibited the growth of DU145, a human prostate tumor cell line, transplanted into BALB/c nude mice.

Several studies supporting the relationship between consumption of tomato products and a reduced incidence of PC have come from the Health Professionals Follow-Up Study. In a randomized two-arm clinical trial, patients who have diagnosed PC and scheduled to undergo radical prostatectomy were randomly assigned to either 30 mg of oral LYC supplementation or no intervention for 3 weeks prior to surgery. The study reported that the plasma prostate-specific antigen (PSA) level decreased by 18% in the intervention group, while it increased by 14% in the control group over the study period. In the intwervention group, 11 of 15 patients (73%) had no involvement of surgical margins and/or extraprostatic tissues with cancer, compared to 2 of 11 patients (18%) in the control group. Twelve of 15 patients (80%) in the LYC group had tumors that measured 4 cc or less, compared to 5 of 11 (45%) in the control group [108]. In the same study, Kucuk et al. noted that the expression of Cx43 in the malignant part of the prostate glands was higher in LYC group than the control group. Prostatic tissue LYC levels were 47% higher in the intervention group compared to control group [108]. Phase II randomized clinical trial of 15 mg of LYC supplementation twice a day for 3 days before radical prostatectomy showed a decrease in plasma IGF-I levels, but no significant change in Bax and Bcl-2 [109]. Recently, Paur et al. [110] showed that post hoc, exploratory analyses within intermediate risk patients based on tumor classification and grade and Gleason post-surgery revealed that median PSA decreased in the tomato group as compared to controls (−2.9 and +6.5%). Separate post hoc analyses showed that the median PSA values reduced by 1% in patients with the highest increase in plasma LYC, selenium and C20:5 n-3 fatty acid, compared with the 8.5% increase in patients with the lowest increase in LYC, selenium, and C20:5 n-3 fatty acid. In addition, PSA decreased in patients with the highest increase in LYC (= 0.009). In addition, it was showed that neither pre-diagnosis nor post-diagnosis dietary LYC intake was associated with PC-specific mortality (PCSM) (fourth and first quartile HR = 1.00, 95% GA 0.78–1.28, HR = 1.22, 95% GA 0.91–1.64, respectively). Also, neither pre-diagnosis nor post-diagnosis consumption of tomato products was associated with PCSM. Among subjects with high-risk cancers (T3-T4 or Gleason score 8–10 or nodal involvement) consistently reporting LYC intake ≥median on both postdiagnosis surveys was associated with lower PCSM (HR = 0.41, 95% GA 0.17–0.99, based on ten PCSM cases consistently ≥median intake compared to consistently reporting intake <median [111].

4.2. Breast cancer

In vitro and in vivo studies suggest that intake of LYC-containing foods may reduce breast cancer risk. Assar et al. [112] have recently reported that LYC inhibits prostate as well as breast cancer cell growth at physiologically relevant concentrations ≥1.25 µM. Similar concentrations also caused a 30–40% reduction in IκB phosphorylation (which regulates the activity of NF-κB [113] as determined by Western blot analysis. However, immunofluorescence staining of LYC-treated cells showed a significant suppression of NF-κB p65 subunit nuclear translocation (≥25%) caused by TNF. In another in vitro study reported by Gloria et al. [114], a significant decrease in the number of viable breast cancer cells treated with LYC and beta-carotene carotenoids were observed. Carotenoids promoted cell cycle arrest and then decreased cell viability in the majority of cell lines after 96 h from the controls. In addition, when cells were treated with carotenoids, an increase in apoptosis was observed in cell lines. Cui et al. [115] reported that LYC intake was inversely associated with estrogen and progesterone receptor positive breast cancer risk in postmenopausal women ($n = 84,805$), averaging 7.6 years (RR = 0.85 for high quartile of intake as compared with the lowest quartile of intake, P-trend = 0.064). In an animal study, the incidence of breast cancer was found to be inhibited by LYC (70%), genistein (60%) and their combination (40%). Tumor weight was reduced by 48, 61 and 67% with LYC, genistein and LYC + genistein, respectively, and the mean tumor volume decreased by 18, 35, and 65%, respectively. Administration of the combination of LYC and genistein suppressed breast cancer development and was associated with a decrease in malondialdehyde (MDA), 8-isoprostane and 8-OHDG levels, and increase in serum LYC and genistein. Animals treated with DMBA developed breast cancer associated with increased expression of Bcl-2 in breast tissues and decreased expression of Bax, caspase-3, and caspase-9. The combination of genistein and LYC was more effective than either agent alone to inhibit DMBA-induced breast tumors and to modulate the expression of apoptosis-associated proteins [116]. Recently, in a randomized, placebo-controlled, double-blind, cross-over study, Voskuil et al. [117] found that tomato extract supplementation (30 mg/day LYC) for 2 months reduced free insulin-like growth factor-I (IGF-I) in premenopausal women with a high risk of breast cancer ($n = 36$) I) by 7.0%. Al-Malki et al. [118] demonstrated that combined treatment of LYC and tocopherol (LYC-Toco) caused a reduction in MDA and nitric oxide (NO) in serum and breast tissues in LYC-Toco group than the LYC alone group. Superoxide dismutase, catalase, and glutathione peroxidase activities were significantly higher when compared to rats treated with LYC alone. Serum alanine transaminase, aspartate aminotransferase, total bilirubin and malondialdehyde, which increased in the group of rats treated with diethylnitrosamine (DEN), and hepatic antioxidant enzymes (catalase, superoxide dismutase, and glutathione peroxidase) and glutathione, which decreased in the cancerous group, improved in LYC-treated animals [119]. LYC also caused a reversal and reduced NF-κB and cyclooxygenase-2, consequently increasing Nrf2/HO-1 expression and inhibition of inflammatory cascade, thereby activating the antioxidant signaling. LYC also reduced increases in phosphorylated mammalian targets for phosphorylated rapamycin (p-mTOR), phosphorylated p70 ribosomal protein S6 kinase 1, phosphorylated 4E-binding protein 1, and protein kinase B.

4.3. Gastric and colorectal cancer

Studies have also reported a positive correlation between LYC or tomato product consumption and gastric and colorectal cancers [120, 121]. Although there has been a series of epidemiological studies investigating the relationship between LYC or LYC-rich food and serum/plasma LYC concentration and colorectal cancer risk, the results of these studies have not been consistent [79, 122]. Teodoro et al. [123] have demonstrated a significant reduction in the number of viable cells in human colon adenocarcinoma cells (HT-29), human colon carcinoma cells (T-84), and breast cancer cell line (MCF-7) after 48 h of treatment with LYC. LYC stimulated cell cycle arrest followed by reduced cell viability in the majority of cell lines after 96 h as compared to controls. In addition, when cells were treated with LYC, an increase in apoptosis was observed in four cell lines (T-84, HT-29, MCF-7, and DU145). LYC has also been reported to inhibit cell proliferation in human colon cancer HT-29 cells with IC50 value of 10 μM. LYC treatment also suppressed Akt activation and non-phosphorylated β-catenin protein levels in human colon cancer cells. In addition, LYC significantly increased the nuclear cyclin-dependent kinase inhibitor p27(kip) abundance and inhibited the phosphorylation of retinoblastoma tumor suppressor protein in human colon cancer cells [124]. In another study, it was shown that inhibition of cell growth by tomato digestate was dose dependent and resulted from cell cycle arrest at G0/G1 and G2/M phase and progression by apoptosis induction. Down-regulation of Cyclin D1, Bcl-2, and Bcl-x1 expression has also been observed [125]. In a study conducted by our research group [126], we showed that 5% of the tomato powder added to the diet reduced the aberrant crypt foci (ACF) ratio and also reduced adenocarcinoma development and azoxymethane (AOM)-induced colorectal cancer formation in rats. In addition, the addition of tomato powder indicated that it exhibits chemopreventive activity by regulating Nrf2/HO-1 signaling pathway in colorectal tissue while inhibiting cyclooxygenase-2 (COX-2) expression and inducing apoptosis via the NF-κB pathway. Dias et al. [127] reported that treatment with LYC, synbiotics or a combination thereof significantly increased apoptosis, decreased PCNA and p53 labeling indices, and classical ACF and mucin-negative ACF development. In addition, a lower genotoxicity of fecal water was also detected in groups treated with the chemopreventive agents. The additive/synergistic effect of combined treatment with LYC/synbiotics was observed only for the fecal water genotoxicity and mucin-negative ACF parameters. In a study in a mouse xenograft model, Tang et al. [128] reported that LYC suppressed the nuclear expression of PCNA and β-catenin proteins in tumor tissues. LYC consumption may also increase the nuclear levels of the E-cadherin adherent molecule and the cell cycle inhibitor p21 (CIP1/WAF1) protein. The inhibitory effects of LYC were associated with the suppression of COX-2, PGE (2) and phosphorylated ERK1/2 proteins. In addition, the inhibitory effects of LYC were inversely correlated with plasma levels of matrix metalloproteinase 9 (MMP-9) in tumor-bearing mice.

In a randomized, placebo-controlled, double-blind crossover study, the tomato-based LYC supplementation (Lyc-o-Mato®, 30 mg/day LYC) for 8 weeks has been reported to increase serum insulin-like growth factor binding protein-1 (IGFBP-1) concentration in men and women with high risk for colorectal cancer [129]. The group also reported that the serum IGFPB-2 concentration in men and women increased by 8.2 and 7.8%, respectively. In a double-blind, randomized, placebo-controlled trial, Walfisch et al. [130], a reduction of 25% in plasma IGF-I concentration was reported in 30 patients waiting for colectomy surgery, supplemented with Lyc-o-Mato®. In the same study, a 24% reduction in IGF-I/IGFBP-3 ratio was also observed. In another study, 20 healthy individuals participated in a double-blind crossover dietary intervention and consumed a tomato juice drink (250 ml Lyc-o-Mato® beverage, 5.7 mg LYC, 3.7 mg phytoene, 2.7 mg phytoplankton, 1.8 mg α-tocopherol) and a 26-day wash between each placebo drink [131] for 26 days each. The blood plasma levels of IGF-I were found to be inversely correlated with the consumption of LYC. In yet another study, 20 healthy subjects participated in a double-blind crossover dietary intervention and consumed a tomato juice beverage (250 ml of Lyc-o-Mato® drink) and a 26-day wash between each placebo drink, the plasma IGF-I levels were inversely correlated with the intake of LYC [131].

LYC has also been reported to inhibit *Helicobacter pylori*-induced increases in ROS, 8-OH-dG, and apoptosis by increasing Bax and decreasing Bcl-2 expression as well as PARP-1 cleavage, changes in cell cycle distribution, double-stranded DNA breaks, activation of ataxia-telangiectasia-mutated (ATM) and ATM and Rad3-related (ATR)-mediated DNA damage response in gastric epithelial AGS cells [132]. The administration of LYC (50, 100 and 150 mg/kg body weight) in gastric carcinoma-induced rats up-regulated the redox status and immune activities and was useful in reducing the gastric cancer risk [133].

4.4. Liver cancer

The frequent consumption of tomatoes and tomato-based products has been suggested to lower the risk of other cancers, such as the liver, renal and ovarian cancers. LYC can block the growth on human Hep3B hepatoma cells in a dose-dependent manner and at the same time has been shown to inhibit metastasis in SK-Hep 1 human hepatoma cell line [134, 135]. In a study conducted by our research group, we reported a decrease in serum alanine transaminase, aspartate aminotransferase, total bilirubin and malondialdehyde by LYC in the diethylnitrosamine (DEN)-treated animals. LYC increased the hepatic antioxidant enzymes (catalase, superoxide dismutase, and glutathione peroxidase) and glutathione and reduced the NF-κB/cyclooxygenase-2. The Nrf2/HO-1 expression increased, and the inflammatory cascade inhibited by LYC, suggesting an activation of the antioxidant signaling by LYC. In this study, LYC reduced the increases in phosphorylated mammalian targets of phosphorylated rapamycin (p-mTOR), phosphorylated p70 ribosomal protein S6 kinase 1, phosphorylated 4E binding protein 1, and protein kinase B [119]. In another study on DEN-induced hepatocarcinogenesis in rats, LYC was reported to be effective against preneoplastic foci in the liver by decreasing the size of the liver; whereas LYC administration in another animal study did not reduce the risk of spontaneous liver cancer [136, 137]. The LYC-added tomato paste has been reported to be protective against oxidative stress induced by N-nitrosodiethylamine (NDEA) in rats. It decreases the microsomal lipid peroxidation in the liver and significantly reduced plasma protein carbonyl levels [138]. LYC supplementation also prevents liver-specific carcinogenic DEN-induced of hepatic preneoplastic foci and macroscopic nodules in rat hepatic glutathione S-transferase placental-form positive foci in rats that developed spontaneous liver tumors and ameliorated DEN-initiated, HFD (high-fat diet)-promoted precancerous lesions [139, 140]. It was effective in decreasing NASH-promoted, DEN-initiated hepatocarcinogenesis in rats [136]. Apo-10'-lycopenoic acid, a LYC metabolite produced by β-carotene-9',10'-oxygenase (BCO2) inhibited hepatic inflammation and liver inflammation induced by carcinogen-initiated high-fat diets [98, 141] showed that LYC supplementation (100 mg/kg diet) for 24 weeks decreased hepatic proinflammatory signal (phosphorylation of NK-κB p65 and STAT3, IL6 protein) and inflammatory foci in wild-type mice. In contrast, the protective effects of LYC in BCO2-KO were related to reduce hepatic endoplasmic reticulum stress-mediated unfolded protein response, the ER(UPR), through decreasing ER(UPR)-mediated protein kinase RNA-activated like kinase-eukaryotic initiation factor 2α activation, and inositol-requiring 1α-X-box-binding protein 1 signaling. LYC treatment in BCO2-KO mice inhibited carcinogenic signals, including Met mRNA, β-catenin protein and mTOR complex 1 activation associated with increased liver microRNA (miR)-199a/b and miR214 levels [141]. The connection between LYC and aflatoxin B1 (AFB1) initiated HCC has also been examined [142], and in recent studies [143], the hepatocarcinogenesis pathway has been linked to the activation of the oxidative stress-inflammatory pathway in rat liver.

4.5. Renal cancer

Previous research has shown that micronutrients consumed through diet or dietary supplementation, including vitamin E and carotenoids, can inhibit oxidative DNA damage, mutagenesis and tumor growth [144, 145]. However, many studies have shown that there is no significant association between RCC and antioxidant micronutrient intake [146], while others suggest supportive evidence that some micronutrients may have a protective effect [147]. Increased uptake of LYC in postmenopausal women in the Women's Health Initiative (WHI) was inversely associated with RCC risk ($p = 0.015$); compared with the lowest quartile of LYC intake, the highest quartile of intake was associated with a 39% lower risk for RCC (hazard ratio, 0.61, 95% confidence interval, 0.39–0.97) when compared with the lowest quartile of LYC intake [145]. It was also reported that no other micronutrient was significantly associated with RCC risk [145]. Another case-control study reported that the intake of vegetables was associated with a reduction in the risk of RCC (OR 0.5; 95% CI 0.3, 0.7; P trend = 0.002) [148]). In the same study, it was reported that both β-cryptoxanthin and LYC were associated with reduced risks, but when both were included in a mutually adjusted backward stepwise regression model, only β-cryptoxanthin remained significant (OR 0.5; 95% CI 0.3, 0.8). When other micronutrients and fiber types were investigated together, only vegetable fiber and β-cryptoxanthin showed significant trends. They also reported that these findings are stronger for people over 65 years of age. Additionally, among nonsmokers, low intake of cruciferous vegetables and fruit fiber was also associated with increased risk of RCC (P interaction = 0.03); similar reverse relationships were found for β-cryptoxanthin, LYC and vitamin C [148]. LYC has also been found to decrease the tumor presence and the average number of renal carcinomas in a small animal model (rat) for studying renal cell carcinoma (RCC) [149]. In the LYC group, the tumor counts decreased and as the LYC supplement increased from 0 to 200, the numbers tended to decrease linearly. Control rats fed only on a basal diet had a greater length of tumors (23.98 mm) than those fed to LYC supplementation groups (12.90 and 2.90 mm) (11.07 mm). In addition, when LYC increased from 0 to 200 mg/kg, tumor length decreased. It tended to decrease linearly. All tumors showed strong staining with antibodies to mTOR, phospho-S6, and EGFR.

4.6. Bladder cancer

LYC supplementation has been reported to exhibit a non-significant trend after administration of N-butyl-N-(4-hydroxybutyl) nitrosamine to reduce the number of bladder transitional cell carcinomas in rats [150]. In a case-control study involving 569 bladder cancer cases and 3123 controls, the relative risk for bladder cancer was 1.08, which compared the highest and lowest rates of LYC uptake [151]. However, in a cohort study, serum LYC levels in bladder cancer cases were found to be lower than those of compatible controls [152]. In another case-control study with 84 cases and 173 controls, OR for bladder cancer was 0.94 (95% CI 0.89–0.99) in the highest quartile of plasma LYC intake when compared to lowest after controlling for age, sex, education, and pack-years of smoking [153].

4.7. Lung cancer

Many studies have shown that smokers and lung cancer patients tend to be lower plasma concentrations of b-carotene, retinol, LYC, b-cryptoxanthin and a-tocopherol [154]. Graham et al. [155] have treated LYC solutions with human plasma and isolated LDL with cigarette smoke and observed the depletion of all(E)-chylopen, 5 (Z)-chylonopen and beta-carotene. Depletion of all-(E)-lycopenin (15.0 ± 11.0%, $n = 10$) was greater than 5 (Z)-lycopenin (10.4 ± 9.6%) or beta-carotene (12.4 ± 10.5%) in plasma. LDL was found to be more sensitive to both all(E)- and 5 (Z)-clycopenia than beta-carotene (20.8 ± 11.8, 15.4 ± 11.5 and 11.5 ± 12.5%, $n = 3$). It was also reported that smoke exposure reduced the concentrations of LYC in plasma and lung tissue of LYC supplemented ferrets, which was consistent with the National Health and Nutrition Examination survey III finding that smokers had lower serum levels of LYC compared to nonsmokers [156]. In one study, the concentration of LYC in lungs was 1.2 μmol/kg lung tissue in ferrets fortified with LYC at a dose of 60 mg/day, and this did not cause a harmful effect, instead it prevented the induction of lung squamous metaplasia and cell proliferation induced by smoke exposure [157]. On the other hand, intake of tomato or tomato products including LYC has been associated with a lower risk of lung cancer [158]. In cell culture, LYC has been shown to inhibit the nitration of proteins and DNA strand breakage caused by peroxynitrite treatment of hamster lung fibroblasts [159]. Apo-100-lycopenoic acid has been reported to inhibit the growth of the normal human bronchial epithelial cells, BEAS-2B immortalized normal bronchial epithelial cells, and A549 non-small cell lung cancer cells [158]. LYC dissolved in drinking water at a dose of 50 ppm significantly reduced diethylnitrosamine (DEH), methylnitrosourea (MNU), and dimethylhydrazine (DMD)-induced lung adenomas along with carcinomas in male mice [160]. The inhibitory effect of apo-100-lycopenoic acid was associated with decreased cyclin E, inhibition of cell cycle progression and an increase in cell cycle regulator p21 and p27 protein levels. In addition, apo-100-lycopenoic acid trans-activated the retinoic acid receptor β (RARβ) promoter and initiated the expression of RARβ. In another animal study, the incidence of lung adenomas and carcinomas in male mice receiving 50 ppm LYC in addition to diethylnitrosamine (DEN), N-methyl-N-(MNU) and 1,2-dimethylhydrazine (DMH) was lower than the incidence seen in non-LYC recipients (18.8 versus 75.0%) [161].

5. Concluding remarks

Some plant and plant-based products and their active ingredients exhibit significant anti-tumor properties. They may act by blocking the cell cycle checkpoints (paclitaxel) and specific enzymes, such as the S-phase specific topoisomerase-I (camptothecins) and S and G2 phase-specific topoisomerase-II (etoposide), and by preventing the microtubule polymerization (vinblastine), as well as by various other mechanisms. Diallyl disulfide, limonoids, azadirachtin, pentacyclic triterpenediol, theaflavins, curcumin, lupeol, and AECHL-1 [162–169], for example, modulate the p53-regulated pathways. Bromelain, theaflavin, thearubigin, curcumin, E-piplartine (trans-piplartine), 3β-hydroxylup-20(29)-ene-27,28-dioic acid, withanolide D, withaferin A [70, 170–176] affect MAPK-regulated pathways. The other pathways include death receptors (example, theaflavins [177] and ROS-mediated pathways (isointermedeol, mahanine, chlorogenic acid, withaferin A [50, 51, 178]. The β-sitosterol, which has a significant anticancer activity against colon cancer, acts by scavenging ROS and suppressing the expression of PCNA [62]. Sesquiterpene isointermedeol (ISO), which is a major constituent of *Cymbopogon flexuosus* (lemon grass) and inhibitor of proliferation of human leukaemia HL-60 cells, also induces ROS production with the concomitant loss of mitochondrial membrane potential, DNA laddering, and apoptotic body formation.

LYC, which is a highly unsaturated, straight-chain hydrocarbon, is reported to be beneficial in cancers, especially the prostate cancer. It can reduce oxidative stress by modulating ROS-producing enzymes (CYP-P450 enzymes, NADPH oxidase, iNOS, COX-2, and 5-LOX) and inducing antioxidant/detoxifying phase II enzymes [98]. These phase II enzymes are regulated by the nuclear factor E2-related factor 2-antioxidant response element (Nrf2-ARE) system. The Nrf2/HO-1 signaling is suggested to be an important primary target for chemoprevention (cisplatin-induced nephrotoxicity) by LYC. LYC can also decrease inflammation by inhibiting NF-κB [99]. It can inhibit the proliferation and induction of differentiation of cancer cells by modulating the expression of cell cycle regulatory proteins, modulating the IGF-1/IGFBP-3 system and other mechanisms including the prevention of oxidative DNA damage and modulation of the immune function, as well as the inactivation of growth factor (PDGF, VEGF, and IGF) induced PI3K/AKT/PKB and Ras/RAF/MAPK signaling pathways [100].

6. Future perspective

Overall, the research articles reviewed in this chapter provide convincing evidence suggesting a role for LYC in cancer, particularly in prostate cancer. LYC may act by a variety of mechanisms, some of which could be linked to the antioxidant activity of this non-pro-vitamin-A carotenoid. Lycopene supplementation could be a potential candidate for future clinical trials in prostate cancer and other cancers both as a preventive and therapeutic agent and in combination with other therapies. This phytochemical offers great promise in integrative oncology and warrants further clinical evaluation with careful attention to individualized dose escalation until an effective and safe dose is found.

Acknowledgements

This work was supported by the Turkish Academy of Sciences (KS).

Author details

Kazim Sahin[1]*, Shakir Ali[2], Nurhan Sahin[1], Cemal Orhan[1] and Omer Kucuk[3]

*Address all correspondence to: nsahinkm@yahoo.com

1 Veterinary Faculty, Firat University, Elazig, Turkey

2 Department of Biochemistry, School of Chemical and Life Sciences, Jamia Hamdard, New Delhi, India

3 Winship Cancer Institute, Emory University, Atlanta, Georgia, USA

References

[1] Newman DJ. Natural products as leads to potential drugs: an old process or the new hope for drug discovery?. Journal of Medicinal Chemistry. 2008;**51**:2589-2599. DOI: 10.1021/jm0704090

[2] Mondal S, Bandyopadhyay S, Ghosh MK, Mukhopadhyay S, Roy S, Mandal C. Natural products: promising resources for cancer drug discovery. Anti-Cancer Agents in Medicinal Chemistry. 2012;**12**:49-75. DOI: 10.2174/187152012798764697

[3] Singh BN, Singh BR, Sarma BK, Singh HB. Potential chemoprevention of N-nitroso-diethylamine-induced hepatocarcinogenesis by polyphenolics from *Acacia nilotica* bark. Chemico-Biological Interactions. 2009;**181**:20-28. DOI: 10.1016/j.cbi.2009.05.007

[4] Meena PD, Kaushik P, Shukla S, Soni AK, Kumar M, Kumar A. Anticancer and antimu-tagenic properties of *Acacia nilotica* (Linn.) on 7,12-dimethylbenz(a)anthracene-induced skin papillomagenesis in Swiss albino mice. Asian Pacific Journal of Cancer Prevention. 2006;**7**:627-632

[5] Jagetia GC, Venkatesh P, Baliga MS. *Aegle marmelos* (L.) Correa inhibits the prolifera-tion of transplanted Ehrlich ascites carcinoma in mice. Biological and Pharmaceutical Bulletin. 2005;**28**:58-64

[6] Saini M, Goyal PK, Chaudhary G. Anti-tumor activity of *Aloe vera* against DMBA/cro-ton oil-induced skin papillomagenesis in Swiss albino mice. Journal of Environmental Pathology, Toxicology and Oncology. 2010;**29**:127-135

[7] Jahan S, Goyal PK. Protective effect of *Alstonia scholaris* against radiation-induced clastogenic and biochemical alterations in mice. Journal of Environmental Pathology, Toxicology and Oncology. 2010;**29**:101-111

[8] Jahan S, Chaudhary R, Goyal PK. Anticancer activity of an Indian medicinal plant, *Alstonia scholaris*, on skin carcinogenesis in mice. Integrative Cancer Therapies. 2009;**8**:273-279. DOI: 10.1177/1534735409343590

[9]   Gupta U, Jahan S, Chaudhary R, Goyal PK. Amelioration of radiation-induced hematological and biochemical alterations by *Alstonia scholaris* (a medicinal plant) extract. Integrative Cancer Therapies. 2008;7:155-161. DOI: 10.1177/1534735408322850

[10] Vinothini G, Manikandan P, Anandan R, Nagini S. Chemoprevention of rat mammary carcinogenesis by *Azadirachta indica* leaf fractions: modulation of hormone status, xenobiotic-metabolizing enzymes, oxidative stress, cell proliferation and apoptosis. Food and Chemical Toxicology. 2009;47:1852-1863. DOI: 10.1016/j.fct.2009.04.045

[11] Kumar S, Suresh PK, Vijayababu MR, Arunkumar A, Arunakaran J. Anticancer effects of ethanolic neem leaf extract on prostate cancer cell line (PC-3). Journal of Ethnopharmacology. 2006;105:246-250. DOI: 10.1016/j.jep.2005.11.006

[12] Guruvayoorappan C, Kuttan G. Immunomodulatory and antitumor activity of *Biophytum sensitivum* extract. Asian Pacific Journal of Cancer Prevention. 2007;8(1):27-32

[13] Bhushan S, Kumar A, Malik F, Andotra SS, Sethi VK, Kaur IP, Taneja SC, Qazi GN, Singh J. A triterpenediol from *Boswellia serrata* induces apoptosis through both the intrinsic and extrinsic apoptotic pathways in human leukemia HL-60 cells. Apoptosis. 2007;12(10):1911-1926. DOI: 10.1007/s10495-007-0105-5

[14] Choedon T, Shukla SK, Kumar V. Chemopreventive and anticancer properties of the aqueous extract of flowers of *Butea monosperma*. Journal of Ethnopharmacology. 2010;129(2):208-213. DOI: 10.1016/j.jep.2010.03.011

[15] Prasanna R, Harish CC, Pichai R, Sakthisekaran D, Gunasekaran P. Anti-cancer effect of *Cassia auriculata* leaf extract in vitro through cell cycle arrest and induction of apoptosis in human breast and larynx cancer cell lines. Cell Biology International. 2009;33(2):127-134. DOI: 10.1016/j.cellbi.2008.10.006

[16] Bhagat M, Saxena AK. Evaluation of *Cassia occidentalis* for in vitro cytotoxicity against human cancer cell lines and antibacterial activity. Indian Journal of Pharmacology. 2010;42(4):234-237. DOI: 10.4103/0253-7613.68428

[17] Rejiya CS, Cibin TR, Abraham A. Leaves of *Cassia tora* as a novel cancer therapeutic—an in vitro study. Toxicology in Vitro. 2009;23(6):1034-1038. DOI: 10.1016/j.tiv.2009.06.010

[18] Saxena A, Saxena AK, Singh J, Bhushan S. Natural antioxidants synergistically enhance the anticancer potential of AP9-cd, a novel lignan composition from *Cedrus deodara* in human leukemia HL-60 cells. Chemico-Biological Interactions. 2010;188(3):580-590. DOI: 10.1016/j.cbi.2010.09.029

[19] Radhika NK, Sreejith PS, Asha VV. Cytotoxic and apoptotic activity of *Cheilanthes farinosa* (Forsk.) Kaulf. against human hepatoma, Hep3B cells. Journal of Ethnopharmacology. 2010;128(1):166-171. DOI: 10.1016/j.jep.2010.01.002

[20] Koppikar SJ, Choudhari AS, Suryavanshi SA, Kumari S, Chattopadhyay S, Kaul GR. Aqueous cinnamon extract (ACE-c) from the bark of *Cinnamomum cassia* causes apoptosis in human cervical cancer cell line (SiHa) through loss of mitochondrial membrane potential. BMC Cancer. 2010;10:210. DOI: 10.1186/1471-2407-10-210

[21] Kumar S, Chattopadhyay SK, Darokar MP, Garg A, Khanuja SP. Cytotoxic activities of xanthochymol and isoxanthochymol substantiated by LC-MS/MS. Planta Medica. 2007;**73**(14):1452-1456. DOI: 10.1055/s-2007-990255

[22] Pal HC, Sehar I, Bhushan S, Gupta BD, Saxena AK. Activation of caspases and poly (ADP-ribose) polymerase cleavage to induce apoptosis in leukemia HL-60 cells by *Inula racemosa*. Toxicology in Vitro. 2010;**24**(6):1599-1609. DOI: 10.1016/j.tiv.2010.06.007

[23] Wills PJ, Asha VV. Chemopreventive action of *Lygodium flexuosum* extract in human hepatoma PLC/PRF/5 and Hep 3B cells. Journal of Ethnopharmacology. 2009;**122**(2):294-303. DOI: 10.1016/j.jep.2009.01.006

[24] Sharma M, Agrawal SK, Sharma PR, Chadha BS, Khosla MK, Saxena AK. Cytotoxic and apoptotic activity of essential oil from Ocimumviride towards COLO 205 cells. Food and Chemical Toxicology. 2010;**48**(1):336-344. DOI: 10.1016/j.fct.2009.10.021

[25] Rao AS, Reddy SG, Babu PP, Reddy AR. The antioxidant and antiproliferative activities of methanolic extracts from Njavara rice bran. BMC Complementary and Alternative Medicine. 2010;**10**:4. DOI: 10.1186/1472-6882-10-4

[26] Sharma P, Parmar J, Verma P, Sharma P, Goyal PK. Antitumor activity of *Phyllanthus niruri* (a medicinal plant) on chemicalinduced skin carcinogenesis in mice. Asian Pacific Journal of Cancer Prevention. 2009;**10**(6):1089-1094

[27] Nalini N, Manju V, Menon VP. Effect of spices on lipid metabolism in 1,2-dimethylhydrazine-induced rat colon carcinogenesis. Journal of Medicinal Food. 2006;**9**(2):237-245. DOI: 10.1089/jmf.2006.9.237

[28] Manjula SN, Kenganora M, Parihar VK, Kumar S, Nayak PG, Kumar N. Ranganath Pai KS, Rao CM. Antitumor and antioxidant activity of *Polyalthia longifolia* stem bark ethanol extract. Pharmaceutical Biology. 2010;**48**(6):690-696. DOI: 10.3109/13880200903257974

[29] Mishra KP, Padwad YS, Dutta A, Ganju L, Sairam M, Banerjee PK, Sawhney RC. Aqueous extract of Rhodiola imbricata rhizome inhibits proliferation of an erythroleukemic cell line K-562 by inducing apoptosis and cell cycle arrest at G2/M phase. Immunobiology. 2008;**213**(2):125-131. DOI: 10.1016/j.imbio.2007.07.003

[30] Sugapriya D, Shanthi P, Sachdanandam P. Restoration of energy metabolism in leukemic mice treated by a siddha drug *Semecarpus anacardium* Linn. nut milk extract. Chemico-Biological Interactions. 2008;**173**(1):43-58. DOI: 10.1016/j.cbi.2008.01.013

[31] Mathivadhani P, Shanthi P, Sachdanandam P. Apoptotic effect of *Semecarpus anacardium* nut extract on T47D breast cancer cell line. Cell Biology InternationalCell Biology International. 2007;**31**(10):1198-1206

[32] Laladhas KP, Cheriyan VT, Puliappadamba VT, Bava SV, Unnithan RG, Vijayammal PL, Anto RJ. A novel protein fraction from *Sesbania grandiflora* shows potential anticancer and chemopreventive efficacy, in vitro and in vivo. Journal of Cellular and Molecular Medicine. 2010;**14**(3):636-646 . DOI: 10.1111/j.1582-4934.2008.00648.x

[33] Sivalokanathan S, Ilayaraja M, Balasubramanian MP. Antioxidant activity of *Terminalia arjuna* bark extract on Nnitrosodiethylamine induced hepatocellular carcinoma in rats. Molecular and Cellular Biochemistry. 2006;**281**(1-2):87-93

[34] Chaudhary R, Jahan S, Goyal PK. Chemopreventive potential of an Indian medicinal plant (*Tinospora cordifolia*) on skin carcinogenesis in mice. Journal of Environmental Pathology, Toxicology and Oncology. 2008;**27**(3):233-243

[35] Singh B, Kale RK. Chemomodulatory effect of *Trachyspermum ammi* on murine skin and forestomach papillomagenesis. Nutrition and Cancer. 2010;**62**(1):74-84 . DOI: 10.1080/01635580903191478

[36] Muralikrishnan G, Amanullah S, Basha MI, Dinda AK, Shakeel F. Modulating effect of *Withania somnifera* on TCA cycle enzymes and electron transport chain in azoxymethane-induced colon cancer in mice. Immunopharmacology and Immunotoxicology. 2010;**32**(3):523-527. DOI: 10.3109/08923970903581540

[37] Mathur R, Gupta SK, Singh N, Mathur S, Kochupillai V, Velpandian T. Evaluation of the effect of *Withania somnifera* root extracts on cell cycle and angiogenesis. Journal of Ethnopharmacology. 2006;**105**(3):336-341

[38] Vijaya PV, Arul DCS, Ramkuma KM. Induction of apoptosis by ginger in HEp-2 cell line is mediated by reactive oxygen species. Basic & Clinical Pharmacology & Toxicology. 2007;**100**(5):302-307

[39] Horwitz SB. Taxol (paclitaxel): mechanisms of action. Annals of Oncology. 1994;**5**(Suppl 6):S3-6

[40] Chin YW, Balunas MJ, Chai HB, Kinghorn AD. Drug discovery from natural sources. The AAPS Journal. 2006;**8**(2):E239-253

[41] Serafim TL, Oliveira PJ, Sardao VA, Perkins E, Parke D, Holy J. Different concentrations of berberine result in distinct cellular localization patterns and cell cycle effects in a melanoma cell line. Cancer Chemotherapy and Pharmacology. 2008;**61**(6):1007-1018

[42] Pinto-Garcia L, Efferth T, Torres A, Hoheisel JD, Youns M. Berberine inhibits cell growth and mediates caspase-independent cell death in human pancreatic cancer cells. Planta Medica. 2010;**76**(11):1155-1161. DOI: 10.1055/s-0030-1249931

[43] Auyeung KK, Ko JK. *Coptis chinensis* inhibits hepatocellular carcinoma cell growth through nonsteroidal anti-inflammatory drug-activated gene activation. International Journal of Molecular Medicine. 2009;**24**(4):571-577

[44] Sun Y, Xun K, Wang Y, Chen X. A systematic review of the anticancer properties of berberine, a natural product from Chinese herbs. Anticancer Drugs. 2009;**20**(9):757-769. DOI: 10.1097/CAD.0b013e328330d95b

[45] Sindhu G, Manoharan S. Anti-clastogenic effect of berberine against DMBA-induced clastogenesis. Basic & Clinical Pharmacology & Toxicology. 2010;**107**(4):818-824. DOI: 10.1111/j.1742-7843.2010.00579.x.

[46] Kim S, Choi JH, Kim JB, Nam SJ, Yang JH, Kim JH, Lee JE. Berberine suppresses TNF-alpha-induced MMP-9 and cell invasion through inhibition of AP-1 activity in MDA-MB-231 human breast cancer cells. Molecules. 2008;**13**(12):2975-2985. DOI: 10.3390/molecules13122975

[47] Choi MS, Oh JH, Kim SM, Jung HY, Yoo HS, Lee YM, Moon DC, Han SB, Hong JT. Berberine inhibits p53-dependent cell growth through induction of apoptosis of prostate cancer cells. International Journal of Oncology. 2009;**34**(5):1221-1230

[48] Lin CC, Lin SY, Chung JG, Lin JP, Chen GW, Kao ST. Down-regulation of cyclin B1 and up-regulation of Wee1 by berberine promotes entry of leukemia cells into the G2/M-phase of the cell cycle. Anticancer Research. 2006;**26**(2A):1097-1104

[49] Tang J, Feng Y, Tsao S, Wang N, Curtain R, Wang Y. Berberine and *Coptidis rhizoma* as novel antineoplastic agents: a review of traditional use and biomedical investigations. Journal of Ethnopharmacology. 2009;**126**(1):5-17. DOI: 10.1016/j.jep.2009.08.009

[50] Rakshit S, Mandal L, Pal BC, Bagchi J, Biswas N, Chaudhuri J, Chowdhury AA, Manna A, Chaudhuri U, Konar A, Mukherjee T, Jaisankar P, Bandyopadhyay S. Involvement of ROS in chlorogenic acid-induced apoptosis of Bcr-Abl+ CML cells. Biochemical Pharmacology. 2010;**80**(11):1662-1675. DOI: 10.1016/j.bcp.2010.08.013

[51] Malik F, Kumar A, Bhushan S, Khan S, Bhatia A, Suri KA, Qazi GN, Singh J. Reactive oxygen species generation and mitochondrial dysfunction in the apoptotic cell death of human myeloid leukemia HL-60 cells by a dietary compound withaferin A with concomitant protection by N-acetyl cysteine. Apoptosis. 2007;**12**(11):2115-2133

[52] Fulda S. and Kroemer G. Targeting mitochondrial apoptosis by betulinic acid in human cancers. Drug Discovery Today. 2009;**14**(17-18):885-890. DOI: 10.1016/j.drudis.2009.05.015

[53] Athar M, Back JH, Tang X, Kim KH, Kopelovich L, Bickers DR and Kim AL. Resveratrol: a review of preclinical studies for human cancer prevention. Toxicology and Applied Pharmacology. 2007;**224**(3):274-283.

[54] Reddy KP, Bid HK, Nayak VL, Chaudhary P, Chaturvedi JP, Arya KR, Konwar R, Narender T. In vitro and in vivo anticancer activity of 2-deacetoxytaxinine J and synthesis of novel taxoids and their in vitro anticancer activity. European Journal of Medicinal Chemistry. 2009;**44**(10):3947-3953. DOI: 10.1016/j.ejmech.2009.04.022

[55] Singh M, Pandey A, Karikari CA, Singh G, Rakheja D. Cell cycle inhibition and apoptosis induced by curcumin in Ewing sarcoma cell line SK-NEP-1. Medical Oncology. 2009;**27**(4):1096-1101. DOI: 10.1007/s12032-009-9341-6

[56] Samanta SK, Bhattacharya K, Mandal C, Pal BC. Identification and quantification of the active component quercetin 3-Orutinoside from Barringtonia racemosa, targets mitochondrial apoptotic pathway in acute lymphoblastic leukemia. Journal of Asian Natural Products Research. 2010;**12**(8):639-648. DOI: 10.1080/10286020.2010.489040

[57] Sashidhara KV, Rosaiah JN, Kumar A, Bid HK, Konwar R, Chattopadhyay N. Cell growth inhibitory action of an unusual labdane diterpene, 13-epi-sclareol in breast and uterine cancers in vitro. Phytotherapy Research. 2007;**21**(11):1105-1108

[58] Mallick S, Ghosh P, Samanta SK, Kinra S, Pal BC, Gomes A, Vedasiromoni JR. Corchorusin-D, a saikosaponin-like compound isolated from *Corchorus acutanglus* Lam., targets mitochondrial apoptotic pathways in leukemic cell lines (HL-60 and U937). Cancer Chemotherapy and Pharmacology. 2010;**66**(4):709-719. DOI: 10.1007/s00280-009-1214-3

[59] Chiruvella KK, Kari V, Choudhary B, Nambiar M, Ghanta RG, Raghavan SC. Methyl angolensate, a natural tetranortriterpenoid induces intrinsic apoptotic pathway in leukemic cells. FEBS Letters. 2008;**582**(29):4066-4076. DOI: 10.1016/j.febslet.2008.11.001

[60] Ghosh S, Das Sarma M, Patra A, Hazra B. Anti-inflammatory and anticancer compounds isolated from Ventilago madraspatana Gaertn., *Rubia cordifolia* Linn. and *Lantana camara* Linn. Journal of Pharmacy and Pharmacology. 2010;**62**(9):1158-1166. DOI: 10.1111/j.2042-7158.2010.01151.x

[61] Sashidhara KV, Singh SP, Kant R, Maulik PR, Sarkar J, Kanojiya S, Ravi KK. Cytotoxic cycloartane triterpene and rare isomeric bisclerodane diterpenes from the leaves of *Polyalthia longifolia* var. pendula. Bioorganic & Medicinal Chemistry Letters. 2010;**20**(19):5767-5771. DOI: 10.1016/j.bmcl.2010.07.141

[62] Lajkó E, Bányai P, Zámbó Z, Kursinszki L, Szőke É, Kőhidai L. Targeted tumor therapy by *Rubia tinctorum* L.: analytical characterization of hydroxyanthraquinones and investigation of their selective cytotoxic, adhesion and migration modulator effects on melanoma cell lines (A2058 and HT168-M1). Cancer Cell International. 2015;**18**(15):119. DOI: 10.1186/s12935-015-0271-4

[63] Nair PK, Melnick SJ, Wnuk SF, Rapp M, Escalon E, Ramachandran C. Isolation and characterization of an anticancer catechol compound from *Semecarpus anacardium*. Journal of Ethnopharmacology. 2009;**122**(3):450-456. DOI: 10.1016/j.jep.2009.02.001

[64] Baskar AA, Ignacimuthu S, Paulraj GM, Al Numair KS. Chemopreventive potential of beta-Sitosterol in experimental colon cancer model—an in vitro and in vivo study. BMC Complementary and Alternative Medicine. 2010;**10**:24. DOI: 10.1186/1472-6882-10-24

[65] Chatterjee R, Singh O, Pachuau L, Malik SP, Paul M, Bhadra K, Paul S, Kumar GS, Mondal NB, Banerjee S. Identification of a sulfonoquinovosyldiacylglyceride from *Azadirachta indica* and studies on its cytotoxic activity and DNA binding properties. Bioorganic & Medicinal Chemistry Letters. 2010;**20**(22):6699-6702. DOI: 10.1016/j.bmcl.2010.09.007

[66] Arunkumar A, Vijayababu MR, Kanagaraj P, Balasubramanian K, Aruldhas MM, Arunakaran J. Growth suppressing effect of garlic compound diallyl disulfide on prostate cancer cell line (PC-3) in vitro. Biological and Pharmaceutical Bulletin. 2005;**28**(4):740-743

[67] Joo H, Lee HJ, Shin EA, Kim H, Seo KH, Baek NI, Kim B, Kim SH. c-Jun N-terminal kinase-dependent endoplasmic reticulum stress pathway is critically involved in arjunic acid induced apoptosis in non-small cell lung cancer cells. Phytotherapy Research. 2016;**30**(4):596-603. DOI: 10.1002/ptr.5563

[68] Puliyappadamba VT, Cheriyan VT, Thulasidasan AK, Bava SV, Vinod BS, Prabhu PR, Varghese R, Bevin A, Venugopal S, Anto RJ. Nicotine-induced survival signaling in lung

cancer cells is dependent on their p53 status while its downregulation by curcumin is independent. Molecular Cancer. 2010;**9**:220. DOI: 10.1186/1476-4598-9-220

[69] Ravindran J, Prasad S, Aggarwal BB. Curcumin and cancer cells, how many ways can curry kill tumor cells selectively?. The AAPS Journal. 2009;**11**(3):495-510. DOI: 10.1208/s12248-009-9128-x

[70] Bhui K, Tyagi S, Prakash B, Shukla Y. Pineapple bromelain induces autophagy, facilitating apoptotic response in mammary carcinoma cells. Biofactors. 2010;**36**(6):474-482. DOI: 10.1002/biof.121

[71] Babica P, Čtveráčková L, Lenčešová Z, Trosko JE, Upham BL. Chemopreventive agents attenuate rapid inhibition of gap junctional intercellular communication induced by environmental toxicants. Nutrition and Cancer. 2016;**68**(5):827-837. DOI: 10.1080/01635581.2016.1180409

[72] Velmurugan B, Mani A, Nagini S. Combination of Sallylcysteine and lycopene induces apoptosis by modulating Bcl-2, Bax, Bim and caspases during experimental gastric carcinogenesis. European Journal of Cancer Prevention. 2005;**14**(4):387-393.

[73] Deepak AV, Salimath BP. Antiangiogenic and proapoptotic activity of a novel glycoprotein from *U. indica* is mediated by NFkappaB and Caspase activated DNase in ascites tumor model. Biochimie. 2006;**88**(3-4):297-307

[74] U.S. National Research Council, Committee on Diet and Health. Diet and health: implications for reducing chronic disease risk. Washington (DC): National Academy Press. 1989

[75] American Cancer Society. Nutrition and cancer: causation and prevention. An American Cancer Society special report. CA: A Cancer Journal for Clinicians. 1984;**34**:5-10

[76] Steinmetz KA, Potter JD. Vegetables, fruit, and cancer. I. Epidemiology. Cancer Causes Control. 1991;**2**(5):325-357

[77] Block G, Patterson B, Subar A. Fruit, vegetables, and cancer prevention: a review of the epidemiological evidence. Nutrition and Cancer. 1992;**18**(1):1-29

[78] Glade MJ. Food, nutrition, and the prevention of cancer: a global perspective. American Institute for Cancer Research/World Cancer Research Fund, American Institute for Cancer Research, 1997. Nutrition. 1999;**15**(6):523-526

[79] Giovannucci E. Tomatoes, tomato-based products, lycopene, and cancer: review of the epidemiologic literature. Journal of the National Cancer Institute. 1999;**91**(4):317-331

[80] Eroglu A, Harrison EH. Carotenoid metabolism in mammals, including man: formation, occurrence, and function of apocarotenoids. The Journal of Lipid Research. 2013;**54**(7):1719-1730. DOI: 10.1194/jlr.R039537

[81] Rao AV, Agarwal S. Role of antioxidant lycopene in cancer and heart disease. The Journal of the American College of Nutrition. 2000;**19**(5):563-569

[82] Nguyen ML, Schwartz SJ. Lycopene: chemical and biological properties. Food Technology. 1999;**53**:38-45

[83] Stahl W, Sies H. Uptake of lycopene and its geometrical isomers is greater from heat-processed than from unprocessed tomato juice in humans. Journal of Nutrition. 1992;**122**:2161-2166

[84] Caris-Veyrat C, Schmid A, Carail M, Böhm V. Cleavage products of lycopene produced by in vitro oxidations: characterization and mechanisms of formation. Journal of Agricultural and Food Chemistry. 2003;**51**(25):7318-7325

[85] Ferreira AL, Yeumb KJ, Russell RM, Krinsky NI, Tang G. Enzymatic and oxidative metabolites of lycopene. The Journal of Nutritional Biochemistry. 2004;**14**(9):531-540

[86] Gajic M, Zaripheh S, Sun F, Erdman JW Jr. Apo-80-lycopenal and apo-120-lycopenal are metabolic products of lycopene in rat liver. Journal of Nutrition. 2006;**136**(6):1552-1557

[87] Kopec RE, Riedl KM, Harrison EH, Curley Jr, RW, Hruszkewycz DP, Clinton SK, Schwartz SJ. Identification and quantification of apolycopenals in fruits, vegetables, and human plasma. Journal of Agricultural and Food Chemistry. 2010;**58**(6):3290-3296. DOI: 10.1021/jf100415

[88] Giovannucci E, Rimm EB, Liu Y, Stampfer MJ, Willett WC. A rospective study of tomato products, lycopene, and prostate cancer risk. Journal of the National Cancer Institute. 2002;**94**(5):391-398

[89] Etminan M, Takkouche B, Caamaño-Isorna F. The role of tomato products and lycopene in the prevention of prostate cancer: a meta-analysis of observational studies. Cancer Epidemiology, Biomarkers & Prevention. 2004;**13**(3):340-345

[90] Talvas J, Caris-Veyrat C, Guy L, Rambeau M, Lyan B, Minet-Quinard R, Lobaccaro JM, Vasson MP, Georgé S, Mazur A, Rock E. Differential effects of lycopene consumed in tomato paste and lycopene in the form of a purified extract on target genes of cancer prostatic cells. The American Journal of Clinical Nutrition. 2010;**91**(6):1716-1724. DOI: 10.3945/ajcn.2009.28666

[91] Nahum A, Hirsch K, Danilenko M, Watts CK, Prall OW, Levy Y, Sharoni Y. Lycopene inhibition of cell cycle progression in breast and endometrial cancer cells is associated with reduction in cyclin D levels and retention of p27Kip1 in the cyclin E-cdk2 complexes. Oncogene. 2001;**20**(26):3428-3436

[92] Livny O, Kaplan I, Reifen R, Polak-Charcon S, Madar Z, Schwartz B. Lycopene inhibits proliferation and enhances gap-junction communication of KB-1 human oral tumor cells. Journal of Nutrition. 2002;**132**(12):3754-3759.

[93] Liu C, Lian F, Smith DE, Russell RM, Wang XD. Lycopene supplementation inhibits lung squamous metaplasia and induces apoptosis via upregulating insulin-like growth factor-binding protein 3 in cigarette smoke exposed ferrets. Cancer Research. 2003;**63**(12):3138-3144

[94] Tang L, Jin T, Zeng X, Wang JS. Lycopene inhibits the growth of human androgen-independent prostate cancer cells in vitro and in BALB/c nude mice. Journal of Nutrition. 2005;135(2):287-290

[95] Herzog A, Siler U, Spitzer V, Seifert N, Denelavas A, Hunziker PB, Hunziker W, Goralczyk R, Wertz K. Lycopene reduced gene expression of steroid targets and inflammatory markers in normal rat prostate. The FASEB Journal. 2005;19(2):272-274

[96] Arathi BA, Sowmya PR, Kuriakose GC, Vijay K, Baskaran V, Jayabaskaran C, Lakshminarayana R. Enhanced cytotoxic and apoptosis inducing activity of lycopene oxidation products in different cancer cell lines. Food and Chemical Toxicology. 2016;97:265-276. DOI: 10.1016/j.fct.2016.09.016

[97] Seren S, Lieberman R, Bayraktar UD, Heath E, Sahin K, Andic F, Kucuk O. Lycopene in cancer prevention and treatment. American Journal of Therapeutics. 2008;15(1):66-81. DOI: 10.1097/MJT.0b013e31804c7120

[98] Ip BC, Wang XD. Non-alcoholic steatohepatitis and hepatocellular carcinoma: implications for lycopene intervention. Nutrients. 2013;6(1):124-162. DOI: 10.3390/nu6010124

[99] Sahin K, Tuzcu M, Sahin N, Ali S, Kucuk O. Nrf2/HO-1 signaling pathway may be the prime target for chemoprevention of cisplatin-induced nephrotoxicity by lycopene. Food and Chemical Toxicology . 2010;48(10):2670-2674. DOI: 10.1016/j.fct.2010.06.038

[100] Trejo-Solís C, Pedraza-Chaverrí J, Torres-Ramos M, Jiménez-Farfán D, Cruz Salgado A, Serrano-García N, Osorio-Rico L, Sotelo J. Multiple molecular and cellular mechanisms of action of lycopene in cancer inhibition. Evidence-Based Complementary and Alternative Medicine. 2013;2013:705121. DOI: 10.1155/2013/705121

[101] Lu QY, Hung JC, Heber D, Go VL, Reuter VE, Cordon-Cardo C, Scher HI, Marshall JR, Zhang ZF. Inverse associations between plasma lycopene and other carotenoids and prostate cancer. Cancer Epidemiology, Biomarkers & Prevention. 2001;10(7):749-756

[102] Hwang ES, Bowen PE. Cell cycle arrest and induction of apoptosis by lycopene in LNCaP human prostate cancer cells. Journal of Medicinal Food. 2004;7:284-289

[103] Ford NA, Elsen AC, Zuniga K, Lindshield BL, Erdman JW Jr. Lycopene and apo-12'-lycopenal reduce cell proliferation and alter cell cycle progression in human prostate cancer cells. Nutrition and Cancer. 2011;63:256-263. DOI: 10.1080/01635581.2011.523494

[104] Li D, Chen L, Zhao W, Hao J, An R. MicroRNA-let-7f-1 is induced by lycopene and inhibits cell proliferation and triggers apoptosis in prostate cancer. Molecular Medicine Reports. 2016;13(3):2708-2714. DOI: 10.3892/mmr.2016.4841

[105] Tan HL, Thomas-Ahner JM, Moran NE, Cooperstone JL, Erdman JW Jr, Young GS, Clinton SK. β-Carotene 9',10' oxygenase modulates the anticancer activity of dietary tomato or lycopene on prostate carcinogenesis in the TRAMP model. Cancer Prevention Research (Phila). 2016;2. DOI: 10.1158/1940-6207.CAPR-15-0402

[106] Gong X, Marisiddaiah R, Zaripheh S, Wiener D, Rubin LP. Mitochondrial β-carotene 9′,10′ oxygenase modulates prostate cancer growth via NF-κB inhibition: a lycopene-independent function. Molecular Cancer Research. 2016;**14**(10):966-975

[107] Yang CM, Yen YT, Huang CS, Hu ML. Growth inhibitory efficacy of lycopene and β-carotene against androgen-independent prostate tumor cells xenografted in nude mice. Molecular Nutrition & Food Research. 2011;**55**(4):606-612. DOI: 10.1002/mnfr.201000308

[108] Kucuk O, Sarkar F, Sakr W, Djuric Z, Khachik F, Pollak M, Bertram J, Grignon D, Banerjee M, Crissman J, Pontes E, Wood DP Jr. Phase II randomized clinical trial of lycopene supplementation before radical prostatectomy. Cancer Epidemiology, Biomarkers & Prevention. 2001;**10**(8):861-868

[109] Gupta S. Review prostate cancer chemoprevention current status and future prospect. Toxicology and Applied Pharmacology. 2007;**224**(3):369-376. DOI: 10.1016/j.taap.2006.11.008

[110] Paur I, Lilleby W, Bøhn SK, Hulander E, Klein W, Vlatkovic L, Axcrona K, Bolstad N, Bjøro T, Laake P, Taskén KA, Svindland A, Eri LM, Brennhovd B, Carlsen MH, Fosså SD, Smeland SS, Karlsen AS, Blomhoff R. Tomato-based randomized controlled trial in prostate cancer patients: effect on PSA. Clinical Nutrition. 2016;**pii: S0261-5614**(16):30147-30149. DOI: 10.1016/j.clnu.2016.06.01

[111] Wang Y, Jacobs EJ, Newton CC, McCullough ML. Lycopene, tomato products and prostate cancer-specific mortality among men diagnosed with nonmetastatic prostate cancer in the Cancer Prevention Study II Nutrition Cohort. International Journal of Cancer. 2016;**138**(12):2846-2855. DOI: 10.1002/ijc.30027

[112] Assar EA, Vidalle MC, Chopra M, Hafizi S. Lycopene acts through inhibition of IκB kinase to suppress NF-κB signaling in human prostate and breast cancer cells. Tumour Biology. 2016;**37**(7):9375-9385. DOI: 10.1007/s13277-016-4798-3

[113] Ali S, Mann DA. Signal transduction via the NF-κB pathway: a targeted treatment modality for infection, inflammation and repair (Review). Cell Biochemistry and Function. 2004;**22**(2):67-79. DOI: 10.1002/cbf.1082

[114] Gloria NF, Soares N, Brand C, Oliveira FL, Borojevic R, Teodoro AJ. Lycopene and beta-carotene induce cell-cycle arrest and apoptosis in human breast cancer cell lines. Anticancer Research. 2014;**34**(3):1377-1386

[115] Cui Y, Shikany JM, Liu S, Shagufta Y, Rohan TE. Selected antioxidants and risk of hormone receptor-defined invasive breast cancers among postmenopausal women in the Women's Health Initiative Observational Study. The American Journal of Clinical Nutrition. 2008;**87**(4):1009-1018

[116] Sahin K, Tuzcu M, Sahin N, Akdemir F, Ozercan I, Bayraktar S, Kucuk O. Inhibitory effects of combination of lycopene and genistein on 7,12-dimethyl benz(a)anthracene-induced breast cancer in rats. Nutrition and Cancer. 2011;**63**(8):1279-1286. DOI: 10.1080/01635581.2011.606955

[117] Voskuil DW, Vrieling A, Korse CM, Beijnen JH, Bonfrer JM, van Doorn J, Kaas R, Oldenburg HS, Russell NS, Rutgers EJ, Verhoef S, van Leeuwen FE, van't Veer LJ, Rookus MA. Effects of lycopene on the insulin-like growth factor (IGF) system in pre-menopausal breast cancer survivors and women at high familial breast cancer risk. Nutrition and Cancer. 2008;**60**(3):342-353. DOI: 10.1080/01635580701861777

[118] Al-Malki AL, Moselhy SS, Refai MY. Synergistic effect of lycopene and tocopherol against oxidative stress and mammary tumorigenesis induced by 7,12-dimethyl[a] benzanthracene in female rats. Toxicology and Industrial Health. 2012;**542**(6):542-548. DOI: 10.1177/0748233711416948

[119] Sahin K, Orhan C, Tuzcu M, Sahin N, Ali S, Bahcecioglu IH, Guler O, Ozercan I, Ilhan N, Kucuk O. Orally administered lycopene attenuates diethylnitrosamine-induced hepato-carcinogenesis in rats by modulating Nrf-2/HO-1 and Akt/mTOR pathways. Nutrition and Cancer. 2014;**66**(4):590-598. DOI: 10.1080/01635581.2014.894092

[120] Kim MJ, Kim H. anticancer effect of lycopene in gastric carcinogenesis. Journal of Cancer Prevention. 2015;**20**(2):92-96. DOI: 10.15430/JCP.2015.20.2.92

[121] Wang X, Yang HH, Liu Y, Zhou Q, Chen ZH. Lycopene consumption and risk of colorectal cancer: a meta-analysis of observational studies. Nutrition and Cancer. 2016;**68**(7):1083-1096. DOI: 10.1080/01635581.2016.1206579

[122] Liu C, Russell RM. Nutrition and gastric cancer risk: an update. Nutrition Reviews. 2008;**66**(5):237-249. DOI: 10.1111/j.1753-4887.2008.00029.x

[123] Teodoro AJ, Oliveira FL, Martins NB, Maia Gde A, Martucci RB, Borojevic R. Effect of lycopene on cell viability and cell cycle progression in human cancer cell lines. Cancer Cell International. 2012;**12**(1):36. DOI: 10.1186/1475-2867-12-36

[124] Tang FY, Shih CJ, Cheng LH, Ho HJ, Chen H. Lycopene inhibits growth of human colon cancer cells via suppression of the Akt signaling pathway. Molecular Nutrition & Food Research. 2008;**52**(6):646-654. DOI: 10.1002/mnfr.200700272

[125] Palozza P, Bellovino D, Simone R, Boninsegna A, Cellini F, Monastra G, Gaetani S. Effect of beta-carotene-rich tomato lycopene beta-cyclase (tlcy-b) on cell growth inhibition in HT-29 colon adenocarcinoma cells. British Journal of Nutrition. 2009;**102**(2):207-214. DOI: 10.1017/S0007114508169902

[126] Tuzcu M, Aslan A, Tuzcu Z, Yabas M, Bahcecioglu IH, Ozercan IH, Kucuk O, Sahin K. Tomato powder impedes the development of azoxymethane-induced colorectal cancer in rats through suppression of COX-2 expression via NF-κB and regulating Nrf2/HO-1 pathway. Molecular Nutrition & Food Research. 2012;**56**(9):1477-1481. DOI: 10.1002/mnfr.20120013

[127] Dias MC, Vieiralves NF, Gomes MI, Salvadori DM, Rodrigues MA, Barbisan LF. Effects of lycopene, synbiotic and their association on early biomarkers of rat colon carcinogenesis. Food and Chemical Toxicology . 2010;**48**(3):772-780. DOI: 10.1016/j.fct.2009.12.003

[128] Tang FY, Pai MH, Wang XD. Consumption of lycopene inhibits the growth and progression of colon cancer in a mouse xenograft model. Journal of Agricultural and Food Chemistry. 2011;**59**(16):9011-9021. DOI: 10.1021/jf2017644

[129] Vrieling A, Voskuil DW, Bonfrer JM, Korse CM, van Doorn J, Cats A, Depla AC, Timmer R, Witteman BJ, van Leeuwen FE, Van't Veer LJ, Rookus MA, Kampman E. Lycopene supplementation elevates circulating insulin-like growth factor binding protein-1 and -2 concentrations in persons at greater risk of colorectal cancer. American Journal of Clinical Nutrition. 2007;**86**(5):1456-1462

[130] Walfisch S, Walfisch Y, Kirilov E, Linde N, Mnitentag H, Agbaria R, Sharoni Y, Levy J. Tomato lycopene extract supplementation decreases insulin-like growth factor-I levels in colon cancer patients. European Journal of Cancer Prevention. 2007;**16**(4):298-303

[131] Riso P, Brusamolino A, Martinetti A, Porrini M. Effect of a tomato drink intervention on insulin-like growth factor (IGF)-1 serum levels in healthy subjects. Nutrition and Cancer. 2006;**55**(2):157-162

[132] Jang SH, Lim JW, Morio T, Kim H. Lycopene inhibits Helicobacter pylori-induced ATM/ ATR-dependent DNA damage response in gastric epithelial AGS cells. Free Radical Biology & Medicine. 2012;**52**(3):607-615. DOI: 10.1016/j.freeradbiomed.2011.11.010

[133] Liu C, Russell RM, Wang XD. Lycopene supplementation prevents smoke-induced changes in p53, p53 phosphorylation, cell proliferation, and apoptosis in the gastric mucosa of ferrets. Journal of Nutrition. 2006;**136**(1):106-111

[134] Park YO, Hwang ES, Moon TW. The effect of lycopene on cell growth and oxidative DNA damage of Hep3B human hepatoma cells. Biofactors. 2005;**23**(3):129-139

[135] Hwang ES, Lee HJ. Inhibitory effects of lycopene on the adhesion, invasion, and migration of SK-Hep1 human hepatoma cells. Experimental Biology and Medicine (Maywood). 2006;**231**(3):322-327

[136] Astorg P, Gradelet S, Berges R, Suschetet M. Dietary lycopene decreases the initiation of liver preneoplastic foci by diethylnitrosamine in the rat. Nutrition and Cancer. 1997;**29**(1):60-68

[137] Watanabe S, Kitade Y, Masaki T, Nishioka M, Satoh K, Nishino H. Effects of lycopene and Sho-saiko-to on hepatocarcinogenesis in a rat model of spontaneous liver cancer. Nutrition and Cancer. 2001;**39**(1):96-101

[138] Kujawska M, Ewertowska M, Adamska T, Sadowski C, Ignatowicz E, Jodynis-Liebert J. Antioxidant effect of lycopene-enriched tomato paste on N-nitrosodiethylamine-induced oxidative stress in rats. Journal of Physiology and Biochemistry. 2014;**70**(4):981-990. DOI: 10.1007/s13105-014-0367-7

[139] Wang Y, Ausman LM, Greenberg AS, Russell RM, Wang XD. Dietary lycopene and tomato extract supplementations inhibit nonalcoholic steatohepatitis-promoted hepatocarcinogenesis in rats. International Journal of Cancer. 2010;**126**(8):1788-1796. DOI: 10.1002/ijc.24689

[140] Toledo LP, Ong TP, Pinho AL, Jordão A Jr, Vanucchi H, Moreno FS. Inhibitory effects of lutein and lycopene on placental glutathione S-transferase-positive preneoplastic lesions and DNA strand breakage induced in Wistar rats by the resistant hepatocyte model of hepatocarcinogenesis. Nutrition and Cancer. 2003;47(1):62-69

[141] Ip BC, Liu C, Ausman LM, von Lintig J, Wang XD. Lycopene attenuated hepatic tumorigenesis via differential mechanisms depending on carotenoid cleavage enzyme in mice. Cancer Prevention Research (Phila). 2014;7(12):1219-1227. DOI: 10.1158/1940-6207.CAPR-14-0154

[142] Nishino H. Cancer prevention by natural carotenoids. Journal of Cellular Biochemistry. 1997;67(27):86-91. DOI: 10.1002/(SICI)1097-4644(1997)27+<86::AID-JCB14>3.0.CO;2-J

[143] Maurya BK, Trigun SK. Fisetin modulates antioxidant enzymes and inflammatory factors to inhibit aflatoxin-B1 induced hepatocellular carcinoma in rats. Oxidative Medicine and Cellular Longevity. 2016;2016:1972793. DOI: .org/10.1155/2016/1972793

[144] Sharoni Y, Linnewiel-Hermoni K, Khanin M, Salman H, Veprik A, Danilenko M, Levy J. Carotenoids and apocarotenoids in cellular signaling related to cancer: a review. Molecular Nutrition & Food Research. 2012;56(2):259-269. DOI: 10.1002/mnfr.201100311

[145] Ho WJ, Simon MS, Yildiz VO, Shikany JM, Kato I, Beebe-Dimmer JL, Cetnar JP, Bock CH. Antioxidant micronutrients and the risk of renal cell carcinoma in the Women's Health Initiative cohort. Cancer. 2015;121(4):580-588. DOI: 10.1002/cncr.29091

[146] Bertoia M, Albanes D, Mayne ST, Männistö S, Virtamo J, Wright ME. No association between fruit, vegetables, antioxidant nutrients and risk of renal cell carcinoma. International Journal of Cancer. 2010;126(6):1504-1512. DOI: 10.1002/ijc.24829

[147] Bosetti C, Scotti L, Maso LD, Talamini R, Montella M, Negri E, Ramazzotti V, Franceschi S, La Vecchia C. Micronutrients and the risk of renal cell cancer: a case-control study from Italy. International Journal of Cancer. 2007;120(4):892-896

[148] Brock KE, Ke L, Gridley G, Chiu BC, Ershow AG, Lynch CF, Graubard BI, Cantor KP. Fruit, vegetables, fibre and micronutrients and risk of US renal cell carcinoma. British Journal of Nutrition. 2012;108(6):1077-1085. DOI: 10.1017/S0007114511006489

[149] Sahin K, Cross B, Sahin N, Ciccone K, Suleiman S, Osunkoya AO, Master V, Harris W, Carthon B, Mohammad R, Bilir B, Wertz K, Moreno CS, Walker CL, Kucuk O. Lycopene in the prevention of renal cell cancer in the TSC2 mutant Eker rat model. Archives of Biochemistry and Biophysics. 2015;572:36-39. DOI: 10.1016/j.abb.2015.01.006

[150] Okajima E, Ozono S, Endo T, Majima T, Tsutsumi M, Fukuda T, Akai H, Denda A, Hirao Y, Okajima E, Nishino H, Nir Z, Konishi Y. Chemopreventive efficacy of piroxicam administered alone or in combination with lycopene and ß-carotene on the development of rat urinary bladder carcinoma after N-butyl-N-(4-hydroxybutyl) nitrosamine treatment. Japanese Journal of Cancer Research. 1997;88(6):543-552

[151] Zeegers MP, Goldbohm RA, van den Brandt PA. Are retinol, vitamin C, folate and carotenoids intake associated with bladder cancer risk? Results from the Netherlands Cohort Study. British Journal of Cancer. 2001;28(7):977-983.

[152] Helzlsouer KJ, Comstock GW, Morris JS. Selenium, lycopene, alpha-tocopherol, beta-car-otene, retinol, and subsequent bladder cancer. Cancer Research. 1989;**49**(21):6144-6148

[153] Hung RJ, Zhang ZF, Rao JY, Pantuck A, Reuter VE, Heber D, Lu QY. Protectivev effects of plasma carotenoids on the risk of bladder cancer. Journal of Urology. 2006; **176**(3):1192-1197

[154] Klarod K, Hongsprabhas P, Khampitak T, Wirasorn K, Kiertiburanakul S, Tangrassameeprasert R, Daduang J, Yongvanit P, Boonsiri P. Serum antioxidant lev-els and nutritional status in early and advanced stage lung cancer patients. Nutrition. 2011;**27**(11-12):1156-1160. DOI: 10.1016/j.nut.2010.12.019

[155] Graham DL, Carail M, Caris-Veyrat C, Lowe GM. Cigarette smoke and human plasma lycopene depletion. Food and Chemical Toxicology. 2010;**48**(8-9):2413-2420. DOI: 10.1016/j.fct.2010.06.001

[156] Liu C, Russell RM, Seitz HK, Wang XD. Ethanol enhances retinoic acid metabolism into polar metabolites in rat liver via induction of cytochrome P4502E1. Gastroenterology. 2001;**120**(1):179-189

[157] Liu C, Russell RM, Wang XD. Exposing ferrets to cigarette smoke and a pharmaco-logical dose of beta-carotene supplementation enhance in vitro retinoic acid catabo-lism in lungs via induction of cytochrome P450 enzymes. Journal of Nutrition. 2003;**133**(1):173-179

[158] Lian F, Smith DE, Ernst H, Russell RM, Wang XD. Apo–100–lycopenoic acid inhibits lung cancer cell growth in vitro, and suppresses lung tumorigenesis in the A/J mouse model in vivo. Carcinogenesis. 2007;**28**(7):1567-1574

[159] Muzandu K, Ishizuka M, Sakamoto KQ, Shaban Z, El Bohi K, Kazusaka A, Fujita S. Effect of lycopene and beta-carotene on peroxynitrite-mediated cellular modifications. Toxicology and Applied Pharmacology. 2006;**215**(3):330-340

[160] Kim DJ, Takasuka N, Kim JM, Sekine K, Ota T, Asamoto M, Murakoshi M, Nishino H, Nir Z, Tsuda H. Chemoprevention by lycopene of mouse lung neoplasia after combined initiation treatment with DEN, MNU and DMH. Cancer Letters. 1997;**120**(1):15-22

[161] Kim DJ, Takasuka N, Nishino H, Tsuda H. Chemopreventiopn of lung cancer by 1319 lycopene. Biofactors. 2000;**13**:95-102

[162] Pratheeshkumar P, Thejass P, Kutan G. Diallyl disulfide induces caspase-dependent apoptosis via mitochondria-mediated intrinsic pathway in B16F-10 melanoma cells by up-regulating p53, caspase-3 and down-regulating pro-inflammatory cytokines and nuclear factor-κβ-mediated Bcl-2 activation. Journal of Environmental Pathology, Toxicology and Oncology. 2010;**29**(2):113-125.

[163] Priyadarsini RV, Murugan RS, Sripriya P, Karunagaran D, Nagini S. The neem limonoids azadirachtin and nimbolide induce cell cycle arrest and mitochondria-mediated apop-tosis in human cervical cancer (HeLa) cells. Free Radical Research. 2010;**44**(6):624-634. DOI: 10.3109/10715761003692503

[164] Kumar HG, Priyadarsini VR, Vinothini G, Letchoumy VP, Nagini S. The neem limonoids azadirachtin and nimbolide inhibit cell proliferation and induce apoptosis in an animal model of oral oncogenesis. Investigational New Drugs. 2010;28(4):392-401. DOI: 10.1007/s10637-009-9263-3

[165] Bhushan S, Malik F, Kumar A, Isher HK, Kaur IP, Taneja SC, Singh J. Activation of p53/ p21/PUMA alliance and disruption of PI-3/Akt in multimodal targeting of apoptotic signaling cascades in cervical cancer cells by a pentacyclic triterpenediol from *Boswellia serrata*. Molecular Carcinogenesis. 2009;48(12):1093-1108. DOI: 10.1002/mc.20559

[166] Adhikary A, Mohanty S, Lahiry L, Hossain DM, Chakraborty S, Das T. Theaflavins retard human breast cancer cell migration by inhibiting NF-kappaB via p53-ROS cross-talk. FEBS Letters. 2010;584(1):7-14. DOI: 10.1016/j.febslet.2009.10.081

[167] Singh M, Singh N. Curcumin counteracts the proliferative effect of estradiol and induces apoptosis in cervical cancer cells. Molecular and Cellular Biochemistry. 2010;347(1-2):1-11. DOI: 10.1007/s11010-010-0606-3

[168] Banerjee M, Singh P, Panda D. Curcumin suppresses the dynamic instability of microtubules, activates the mitotic checkpoint and induces apoptosis in MCF-7 cells. The FEBS Journal. 2010;277(16):3437-3448. DOI: 10.1111/j.1742-4658.2010.07750.x

[169] Lavhale MS, Kumar S, Mishra SH, Sitasawad SL. A novel triterpenoid isolated from the root bark of Ailanthus excelsa Roxb (Tree of Heaven), AECHL-1 as a potential anti-cancer agent. PLoS One. 2009;4(4):e5365. DOI: 10.1371/journal.pone.0005365

[170] Bhattacharya U, Halder B, Mukhopadhyay S, Giri AK. Role of oxidation-triggered activation of JNK and p38 MAPK in black tea polyphenols induced apoptotic death of A375 cells. Cancer Science. 2009;100(10):1971-1978. DOI: 10.1111/j.1349-7006.2009.01251.x

[171] Patel R, Krishnan R, Ramchandani A, Maru G. Polymeric black tea polyphenols inhibit mouse skin chemical carcinogenesis by decreasing cell proliferation. Cell Proliferation. 2008;41(3):532-553. DOI: 10.1111/j.1365-2184.2008.00528.x

[172] Prasad CP, Rath G, Mathur S, Bhatnagar D, Ralhan R. Potent growth suppressive activity of curcumin in human breast cancer cells: modulation of Wnt/beta-catenin signaling. Chemico-Biological Interactions. 2009;181(2):263-271. DOI: 10.1016/j.cbi.2009.06.012

[173] Jyothi D, Vanathi P, Mangala Gowri P, Rama Subba Rao V, Madhusudana Rao J, Sreedhar AS. Diferuloylmethane augments the cytotoxic effects of piplartine isolated from *Piper chaba*. Toxicology in Vitro. 2009;23(6):1085-1091. DOI: 10.1016/j.tiv.2009.05.023

[174] Sathya S, Sudhagar S, Vidhya Priya M, Bharathi Raja R, Muthusamy VS, Niranjali Devaraj S, Lakshmi BS. 3β-Hydroxylup-20(29)-ene-27,28-dioic acid dimethyl ester, a novel natural product from Plumbago zeylanica inhibits the proliferation and migration of MDA-MB-231 cells. Chemico-Biological Interactions. 2010;188(3):412-420. DOI: 10.1016/j.cbi.2010.07.019

[175] Mondal S, Mandal C, Sangwan R, Chandra S, Mandal C. Withanolide D induces apoptosis in leukemia by targeting the activation of neutral sphingomyelinase-ceramide

cascade mediated by synergistic activation of c-Jun N-terminal kinase and p38 mitoge-nactivated protein kinase. Molecular Cancer. 2010;**9**:239. DOI: 10.1186/1476-4598-9-239

[176] Mandal C, Dutta A, Mallick A, Chandra S, Misra L, Sangwan RS, Mandal C. Withaferin A induces apoptosis by activating p38 mitogen-activated protein kinase signaling cascade in leukemic cells of lymphoid and myeloid origin through mitochondrial death cascade. Apoptosis. 2008;**13**(12):1450-1464. DOI: 10.1007/s10495-008-0271-0

[177] Lahiry L, Saha B, Chakraborty J, Adhikary A, Mohanty S, Hossain DM, Banerjee S, Das K, Sa G, Das T. Theaflavins target Fas/caspase-8 and Akt/pBad pathways to induce apoptosis in p53-mutated human breast cancer cells. Carcinogenesis. 2010;**31**(2):259-268. DOI: 10.1093/carcin/bgp240

[178] Kumar A, Malik F, Bhushan S, Sethi VK, Shahi AK, Kaur J, Taneja SC, Qazi GN, Singh J. An essential oil and its major constituent isointermedeol induce apoptosis by increased expression of mitochondrial cytochrome c and apical death receptors in human leukaemia HL-60 cells. Chemico-Biological Interactions. 2008;**171**(3):332-347

8

Application of Computer Modeling to Drug Discovery: Case Study of PRK1 Kinase Inhibitors as Potential Drugs in Prostate Cancer Treatment

Abdulkarim Najjar, Fidele Ntie-Kang and

Wolfgang Sippl

Abstract

Computer modeling of natural products (NPs) and NP scaffolds is increasingly gaining importance in drug discovery, particularly in hit/lead discovery programs and at the lead optimization stage. Even though industry had lost interest in the implication of NPs in hit/lead searches, recent reports still show that computer modeling could be a useful assert for the identification of starting scaffolds from nature, which could be further exploited by synthetic modifications. In this chapter, the focus is on some useful tools for computer modeling aimed at the discovery of anticancer drugs from NP scaffolds. We also focus on some recent developments toward the identification of potential anticancer agents by the application of computer modeling. The chapter will lay emphasis on natural sources of anticancer compounds, present some useful databases and computational tools for anticancer drug discovery, and show some recent case studies of the application of computational modeling in anticancer drug discovery, as well as some success stories in virtual screening applications in anticancer drug discovery, highlighting some useful results on the application of on lead discovery (including promising NP scaffolds) against an interesting anticancer drug target, the protein kinase C-related kinase (PRK1).

Keywords: anticancer, molecular modeling, natural products, virtual screening, QSAR

1. Introduction

1.1. Cancer and natural products

Cancer is one of the most feared causes of death, as it represents several disease forms and treatments possibilities are still limited for late stages of the disease [1]. Among the known drugs for cancer treatment, camptothecin, vinblastine, vincristine, podophyllotoxin, and taxol are of natural origin [2]. Nature is known to be an immense repository of natural products (NPs), constituting the source of about half of the anticancer drugs currently in the market [3]. Inspite of the drop in interest for NPs in drug discovery projects, from an industrial point of view, recent reports still show that NPs could constitute a useful assert for the identification of starting scaffolds for further discovery [4–6]. The quest for anticancer drugs of natural origin or with NP scaffolds has resulted in the development of NP databases, the most promising one being the naturally occurring plant-based anti-cancer compound activity-target database (NPACT), with ~1500 NPs, including experimentally verified *in vitro* and *in vivo* biological activities (in the form of IC_{50}s, ED_{50}s, EC_{50}s, GI_{50}s, etc.), along with physical, elemental, and topological properties of the compounds, the tested cancer types, cell lines, protein targets, commercial suppliers, and drug-likeness classification for each compound [7].

1.2. Prostate cancer

Among the many diverse cancer forms, prostate cancer is the second leading cause of cancer deaths in men worldwide [8]. Two different types of prostate cancer were identified: androgen-dependent prostate cancer and androgen-independent prostate cancer [9]. Androgen hormones (testosterone or dihydrotestosterone) are known to activate the androgen receptors located in the cell nucleus. The main function of these receptors is to modify gene expressions, thus controlling several biological activities in the cells, including cell growth and differentiation, development, and function of male reproductive and accessory sex tissues [10, 11]. It was found that the androgen receptors signaling pathway plays an important role in the progress and development of prostate cancer. In the first stage of androgen-dependent prostate cancer, the survival and growth of the cancer cells are mainly dependent on androgen hormones [11]. The initial treatment of androgen-dependent cancer, based on androgen ablation, is called hormone therapy. This procedure aims to stop the cell growth of cancer cells, which, in most cases, respond to this therapy. The recurring prostate cancer cells from hormone therapy would further not respond to androgen ablation, thus leading to the development of androgen-independent prostate cancer, which can further progress to metastasis [11]. The molecular mechanism of tumor recurrence is not completely clear. For the second stage of prostate cancer, there is no efficient therapy available.

1.3. Protein kinase C–related kinase

Protein kinase C–related kinase (PRK1, also known as PKN1) is a serine/threonine kinase known to play a role in controlling the activity of androgen receptors in prostate cancer.

It was shown that the activation of PRK1 stimulates the activity of androgen receptors and is involved in tumorigenesis [12]. In 2008, Schüle et al. showed that PRK1 phosphorylates histone H3 upon ligand-dependent recruitment to androgen receptor target genes [12]. The phosphorylation of histone H3 at threonine 11 (H3T11) increases demethylation of Lys-9 by Jumonji C (JmjC)-domain-containing protein (JMJD2C), which promotes androgen receptor-dependent gene expression and tumor cell proliferation [13]. Additionally, PRK1 may directly phosphorylate JMJD2C, thereby stimulating its activity [14]. Meanwhile, the role of PRK1 in androgen-independent prostate cancer is unknown. PRK1 can be activated by the Rho family GTPases, thus mediating several processes related to the migration and cancer cell invasion and consequently playing a major role in the formation of metastases [15, 16]. Thus, PRK1 is considered to be a promising therapeutic target, and the discovery of novel potent and selective inhibitors could supply a meaningful tool for the treatment of prostate cancer. On the other hand, the discovery of selective and potent inhibitors would provide a tool for understanding particular biological roles of PRK1. In spite of the importance of PRK1 in the targeted therapy of cancer, only a few known inhibitors have been identified. The known PKC inhibitors (**Figures 1** and **2**) include staurosporine (PubChem CID: 44259) and its analogue (Ro-318220; PubChem CID: 5083), bisindolylmaleimide I (BIM I; PubChem CID: 2396), and lestaurtinib (PubChem CID: 126565), as well as the nonselective Akt inhibitor GSK-690693 (PubChem CID: 16725726) and Pfizer's JAK nonselective inhibitor CP-690550 (tofacitinib; PubChem CID: 9926791) [17, 18]. In a previous work, several novel PRK1 inhibitors were identified containing different scaffolds, using a homology model, with varying potencies [19]. In the present work, the focus is to search for new small molecules and natural products, which could inhibit PRK1 by using the recently published crystal structures.

1.4. Structural analysis of PRK1

PRK1 kinase belongs to the protein kinase C (PKC) superfamily and was first identified in 1994 from a human hippocampal cDNA library [20]. Three isoforms are found in mammals (called PRK1, PRK2, and PRK3). They possess different enzymatic properties and are distributed among different tissues [21]. The PRK1 structure is divided into three conserved regions:

- an N-terminal lobe (which includes a regulatory region containing three homologous stretches and is rich in charged amino acids),

- an auto-inhibitory domain called C2-like region (which is sensitive to arachidonic acids), and

- a C-terminal lobe (which contains the catalytic domains or called kinase domain).

    Both lobes are connected by a hinge region. The catalytic domain is located between both terminal lobes and shows high conservation and similarity to the PKC family kinase domain [21, 22]. Moreover, PRK1 and PKC are members of AGC kinase family [23]. The characteristic feature of these kinases is a C-terminal regulatory region (C-tail). The C-tails regulate the enzymatic activity and insert conserved phenylalanine residues into the ATP-binding site [23–25].

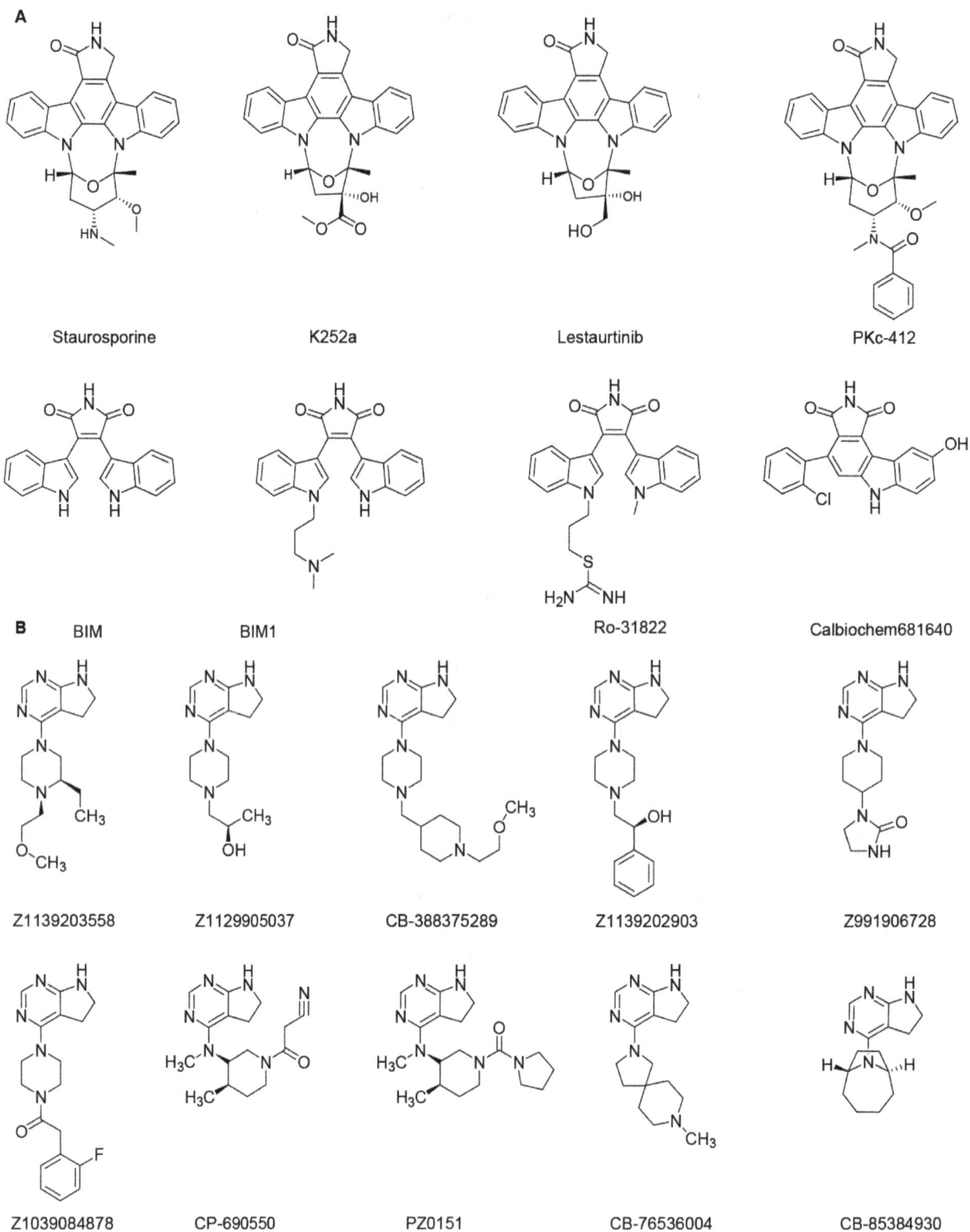

Figure 1. Chemical structures of PRK1 active compounds: (A) staurosporine and derivatives, (B) tofacitinib and other pyrrolopyrimidine derivatives [18].

1.5. Computational approaches in drug discovery

Virtual screening (VS) was first used at the end of the last century to refer to computational algorithms and techniques used to identify novel hit/lead compounds for biological target

A

H-7	HA-1077	F2457-0067	F2458-0011	Ambnee93542761

B

CB-5743914	CB6046000	PD-0166285

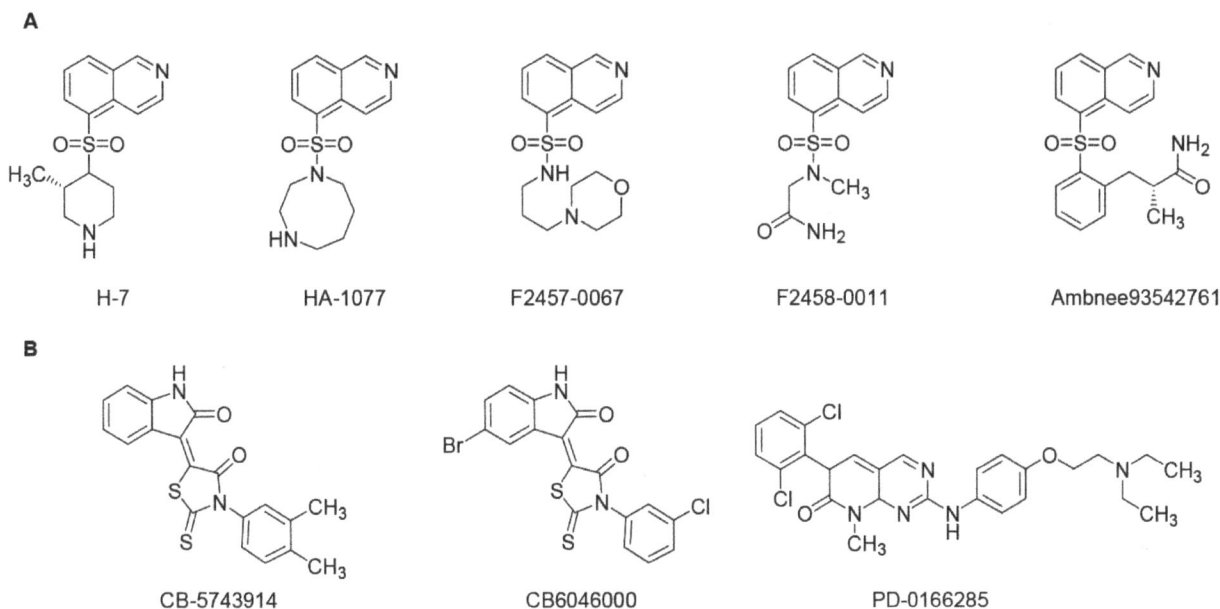

Figure 2. Chemical structures of more PRK1 active compounds. (A) Isoquinoline derivatives, (B) PD-0166285 and structurally diverse compounds identified by VS [18].

from large chemical libraries, depending on the known structure or the drug target or active ligands [26–29]. The VS approach is considered as a complementary approach to experimental or physical screening or high-throughput screening (HTS). VS has been fully integrated to most modern day drug discovery projects [30]. However, VS does not require the physical existence of the compounds to be tested. It is only based on computer models or the three-dimensional (3D) structures of the drug target, also known as structure-based VS (SBVS) or on the chemical structure of known active ligand(s), also known as ligand-based VS (LBVS) [31]. The fundamentals of the SBVS approach depend on the availability of the 3D structure of the biological target and a database of small molecules. The SBVS approach often uses molecular docking to generate the protein-ligand complexes of small molecules from a database into the target active site. The aim is to identify the compounds, which interact favorably with the target binding site [32]. Meanwhile, LBVS methods utilize chemical similarity analysis of structurally diverse or known active ligands, with the view of identifying novel small molecules, which could show similar biological activities [33–35]. However, both approaches have practical limitations. Therefore, researchers often combine SBVS and LBVS, with the aim that this might improve the efficiency of the VS results [36, 37]. Computational approaches for the prediction of biological activity also include quantitative structure-activity relationships (QSAR) analysis, which is aimed at finding a correlation between predicted and experimental biological activities of small molecules. This approach incorporates the influence of the molecular descriptors. QSAR models can be used initially to predict the activity of untested hits from a virtual screening campaign [38]. On other hand, QSAR modeling is useful tool during lead optimization, which is aimed at the improvement of the biological activities of the identified hits [39]. Recently, many crystal structures of the PRK1 drug target have been published [24]. Due to the flexibility of the biding site of the PRK1 structure, which adapts to different conformations, each protein-ligand complex was individually analyzed to reveal the important intermolecular interactions responsible for ligand binding that are useful for the identification new hits. The aim of this research project is to analyze ligand binding to PRK1 and to identify novel-specific inhibitors that could block the activity of PRK1, using structure-based VS. In a preliminary study, the applied docking methods were validated and used to investigate its ability to predict the experimental conformations of the co-crystallized ligands. Second, several QSAR models were generated in order to find the significant correlations between the computational and experimental biological activity data. The constructed QSAR models contain different scoring functions, including computed binding-free energy (BFE) values for the protein-ligand complexes, in addition to molecular descriptors of the isolated ligands. To investigate the predictive ability of the generated QSAR models, internal and external methods were performed. Moreover, an enrichment study was performed, in order to assess the ability of the scoring functions to identify known binders or actives in large databases containing actives and inactives. By focusing on kinase data sets, GSK data sets 1 and 2 were screened to search for novel lead compounds, employing virtual screening methods. A NP library including compounds isolated from African flora was also screened. This chapter begins by presenting database tools (small molecule libraries) useful in VS campaigns, with a focus on small molecule libraries and NPs with anticancer properties. This is followed by some recent success stories on VS for the identification of inhibitors and/or modulators of some anticancer drug targets. The end of the chapter shows the case study of VS for the identification of PRK1 inhibitors.

2. Databases of small molecule libraries and some recent success stories in anticancer drug discovery using computer-based methods

2.1. Small molecule databases for virtual screening

A summary of small molecule libraries utilizable in virtual screening experiments has been provided in **Table 1**. Known cancer drugs have been included in several databases, including ChEBI [43], ChEMBL [44], DrugBank [46], EpiDBase [48], NANPDB [51], NCI-DIS, NCI-DTP, and NCI-FDA [52], along with SANCDB [54], SuperDrug [55], p-ANAPL [58], PubChem [59], and ZINC15 [60]. However, those with tested and proven *in vitro* activities against known cancer cell lines and/or with known *in vivo* activities only include CancerDR [41], OAA [53], and SYFPEITHI [56], along with the NP libraries: AfroCancer [40], CancerHSP [42], CHMIS-C [43], InPACdb [49], MAPS [50], NPACT [7], and TIPdb [57].

2.2. Some recent success stories

Computational modeling has been applied to understand drug-target interactions in several validated anticancer drug targets, for the identification of novel inhibitors from small molecule databases and/or for the elucidation of modes of action. We here present some few recent cases. A typical example is the recent discovery of new inhibitors of CXC chemokine receptor 2 (CXCR2) by applying ligand-based pharmacophore models [61]. It should be mentioned that CXCR2 and its ligand, CXCL8, are known to be implicated in a number of inflammation-mediated diseases, including cancer [62–65]. In the study, Ha et al. generated a pharmacophore

Database	Description	Web accessibility	Reference
AfroCancer	A data set of natural anticancer products from African flora	http://www.african-compounds.org/about/afrocancer/	[40]
Cancer drug resistance database (CancerDR)	A database of 148 anticancer drugs and their effectiveness against around 1000 cancer cell lines	http://crdd.osdd.net/raghava/cancerdr/#thumb	[41]
CancerHSP	An anticancer herbs database of systems pharmacology	http://lsp.nwsuaf.edu.cn/CancerHSP.php/	[42]
ChEBI	A database for chemical entities of biological interest	http://www.ebi.ac.uk/chebi/	[43]
ChEMBL	An open large-scale bioactivity compound database	https://www.ebi.ac.uk/chembl/	[44]
CHMIS-C	A herbal medicines database for cancer	http://sw16.im.med.umich.edu/chmis-c/	[45]
DrugBank	A resource that combines detailed drug data with comprehensive drug target information	https://www.drugbank.ca/	[46]
DUDE datasets	Benchmarking data sets of actives and decoys for diverse targets, including proteins, GPCRs and ion channels, clustered ligands, etc. drawn from ChEMBL	http://dude.docking.org/	[47]
EpiDBase	A database for small molecule epigenetic modulators	http://www.epidbase.org/	[48]
InPACdb	Indian plant anticancer compounds database	http://www.inpacdb.org/	[49]
MAPS Database	A database of phytochemicals, including the data of >500 medicinal plants	http://www.mapsdatabase.com/	[50]
NANPDB	A natural products database for compounds of Northern African origin, with a significant number of bioactive metabolites exhibiting anticancer activity	http://www.african-compounds.org/nanpdb/	[51]
NCI Drug Information System (DIS)	A searchable database of 3D structures (mainly organic compounds) from the NCI Drug Information System (DIS)	https://cactus.nci.nih.gov/ncidb2.2/ http://dtp.nci.nih.gov/docs/3d_database/dis3d.html	[52]
NCI-DTP database	Tested compounds from the National Cancer Institute (NCI) Developmental Therapeutics Program (DTP)	https://dtp.cancer.gov/databases_tools/data_search.htm	[52]
NCI-FDA	Several sets of FDA-approved anticancer drugs to enable cancer research	https://wiki.nci.nih.gov/display/NCIDTPdata/Compound+Sets	[52]
NPACT	A database for plant-based anticancer compounds	http://crdd.osdd.net/raghava/npact/	[7]
Oral anticancer agents (OAA) from Singapore	A database of 39,772 oral anticancer agents prescribed to 8837 patients in Singapore, with 55 clinically significant drug-drug interactions for the evaluation of drug interaction facts	https://www.ncbi.nlm.nih.gov/pubmed/22795926/	[53]

Database	Description	Web accessibility	Reference
SANCDB	A database of natural products from South Africa, containing also anticancer agents from the flora and fauna of this ecologically diverse country	https://sancdb.rubi.ru.ac.za/	[54]
SuperDrug	A database of 3D-structures of active ingredients of essential marketed drugs	http://bioinf.charite.de/superdrug/	[55]
SYFPEITHI	A database of major histocompatibility complex (MHC) ligands and peptide motifs	http://www.syfpeithi.de/	[56]
TIPdb	A database of anticancer, antiplatelet, and antituberculosis phytochemicals from indigenous plants in Taiwan	http://cwtung.kmu.edu.tw/tipdb/	[57]
p-ANAPL	A collection of samples of natural products from African sources	http://www.african-compounds.org/about/p-anapl/	[58]
PubChem	A public repository for information on chemical substances and their biological activities	https://pubchem.ncbi.nlm.nih.gov/	[59]
ZINC15	A free database of over 100 million purchasable compounds for virtual screening	http://zinc15.docking.org/	[60]

Table 1. Summary of some small molecule libraries currently available for anticancer drug discovery.

model based on known CXCR2 antagonists and used it to screen a database of 5 million commercially available compounds from different vendors. The authors were able to identify small molecule hits, which were further tested by *in vitro* screening in a cell-based CXCR2-mediated β-arrestin-2 recruitment assay, followed by several other cell-based assays. *In vivo* studies were conducted by lipopolysaccharide (LPS)-induced lung inflammation in mice. It was also shown that one of the compounds inhibits CXCR2 signaling through down regulation of surface CXCR2.

Moreover, the same compound was shown to inhibit CXCL8-mediated neutrophil migration and LPS-induced lung inflammation in mice significantly. The identified compounds were shown to also inhibit CXCR2/β-arrestin-2 association, cell migration and proliferation, and acute inflammation in mouse models. Another study combined structure-based docking and pharmacophores to design novel indole and chromene analogues, which were cyclin-dependent kinase 2 (CDK2) inhibitors. The identified compounds proved to be active against MCF-7 and HeLa cell lines. The study was conducted by exploiting stereo-specific information obtained from crystal structures of CDK2, substituting the pharmacophores on their moiety and docking the target protein to calculate the binding affinities [66]. Other recent successful cases, where docking, QSAR, machine learning, and pharmacophore-based screening were combined to search for small molecules targeting cancer, are abundant in the literature [67–70].

3. Case study: structure-based virtual screening and QSAR studies on PRK1 inhibitors

3.1. Structure-based design studies (X-ray target structures and cross docking)

Four crystal structures of PRK1 are available in the protein data bank (PDB), **Table 2**. The PRK1 binding site is reported to exhibit either intrinsic or induced flexibility [17, 24]. Moreover, different bound inhibitors are known to induce different conformational changes in the binding site residues [71]. Furthermore, chemical characteristics of the co-crystallized ligands play an important role in the applicability of the X-ray structure for virtual screening. Therefore, a cross-docking procedure was carried out, as a retrospective study aimed at determining the appropriate structure for the virtual screening. The selected structure should be able to bind the nonnative ligands with low root mean square deviation (RMSD), with respect to the reference binding conformation. On the other hand, the performance of the docking power and scoring functions is varying for different targets [32]. The docking power measures the ability of docking algorithms to predict the correct conformation of the ligands [72].

The four X-ray structures of PRK1, including the apo-form, were used for a cross-docking study [24]. The co-crystallized ligands were docked toward the target binding sites, using the Glide cross-docking script, implemented in Schrödinger Suite (2014 version) with standard precision (SP) for flexible ligand docking. In order to optimize the docking solution, an option was selected to perform post-docking minimization and includes number of poses up to 5 per ligand. The structures were prepared using the default setting implemented in Protein Preparation Wizard (Schrödinger 2014). The co-crystallized water molecules were deleted. Hydrogen atoms and partial charges were assigned. Finally, the structure energy minimized applying the OPLS 2005 force field. The binding site was defined using Grid Generation of Schrödinger suite 2014 and sets the co-crystallized ligand as a center of the binding pocket. In the case of apo-structure 4OTD, the binding site was defined by applying centroid of selected residues Leu650 and Lys753 with box size 14 Å. A hydrogen bond constraint was defined at PRK1 hinge region reside Ser704. In addition, all ligands were prepared using LigPrep implemented in Schrödinger utility 2014 involving generation of ionization and tautomeric states at pH 7.4 with less than 10 low-energy ring conformations. The ligands were energy minimized using MMFFs force field.

Ligand	4OTD		4OTG		4OTH		4OTI	
	RMSD	SP	RMSD	SP	RMSD	SP	RMSD	SP
Lestaurtinib-4OTG	6.56	−4.29	0.24	−11.67	4.65	−7.82	7.56	−4.29
Ro-318220-4OTH	6.79	−7.01	2.98	−11.4	0.64	−11.76	6.47	−6.55
Tofacitinib-4OTI	3.14	−4.54	6.11	−8.09	2.7	−8.18	0.55	−8.8
Average RMSD	5.5		3.11		2.67		4.86	

Table 2. RMSD values (Å) for the top-ranked docking solutions (using Glide SP as scoring function).

The RMSD values were calculated, with respect to the respective reference ligand conformations. **Table 2** shows the RMSD values and Glide SP scores for the top-ranked poses in the corresponding structures. It was observed that none of the available structures had a binding site conformation, which allowed all the three different ligands to be docked with RMSD < 2.0 Å. Furthermore, the calculated average RMSD values for each structure were high. However, the applied docking method performed well by reproducing the binding mode of the co-crystallized inhibitor in self-docking. Moreover, the docking method correctly scored the co-crystallized inhibitors at the top of the list (**Table 2**), e.g., the X-ray structure of the ligand lestaurtinib was re-docked with an RMSD = 0.24 Å into its co-crystallized structure (PDB: 4OTG), being also ranked as the top scoring pose (Glide SP = −11.67 kcal/mol). Similar results were observed with the other inhibitors when X-ray structures were docked toward their respective co-crystallized target structures. Meanwhile, the binding pocket conformation for the apo-form of PRK1 was not found to be suitable for docking when using any of the current inhibitor structures. RMSD values were high and the docking scores were low when compared with those obtained in the rest PRK1 structures (**Table 2**). Therefore, an ensemble of PRK1 structures was proposed for the further virtual screening study.

3.2. Docking of active inhibitors

The data set DS1 includes 28 active (**Figures 1** and **2** [18]) and 300 inactive compounds. First, the active compounds were docked toward the ensemble of the three PRK1 structures using the previously described docking methods. The docking solutions were first inspected, with the aim of comparing them with the experimental conformations (the co-crystallized ligands in other kinases). The active compounds could be divided into four subsets, the first set being staurosporine derivatives (10 actives, including the co-crystallized inhibitors lestaurtinib and Ro-318220). The second subset is made of the tofacitinib or pyrrolopyrimidine family (nine actives, in addition to the inhibitor tofacitinib in PDB ID: 4OTI). The third set was made of two isoquinoline derivatives, forming a group of five actives. The last subset contains the remaining inhibitors, with diverse scaffolds. The binding mode for each compound was analyzed and compared with the experimental data. As previously seen in the cross-docking for the co-crystallized inhibitors (**Table 2**), the binding modes for lestaurtinib and Ro-318220 were correctly reproduced. The binding modes for the further staurosporine derivatives were compared with these two analogues. Since the ensemble docking procedure was applied to dock the actives, eight compounds were docked toward the 4OTG structure target site, while the others (Ro-318220 and BIM1) were docked toward the 4OTH site. It was interesting to notice that the top-ranked active poses had a quite conserved binding mode, which shares two H bonds, interacting with the hinge region of PRK1. The obtained binding modes for all staurosporine derivatives were identical to the published structure (in the PRK1 X-ray structure 4OTG). Since a part of the C-terminal regulation region (C-tail) is not resolved, resulting in a more open and accessible ATP binding pocket, most of the staurosporine derivatives could be docked into it. Furthermore, all staurosporine derivatives were docked into both PRK1 structures, which are co-crystallized with one of staurosporine derivatives (4OTG or 4OTH). For pyrrolopyrimidine and tofacitinib derivatives, the inhibitors were docked into three X-ray structures of PRK1. Tofacitinib was co-crystallized in the structure 4OTI. The RMSD value of re-docking tofacitinib was 0.55 Å. The binding modes for the other analogues were compared with the experimental data (4OTI). Additionally, several other analogues were co-crystallized with the Akt1 kinase (PDB IDs: 3MV5, 3MVJ, and 3OCB).

Each active compound forms 2 H bonds with the hinge region, besides additional H bonds with the surrounding residues in the binding pocket. There are also some isoquinoline derivatives that were co-crystallized with other kinases, e.g., cAMP-dependent kinase (PDB IDs: 1YDS and 1YDR) and Rho kinase (PDB IDs: 2GNI). This subset of actives interacts with the PRK1 hinge region by mediating 1 H bond. A former virtual screening campaign had identified several actives, including CB-6046000 and CB-5743914, which were docked using the same previously described docking method. The binding mode showed two H bonds between the dihydroindol-2-one and the backbone of the hinge region, mainly Ser704 and Glu702. Furthermore, the binding mode of PD-0166285 matched the experimental data observed for the LCK kinase (PDB ID: 3KMM).

3.3. Scoring power

The rescoring for the derived docking poses was performed by calculating BFEs and using different solvation models implemented in the AMBER12 package. IC_{50} values had been previously determined for 26 of the active compounds (**Table 3**), with only percentage inhibitions available for two others) [19]. Thus, the correlation coefficient (R^2) between the experimental pIC_{50} and the calculated enthalpy changes (ΔH) for protein-ligand binding was calculated (**Table 3** and **Figure 3**). The BFE calculation was carried out using one snapshot after two consecutive minimizations steps and applying the Generalized Born solvation model [73, 74]. First, the minimization was carried out for water and counterion molecules without the ligand-protein complex, which was restrained to their initial coordinates with a force constant of 500 kcal/mol/Å^2. In this step, there were 2000 iterations (beginning with 1000 steepest descent and followed by 1000 conjugate gradient). The second minimization step was applied for the whole system through 10,000 iterations (first 5000 steepest descent and then 5000 conjugate gradients). A significant correlation was found when using the Nguyen and Simmerling (igb = 8) version of the Generalized Born solvation model [73, 74] and applying the two minimizations steps. The cross-validated R^2 was found to be 0.60, with a root mean square error (RMSE) of 0.89. To understand the effect of the chemical modification on the main scaffold, the binding mode of the actives and the interactions in the binding pocket was analyzed. As mentioned previously, PRK1 actives can be divided into four subsets (**Table 3**). The docking score (Glide SP) and the MM/GBSA BFE values were employed to explore the differences in the inhibitory activity. However, there was a weak correlation between the pIC_{50} and Glide SP scores (R^2 of 0.43, see **Table 4**).

It was observed, from docking, that the isoquinoline derivatives are able to form an H bond between the N atom of the isoquinoline motif and the NH backbone of Ser704 located in the hinge region. The isoquinoline motif occupied the adenine binding site; meanwhile, the substituents were located in the sugar-binding site, which is surrounded by several hydrophilic residues (e.g., Asp708, Asp750). Rescoring, using MMGBSA, showed that H-7 (IC_{50} = 658 µM and ΔH = −34.51 kcal/mol) had a higher score than HA-1077 (IC_{50} = 1.95 µM and ΔH = −29.42 kcal/mol), **Table 3**. The more favorable value resulted from the additional

Compound	IC$_{50}$ (nM)	Exp. pIC$_{50}$	Target structure	Glide SP	MM/GBSA**	PEOE_PC-	Pred. pIC$_{50}$*
Ro-318220	78.3	7.11	4OTH	−11.36	−45.97	−2.71	7.16
BIM1	579	6.24	4OTH	−9.82	−46.10	−2.29	6.58
PKC-412	14.2	7.85	4OTG	−10.98	−55.52	−3.26	8.26
Lestaurtinib	8.6	8.07	4OTG	−11.43	−46.92	−2.77	7.30
K252a	3.2	8.49	4OTG	−11.38	−51.40	−2.95	7.80
Staurosporine	0.81	9.10	4OTG	−11.83	−60.86	−2.72	8.59
Calbiochem681640	1441	5.84	4OTG	−10.61	−47.90	−1.96	6.71
BIM	154.2	6.81	4OTG	−9.16	−38.70	−1.96	5.58
K252c			4OTG	−10.53	−40.12		
Quercetin			4OTG	−8.43	−48.23		
CP-690550 (tofacitinib)	129	6.89	4OTI	−8.81	−38.88	−2.01	5.55
Z1139203558	55730	4.25	4OTG	−8.52	−27.91	−1.84	4.41
Z1129905037	53380	4.27	4OTI	−9.61	−35.25	−1.82	5.29
CB-38374289	42560	4.37	4OTI	−10.49	−33.36	−2.11	5.49
CB-85384930	34020	4.47	4OTH	−9.04	−35.48	−1.48	4.98
Z1139202903	31470	4.50	4OTI	−9.37	−37.77	−2.09	5.62
Z991906728	26400	4.58	4OTG	−9.18	−28.92	−2.02	4.75
CB-76536004	13090	4.88	4OTG	−9.43	−33.02	−1.45	4.83
Z1039084878	6210	5.21	4OTG	−8.76	−29.13	−2.10	4.73
PZ0151	1060	5.97	4OTI	−8.54	−43.19	−2.16	5.97
H-7	658.5	6.18	4OTH	−8.68	−34.51	−1.43	4.78
HA-1077	1945	5.71	4OTI	−8.71	−29.42	−1.39	4.31
F2457-0067	70300	4.15	4OTH	−8.49	−36.31	−1.76	5.10
F2458-0011	53730	4.27	4OTI	−8.07	−29.18	−1.70	4.34
Ambnee93542761	29330	4.53	4OTH	−9.12	−30.33	−1.68	4.66
CB-6046000	5350	5.27	4OTG	−7.39	−47.01	−1.57	5.70
CB-5743914	2940	5.53	4OTG	−9.89	−41.07	−1.72	5.81
PD-0166285	5517	5.26	4OTG	−7.48	−39.17	−2.41	5.53

Comparison of experimental pIC50 versus predicted pIC50 values calculated by QSAR_3 for the 26 training set molecules [18].

The BFE values were calculated according to the docked structure (target structure), which are supplied with the PDB ID.

Table 3. Biological activity, calculated BFE and docking scores of the active compounds.

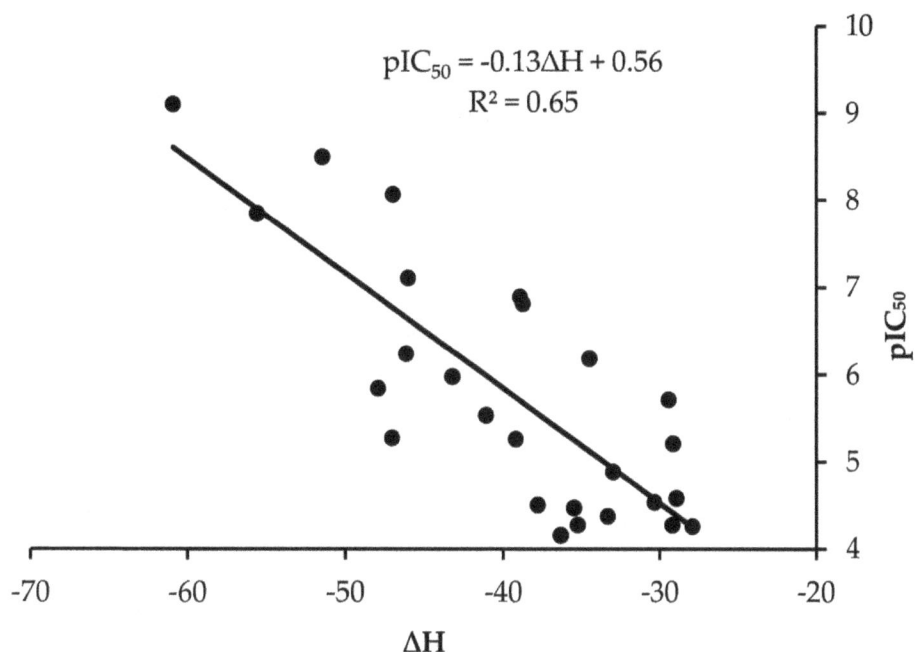

$$pIC_{50} = -0.13\Delta H + 0.56$$
$$R^2 = 0.65$$

Figure 3. Correlation curve of pIC50 versus ΔH scores of actives using MM/GBSA.

hydrophobic interactions between the front hydrophobic pocket residues and Phe910 (from the C-tail) and the methyl substituent on the piperazine ring. Meanwhile, the van der Waals interaction became weaker in the case of HA-1077. This could be explained by the shifting of the position of the substituent, since its seven-membered ring is bulkier. Both derivatives contain a positively charged ring nitrogen, which consequently forms an additional H bond in the ATP-sugar binding pocket (**Figure 4**). Meanwhile, the interaction between Asp708 and the piperazine ring enables the methyl group to get closer to Phe910 and its surrounding residues. Moreover, the sulfonyl moiety of both compounds is located under the P-loop, where it forms hydrophilic and hydrophobic interactions.

			ΔH
	SP	**XP**	**GB8**
R^2	0.43	0.27	**0.65**
EF1%	**100**	**100**	25
EF3%	**30.3**	**33.33**	9.1
AUC*	**0.90**	**0.88**	0.66

*AUC = area under the ROC curve.

Table 4. Enrichment study results using an ensemble of PRK1 structures, where the available scoring functions in Schrödinger and BFE methods were considered. Where **SP**: Standard Precision; **XP**: Extra Precision and ΔH: enthalpy score; GB8: Generalized Born theory model.

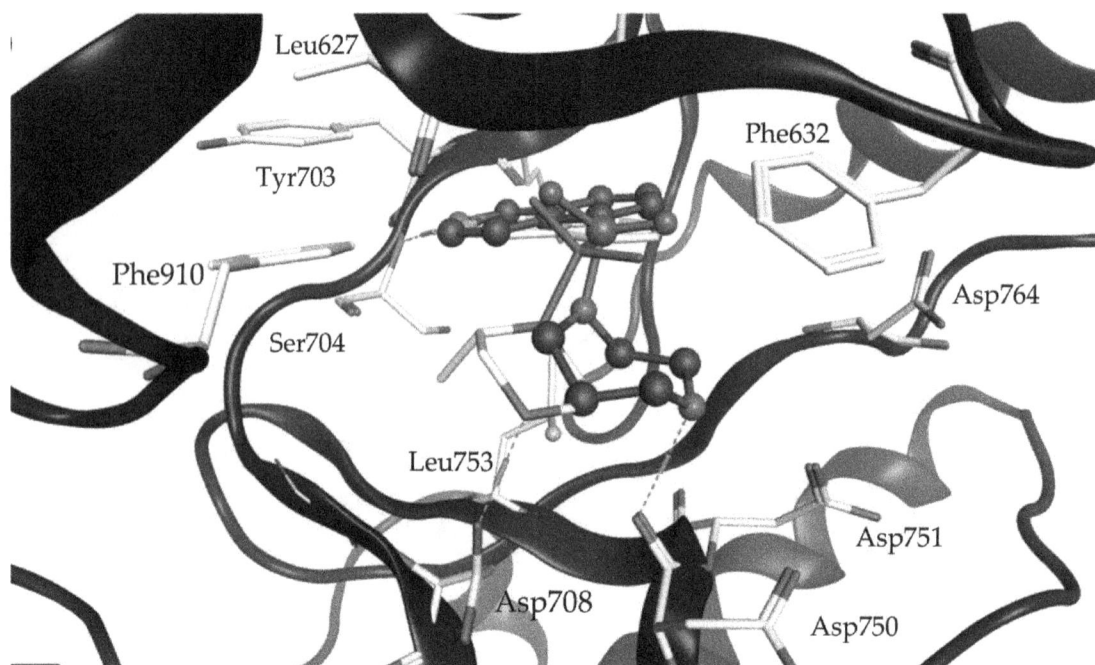

Figure 4. Comparison between the docking poses of two isoquinoline derivatives H-7 (magenta) and HA-1077 shown as green sticks (PRK1 PDB code: 4OTH). The figure was designed using MOE.

The remaining compounds share common interactions (as previously mentioned), but the biological activities of these compounds could not be predicted using the derived BFE model. However, the lower activity of compound ambnee93542761 could be explained by the loss of the interaction between of the sulfonyl moiety and weak hydrophobic interactions with Phe910. Nonetheless, it forms a hydrogen bond with the catalytic Asp764 (IC_{50} = 29.33 μM and ΔH = −30.32 kcal/mol). The results of this subset show the importance of the hydrophobic interactions with the Phe910 of the C-tail and its surrounding residues. However, the BFE values and docking scores failed to predict the affinity of F2457-0067, which shows a favorable BFE value but a low IC_{50} value (**Table 3**). This could probably result from the long linker between the isoquinoline motif and the positively charged morpholine ring. The generated conformations show additional van der Waals interactions. On the other hand, the morpholine ring shows more polar properties compared to the other compounds.

The second subset of actives is made of staurosporine derivatives. Most of these compounds form two H bonds between the pyrrole ring and the hinge backbone (NH of Ser704 and CO of Glu702). The docking results for staurosporine derivatives were compared with two PRK1 crystal structures (4OTG and 4OTH). The favorable BFE values of staurosporine derivatives could be attributed to the strong hydrophobic interactions with residues from the P-loop, e.g., Val635 and Leu627, in addition to the interactions with Leu753. The only observed deviation was with parts of the docked ligand interacting with the sugar pocket, e.g., staurosporine (the most active compound) showed a BFE value of ΔH = −60.85 kcal/mol and an IC_{50} = 0.0008 μM (**Table 3**). The favorable BFE value and activity of staurosporine could be estimated through the targeting of both hydrophobic pocket residues (behind the gatekeeper Met701 and near Phe910); on the other hand, several polar groups occupied the sugar polar pocket. By comparison with lestaurtinib (IC_{50} = 0.0086 μM and ΔH= −46.92 kcal/mol), the differences in the activity and BFE values could be attributed to the smaller ring/shorter linker in lestaurtinib for targeting Asp708 and Asp750 (**Figure 5**).

The third subset of PRK1 inhibitors is made of tofacitinib analogues. Ten compounds belong to this subset (**Table 3**). All derivatives interact with the hinge region by forming two H bonds through the pyrrolopyrimidine scaffold (**Figure 6**). The major substituents, which influence notably the BFE values and the biological activity of tofacitinib, are the N-methyl of the pyridine ring. Any chemical modification changing these interactions will consequently change the BFE value and the activity. A comparison of the calculated BFE values of tofacitinib with those of the other derivatives could clarify the effects of these interactions. As previously mentioned, the loss of the interactions made with the P-loop residues clearly influences the calculated BFE values and, therefore, affects the biological activities. Consequently, Z1129905037 (IC_{50} = 55.73 μM and ΔH = −27.92 kcal/mol) possesses a BFE value lower than tofacitinib (IC_{50} = 0.129 μM and ΔH = −38.88 kcal/mol) (**Table 3**). Furthermore, contrary to tofacitinib, the binding mode of Z1129905037 does not show hydrophobic interactions with the residue located at the bottom of the binding pocket. The ATP-sugar binding site is occupied by non-polar substituents in the case of Z1129905037, which is unfavorable and consequently reduces the activity. The other tofacitinib analogues, which do not contain any tertiary amine as the linker, show higher BFE values and obviously lower biological activities. One exception is PZ0151 (IC_{50} = 1.06 μM and ΔH= −43.19 kcal/mol) which displays the same binding mode with tofacitinib. The pyrrolidine

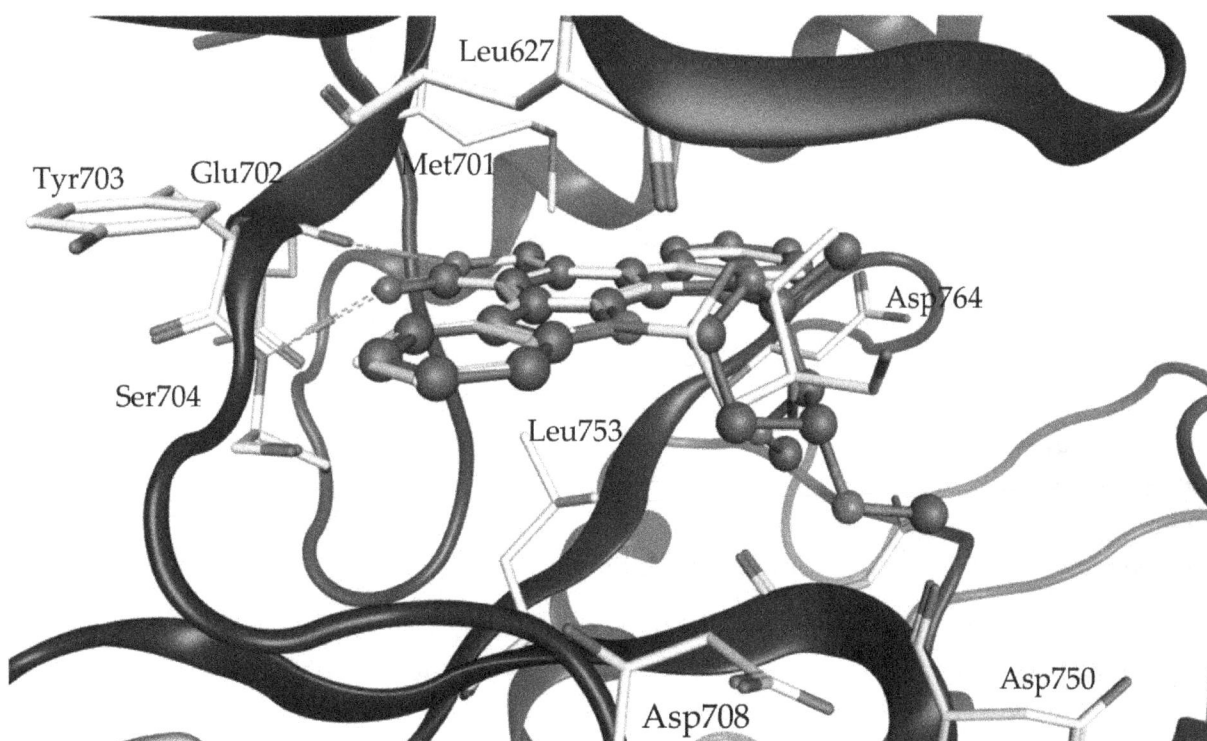

Figure 5. Comparison between the docking pose of staurosporine (seen in cyan sticks) and the binding mode of lestaurtinib (shown in white brown sticks) at PRK1 structure 4OTG. The figure was designed using MOE.

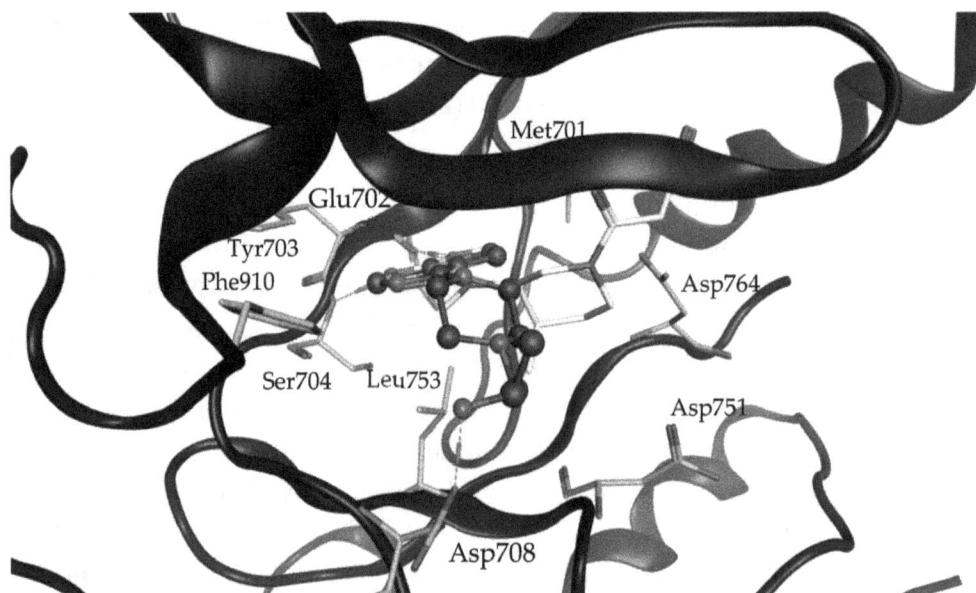

Figure 6. Comparison of the docking pose of Z1129905037 (shown as cyan sticks) and the binding mode of tofacitinib seen in magenta, at the binding site of PRK1 structure 4OTI. The figure was designed using MOE.

ring in PZ0151 takes the position of the CN group of tofacitinib but rather shows a lower activity. This could be as a result of the small size of the binding site under the P-loop residues, which is not suitable for large substituents. In general, it is difficult to explain the changes of the BFE values caused by chemical modification of all compounds under study. The observed correlation coefficient ($R^2 = 0.65$) could only be used to explain major differences in biological activities. However, it could be used as an indicator to identify the interactions, which play major roles in the determination of biological activity.

3.4. Ranking power

An enrichment study was performed in order to measure the ability to identify known binders or actives in large databases of inactives. The previously mentioned data set (named DS1), containing 28 actives and 300 inactives, was used to perform the enrichment study. The ligands were docked using the same ensemble and rescored depending on the previous findings. The results are presented in a BOX-PLOT and receiver operating characteristic (ROC) curves (**Figures 7** and **8**). **Table 4** shows enrichment study results, using an ensemble of PRK1 structures, where the available scoring functions in Schrödinger and BFE methods were considered (ΔH, Glide SP and Glide XP). As seen in **Figure 7**, Glide SP was able to discriminate between actives and inactives better than the BFE scoring (ΔH).

The median values of the pair active/inactive were −9.17/7.23 and −38.79/34.02 for Glide SP and ΔH, respectively. The area under the curve (AUC) and enrichment factors (EF) at two different percentages were calculated. **Table 4** shows the enrichment study results. It is interesting to note that at EF1%, all screened hits were actives when using both Schrödinger's scoring functions (Glide SP and XP). Interesting, it was also observed that for the EF3% (for Glide SP and XP), the rate of true positives was 100% (**Table 4**). The main factor to measure the ranking

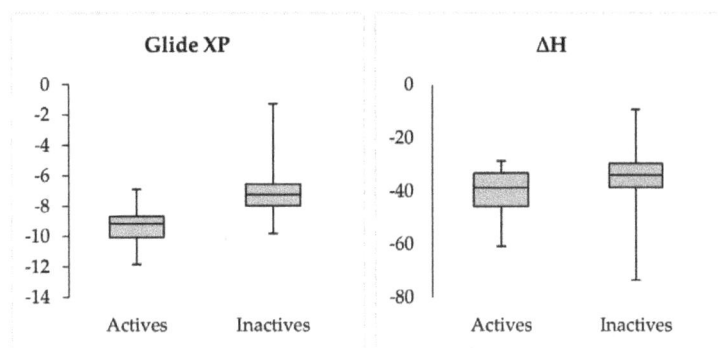

Figure 7. Box plots for the active and inactive compounds using the respective score values.

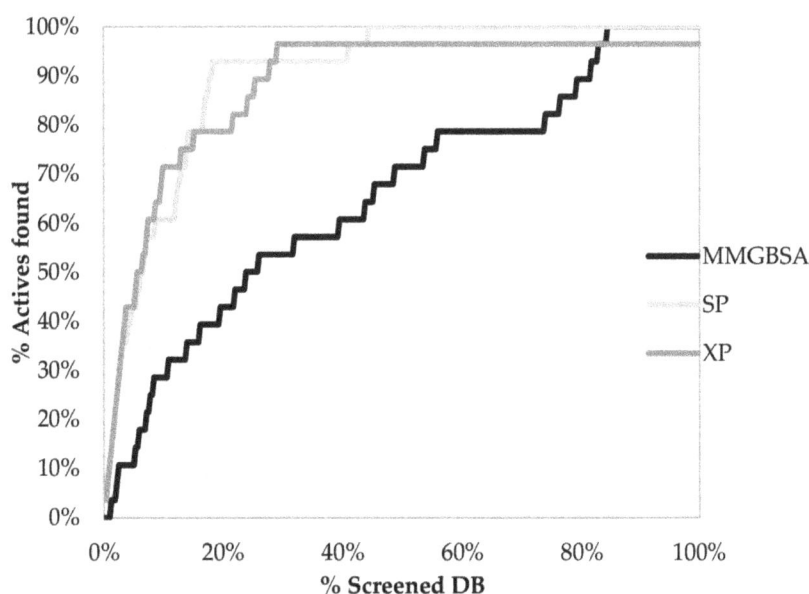

Figure 8. Enrichment plot showing comparison of the % actives found at a given percentage of the ranked database for DS1, using GLIDE SP, XP, and ΔH (MMGBSA).

power of the applied docking methods was the AUC value (**Table 4**). It is clear that the Glide scoring functions performed better to discriminate between the actives of inactives, having AUC = 0.90 and 0.88 for SP and XP, respectively.

3.5. QSAR model generation

Several QSAR models were generated to identify a possible correlation between experimentally obtained pIC_{50} values and calculated BFE or descriptor values (for the compounds on **Figures 1** and **2**). Calculated BFE (obtained by the MM/GBSA approach) from the previous study and 2D molecular descriptors, e.g., different descriptors referring to the partial charge and number of rotatable bonds, were considered. Since the Glide SP score showed a significant discrimination power between the active and inactive compounds, further scoring functions were also tested to optimize the QSAR models.

The best correlation coefficient in the previous study was found by applying Nguyen and Simmerling (igb = 8) Generalized Born solvation model [73, 74], after a minimization step (R^2 = 0.65, RMSE = 0.89 and cross-validated q^2 = 0.60, n = 26). In order to improve the correlation, partial charges of the ligands were calculated to compute several molecular descriptors for generating PLS models [75]. The inclusion of the PEOE_VSA-0 descriptor improved the correlation coefficient value only slightly (model QSAR_, R^2 = 0.68, RMSE = 0.8, and q^2 = 0.61, n = 26). This descriptor indicates the partial equalization of electronegativities with approximated accessible van der Waals surface area (in Å^2) of the molecule [76]. Furthermore, the inclusion of another descriptor based on ligand partial charges (PEOE_PC-) [76], which indicates to the total negative partial charge, was used instead of PEOE_VSA-0 to generate QSAR_2 (R^2 = 0.70, RMSE = 0.78 and q^2 = 0.62, n = 26; Eq. (1)). The model QSAR_3, containing three descriptors, showed a slightly better correlation coefficient (R^2 = 0.71, RMSE = 0.76 and q^2 = 0.63, n = 26; Eq. (2)). The relative importance of the individual descriptors was MM-GBSA: 1, GLIDE_SP: 0.417, and PEOE_PC-: 0.371. The other tested descriptors were not helpful and were not considered for the final models.

Further internal validation of the generated QSAR models was carried out by means of bootstrapping, in which the samples are randomly selected from the used inhibitors to form training and test sets [77, 78]. The respective models are generated, and their statistical parameters (R^2 and q^2) are calculated and compared with those of the original QSAR models (which had been generated from the whole data set). The random selection of the samples was performed within each cluster generated by hierarchical clustering, depending on the structural similarity or within activity distribution clusters of PRK1 inhibitors (low, moderate, and high active inhibitors) [77]. PRK1 inhibitors can be divided into four subsets depending on the chemical scaffolds (**Figures 1** and **2**). In the next step, hierarchical clustering using maximum common substructure (MACCS) keys and calculation of Tanimoto coefficients were carried out using the molecular operator environment (MOE) software tool (chemical computing group, Montreal, Canada, version 2014). Then, several samples within each cluster were taken, considering their activities. From 26 compounds, the sample subset contains only 20 inhibitors. The statistic parameters of the obtained QSAR models are presented in **Table 5**. The goal of the bootstrapping is to perturb the training set while not considering the statistical parameters of the test set. Since the obtained QSAR models were built from subset of the total data set, the values of R^2_{BT} and q^2_{BT} satisfy the minimum acceptable statistical parameters when

	Training set (20 inhibitors)			Test set (6 inhibitors)		
	R^2	RMSE	q^2	R^2_{BT}	RMSE$_{pred}$	q^2_{pred}
QSAR_BT_1	0.71	0.73	0.65	0.43	1.11	0.06
QSAR_BT_2	0.72	0.72	0.63	0.58	0.95	0.19
QSAR_BT_3	0.72	0.71	0.60	0.67	0.84	0.28

Table 5. Statistical parameters of obtained QSAR models in bootstrap validation.

compared with the three original QSAR models. These values also revolve around the values of the original QSAR models, generated from 26 PRK1 inhibitors (**Table 5**). It was observed that the obtained QSAR models possess acceptable statistic parameters ($q^2 > 0.5$) and were comparable with those found in the original QSAR models. However, the QSAR_BT_3 model showed poor correlation when compared with the results found in the whole data set ($q^2 = 0.60$, **Table 5**). The remaining six inhibitors were used as the external test set to verify the ability of the obtained QSAR models (QSAR_BTs) to predict the biological activities of the test set compounds. The values of R^2 between the calculated and measured pIC are 0.43, 0.58, and 0.67 for QSAR_BT_1, QSAR_BT_2, and QSAR_BT_3, respectively (**Table 5**). These results may confirm the ability of the model QSAR_3 and its derivatives (QSAR_BT_3) to predict the biological activities of novel compounds.

Interestingly, QSAR_3 have predicted pIC_{50} values higher or close to 7 for the most potent PRK1 inhibitors ($IC_{50} < 100$ nM). Moreover, QSAR_3 possessed the ability to distinguish between weak, moderate, and highly potent compounds (**Table 3**). Thus, the model could be used as a filter for the prioritization of specific compounds (hits) for synthesis and testing. **Figure 9** displays the graph of the correlation between the observed and predicted pIC_{50} values using QSAR_3 model.

3.6. Validation of the generated QSAR models and GSK databases screening

It has previously been demonstrated that considering only the statistic parameters (R^2, RMSE, and q^2) to validate QSAR models is insufficient and sometimes misleading [78–82]. Therefore, it is important to validate QSAR models by testing the ability to accurately predict the biological activities of ligands not used for QSAR model generation. In the current study, two data

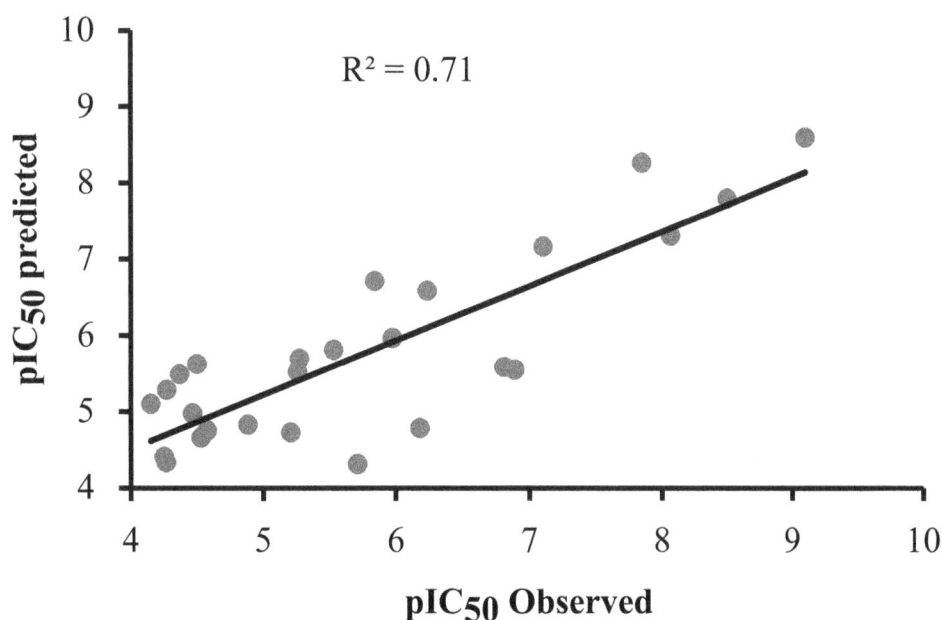

Figure 9. Correlation plot of the observed versus predicted pIC_{50} values of the training set ($n = 26$) using QSAR_3 model.

sets of compounds were available: the first set containing 26 PRK1 inhibitors with IC_{50} values was used as a training set for QSAR model generation (**Figures 1** and **2**). The second set was used as an external test set to validate the QSAR model. These compounds were identified from an *in vitro* screening (GSK PKIS1) and contain 35 compounds including 14 active compounds and 21 inactive compounds (**Figures 10** and **11**) [18]. Seven of the active compounds, for which IC_{50} values were measured (0.04–4.9 μM, **Table 6**), were taken as external test set to further evaluate the predictive power of the QSAR models.

Table 5 provides a comparison of the calculated pIC_{50} versus experimental pIC_{50} values. The calculation of pIC_{50} values was performed by using the QSAR_1, 2, and 3 models. An important statistic parameter to test the predictive power of the QSAR models is the correlation coefficient R^2_{pred} between the predicted and observed pIC_{50} values for the test set [82]. The correlation coefficients between the experimental and predicted pIC_{50} values for the seven test set compounds were quite weak (R^2_{pred} = 0.49, n = 7) when using QSAR_3 model. The predictive power of the QSAR_1 and 2 models was investigated. The correlations of both models were within a similar range (R^2_{pred} = 0.58 and 0.37, n = 7). A further analysis was performed to detect the outliers depending on Z-score values. The Z-score values were calculated using MOE, for QSAR_3. Golbraikh et al. mentioned that at least five compounds are required for a test set to validate a QSAR model [80]. After the analysis of the correlation and Z-scores, compound SB-750140 found to negatively affect the correlation coefficients. The correlation using QSAR_3 shows an improvement (R^2_{pred} = 0.95, RMSD = 0.17 and q^2 = 0.89, n = 6). A similar observation was made for the two other QSAR models (QSAR_1: R^2_{pred} = 0.93, RMSD = 0.21 and q^2 = 0.82, n = 6; QSAR_2: R^2_{pred} = 0.98, RMSD = 0.12 and q^2 = 0.95, n = 6). The outcomes confirm that the generated

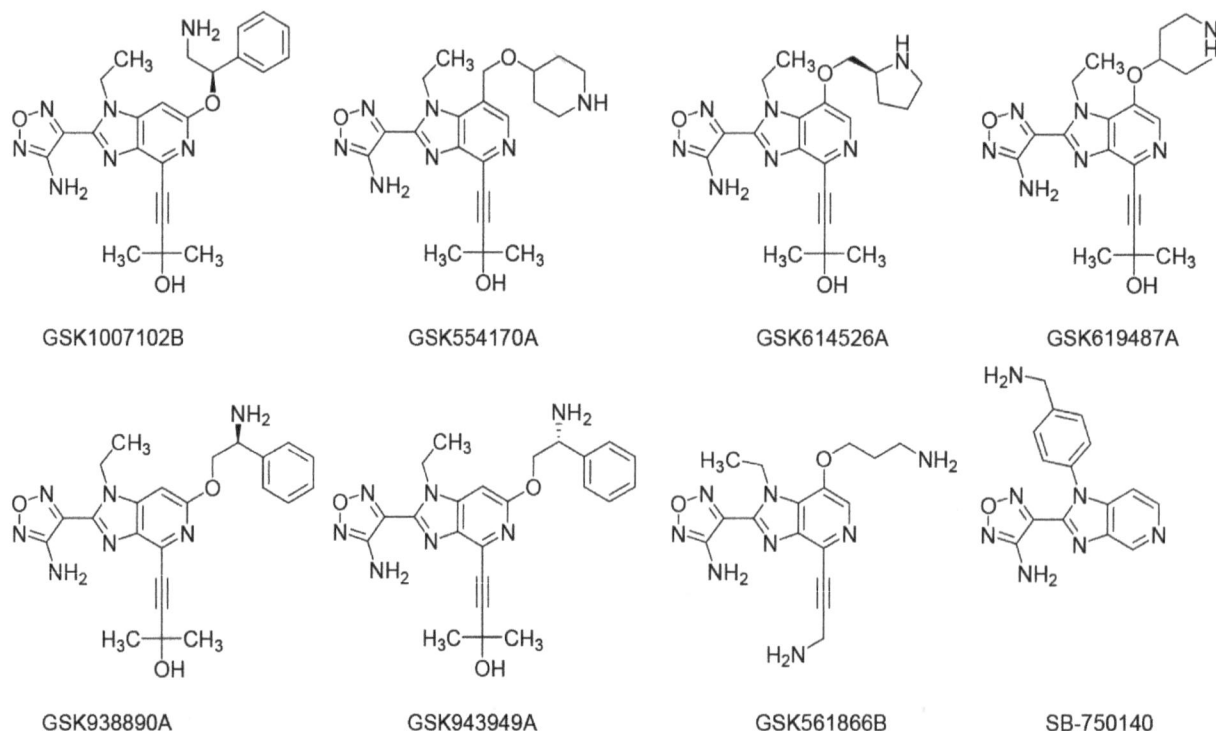

Figure 10. Chemical structures of PRK1 14 actives identified from screening the GSK PKIS1 [18].

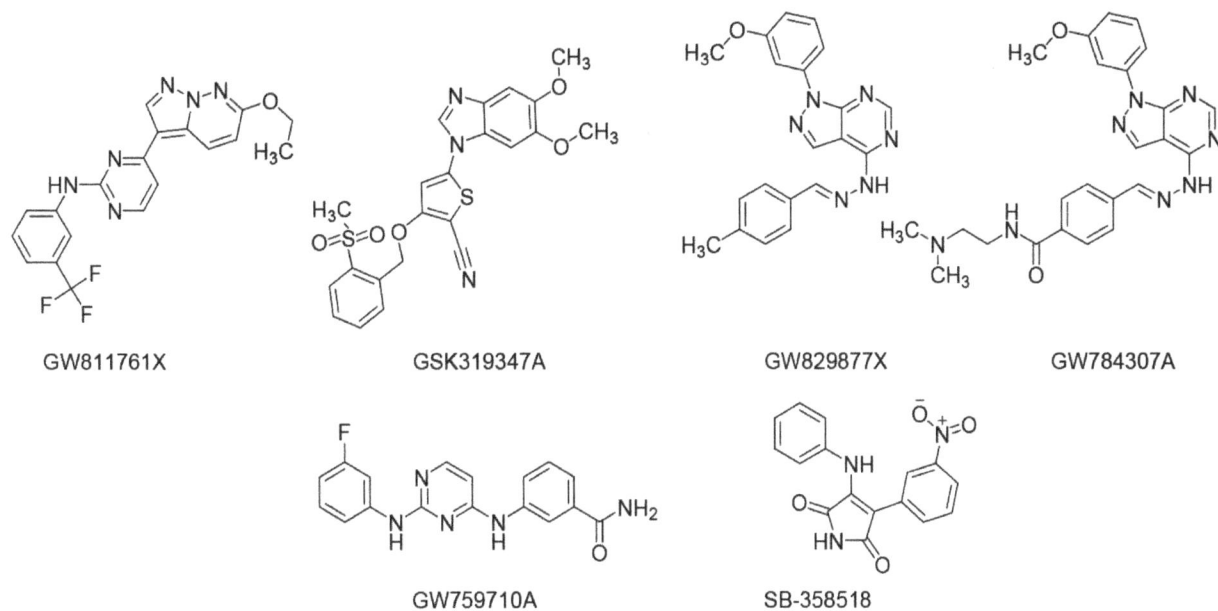

Figure 11. Chemical structures of PRK1 14 actives identified from screening the GSK PKIS1 (continued) [18].

Compound	Binding 1 μM	IC$_{50}$ nM	pIC$_{50}$	Pred. pIC$_{50}$ QSAR_3	Pred.pIC$_{50}$ QSAR_1	Pred. pIC$_{50}$ QSAR_2
GSK943949A	Yes	40	7.40	7.33	7.79	7.99
GSK614526A	Yes	68.1	7.17	7.09	7.68	7.69
SB-750140	Yes	120	6.92	5.70	6.06	5.88
GSK619487A	Yes	181.3	6.74	7.11	7.62	7.65
GSK554170A	Yes	710	6.15	6.34	6.76	7.02
GSK938890A	Yes	3600	5.44	5.67	5.77	6.49
SB-358518	Yes	4900	5.31	5.84	6.16	6.24
GW811761X	Yes	No IC$_{50}$		5.72	5.97	6.05
GW784307A	Yes	No IC$_{50}$		6.86	7.03	7.36
GSK1007102B	Yes	No IC$_{50}$		6.34	6.72	7.21
GSK561866B	Yes	No IC$_{50}$		5.82	6.10	6.45
GSK319347A	Weak	No IC$_{50}$		6.77	6.26	6.96
GW759710A	Weak	No IC$_{50}$		4.99	5.26	5.41
GW829877X	Weak	No IC$_{50}$		5.26	5.52	5.53
GSK1030059A	No			7.66	8.08	7.98
GSK625137A	No			4.16	4.43	4.47
GW290597X	No			6.52	5.67	6.53
GW513184X	No			5.27	5.25	5.55

Compound	Binding 1 μM	IC$_{50}$ nM	pIC$_{50}$	Pred. pIC$_{50}$ QSAR_3	Pred.pIC$_{50}$ QSAR_1	Pred. pIC$_{50}$ QSAR_2
GW643971X	No			5.27	5.19	5.60
GW794607X	No			5.44	5.66	5.71
SB-409514	No			5.13	5.56	5.48
GSK994854A	No			5.93	5.90	6.50
GW874091X	No			5.26	5.65	5.56
GW693481X	No			3.25	3.80	3.92
GSK1000163A	No			6.21	7.02	6.91
GSK1220512A	No			6.03	5.51	6.58
GSK317314A	No			5.94	6.64	6.48
GSK579289A	No			5.14	4.89	5.60
GSK949675A	No			7.20	7.99	7.89
GW580496A	No			6.18	5.37	6.77
SB-476429-A	No			4.68	4.67	4.92
SB-744941	No			4.73	5.52	5.22
GSK571989A	No			6.26	6.42	6.75
GW779439X	No			4.83	4.76	5.35
GSK978744A	No			7.76	7.75	8.10

Table 6. Comparison of the experimental pIC$_{50}$ versus the calculated pIC$_{50}$ using the generated models QSAR_1, 2 and 3 [18].

QSAR models show satisfactory ability to predict the biological activities of the test set compounds. Thus, they could be accepted having an R^2_{pred} value > 0.5 [82]. Moreover, taking the last consideration of the threshold for the predicted pIC$_{50}$ > 7 found in case of actives to refer to potent compounds was clearly in the test set, since the most potent inhibitors in the test set (IC$_{50}$ < 100) were identified with predicted pIC$_{50}$ > 7 (**Table 6**). Meanwhile, the biological activities of the moderately active compounds were predictive with calculated pIC in the range 5.5–7 (**Table 6**). Among the inactive compounds in the test set, three compounds were predicted to be highly potent compounds, but these compounds were inactive in the assay. The visualization of the false positives could not clarify the absence of activity of both compounds. However, GSK978744A and GSK1030059A, which mainly target the PLK kinase, possess the same chemical scaffold, and their binding modes were investigated and compared with the binding modes of analogues co-crystallized with other kinases (CDK2; PDB ID: 2I40, NEK2; PDB ID: 2XNN). However, it is not clear, from structural interactions, why this compound is not active. Additionally, it might possible that the exclusion of entropy changes or solvation of the binding pocket could play a role in the wrong estimation of the biological activity.

Since the QSAR_2 model shows high value of R^2_{pred} in the test set (QSAR_2: R^2_{pred} = 0.98, RMSD = 0.12 and q^2 = 0.95, n = 6), the discrimination performance was therefore discussed. Similar to QSAR_3, the most potent inhibitors in the test set (IC$_{50}$ < 100) were identified with predicted pIC$_{50}$ > 7

(**Table 6**). Furthermore, between the remaining active compounds, two of them were predicted to be high potent inhibitors $pIC_{50} > 7$ (GW784307A: predicted $pIC_{50} = 7.36$; GSK1007102B: predicted $pIC_{50} = 7.21$). However, the IC_{50} values of these two compounds have not been measured yet, but it reported to be active since it binds to PRK1 at 1 μM. Thus, the consideration of the threshold for the predicted $pIC_{50} > 7$ could also be applicable in the QSAR_2 model. The weak active compounds GSK319347A, GW759710A, and GW829877X (shown in **Table 6**) also predicted as moderate or low active compounds where predicted pIC_{50} values were less than 7. Among the inactive compounds, three compounds (the same compounds as in the case of the QSAR_3 model) were predicted to be highly potent compounds, but these compounds were inactive in the assay.

$$QSAR\_2 : pIC_{50} = 0.15509 - 0.09778$$
$$*PEOE\_PC - -0.09778 * MM\text{-}GBSA \tag{1}$$
$$\left(R^2 = 0.70, RMSE = 0.78\, q^2 = 0.62,\ n = 26\right)$$

$$QSAR\_3 : pIC_{50} = -1.37129 - 0.56938 * PEOE\_PC-$$
$$-0.08688 * MM\text{-}GBSA - 0.26312 * GLIDE\_SP \tag{2}$$
$$\left(R^2 = 0.71, RMSE = 0.76 \text{ and } q^2 = 0.63, n = 26\right)$$

By comparing the three generated QSAR models (QSAR_1, 2, and 3) depending on the predicted pIC_{50} values among them to the measured ones, it was found the predicted pIC_{50} values when using QSAR_3 model were closer to the experimental values (**Table 6**), but QSAR_2 model showed the highest value of R^2_{pred} in the test set. Furthermore, in bootstrap validation, it was found that the QSAR_3 model had the ability to predict the biological activity of the test set compounds more accurately than the models QSAR_1 and 2 (**Table 6**). Thus, the QSAR_3 model could be used to predict the biological activities of the highly potent compounds, which should exhibit biological activities power in the nanomolar range and differentiate between the active compounds, according to their activity (low, moderate, and high).

3.7. Virtual screening using the p-ANAPL library

The above protocol was further used to virtually screen for possible PRK1 inhibitors from the p-ANAPL library [58]. As previously applied, ensemble docking was performed to dock the compounds to the X-ray structures of PRK1 stored in the PDB. Both data sets were prepared using Schrödinger 2014.U2, including the generation of several conformations per compound. The docking solutions were visualized using MOE to explore the conserved interactions with residues at the PRK1 hinge region. The selection of the hits was based first on the displayed binding mode, followed by their scoring, then predicting the pIC_{50} values using the generated QSAR models. Depending only on docking scores was insignificant for the selection of promising hit compounds. The docking solutions for the entire data set were visualized and several hits compounds were selected. In the next step, their predicted pIC_{50} values were calculated using QSAR_1, 2, and 3. Depending on the set threshold for the predicted pIC_{50}, several top scoring compounds could be selected as promising hits for the biological assays, e.g., those in **Figure 12**. **Figure 13** displays the binding modes of the selected hits and the interaction with residues at the binding pocket of the corresponding X-ray structure of PRK1.

One of the promising hits, DBT-6b, is Bartericin B (MW = 408.49; PubChem CID: 12136210) from *Dorstenia barteri* [83]. The binding mode of DBT-6b is shown in **Figure 13A**. The compound is predicted to interact with hinge region residue Ser704 with one H bond. The phenol ring forms an additional H bond with the backbone of Asp764 from the DFG-motif. The interaction with the front polar pocket and the ribose binding pocket is mediated by two H bonds between Asp708 and propanol substituent in DBT-6b. The calculated pIC_{50} values were 7.85, 7.64, and 7.45 using the generated QSAR models QSAR_1, 2, and 3, respectively. The second hit (P87), vitexin or apigenin-8-C glucoside (MW = 432.38; PubChem CID: 5280441), is a flavonoid glycoside from diverse sources, e.g., *Hyparrhenia hirta* [84]. The binding mode of P87 (**Figure 13B**) shows that the compound might form one H bond with the hinge region residue Ser704. Additionally, the substituents on the

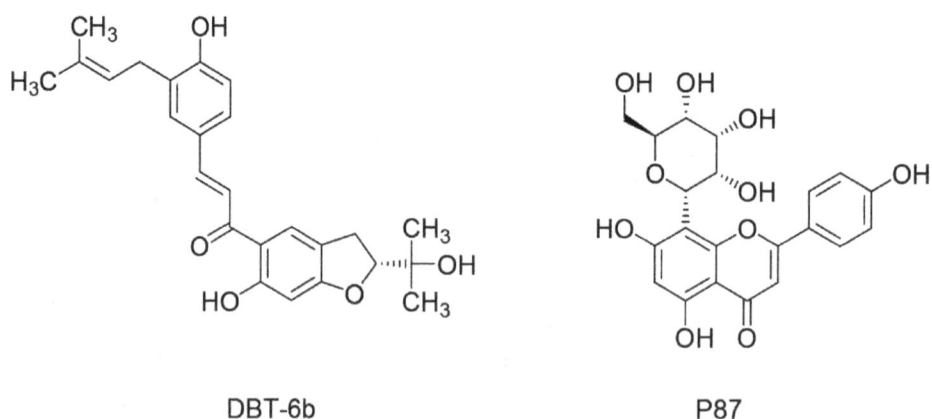

Figure 12. Chemical structures of the selected hits.

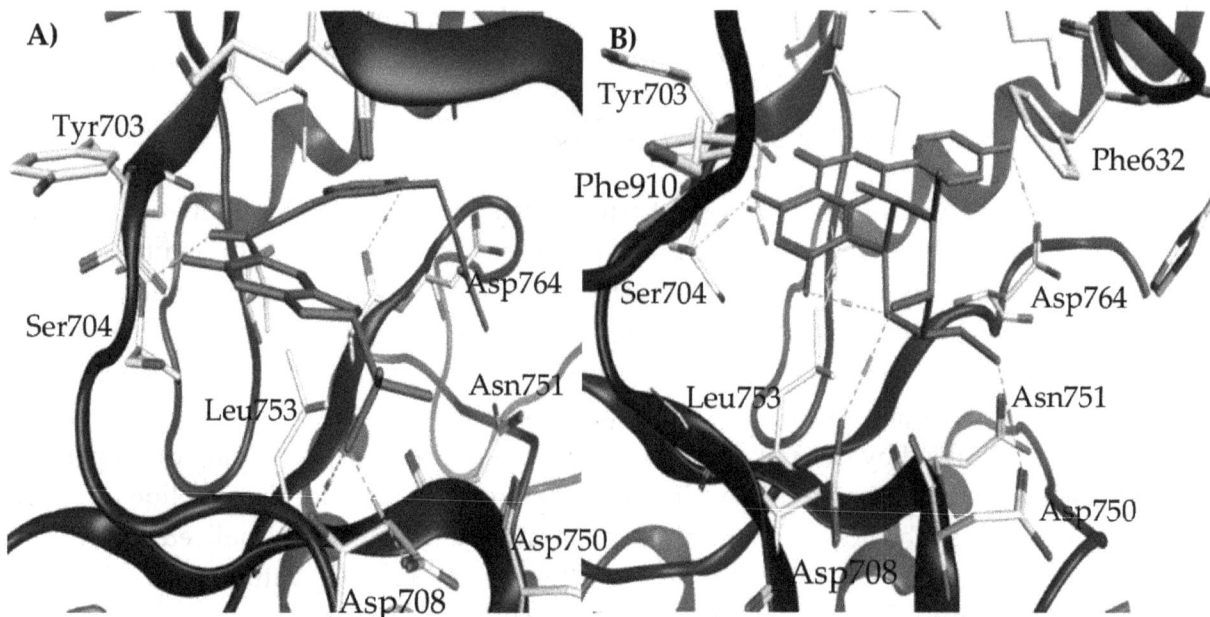

Figure 13. Docking poses of the selected hits in PRK1 binding pocket. (A) Docking poses of DBT-6b in the binding pocket of PRK1 structure 4OTG. (B) Docking pose of P87 in PRK1 structure 4OTH. The figure was designed using MOE.

oxane ring are targeting the front polar pocket and forming two H bonds with Asp708 and Asp750. The phenyl ring interacts with the back hydrophobic pocket and further forms an H bond with Asp764 in the DFG motif. P87 was predicted to be a highly potent compound, with a predicted pIC_{50} value greater than 7, using QSAR models (pred_pIC_{50}= 8.02, 8.6, and 9, respectively). Bartericin B and vitexin are the only two examples of promising compounds from natural products which could target PRK1. Among the screened databases, other hits were selected as promising compounds, which could inhibit PRK1 activity in the nanomolar range. In further investigations, the selected compounds can be submitted for biological assay to figure out their ability to bind into PRK1.

4. Conclusions

This chapter provides a brief summary of database resources for anticancer drug discovery and some recent inputs and success stories for the identification novel inhibitors of selected anticancer drug targets by the use of computer modeling. While the experimental validation of some of the natural product hits identified in the case study is ongoing, the question about the applicability domains of the derived QSAR models reported is still to be answered. Among the identified hits, 50 closely similar compounds to Bartericin B (with cut-off Tanimoto coefficient of 0.7), having reported biological activities in PubChem [59] and ChEMBL [44], with 239 biological activities and 152 published patent data. A similarity search of vitexin in PubChem gives 112 similar compounds, corresponding to 524 biological activities and 208 patents. Bartericin B is known to exhibit antimicrobial activities against *Trichomonas gallinarum*, with minimum lethal concentrations (MLCs) of 0.244 and 0.121 μg/mL after 24 H and 48 H, respectively [83], while its analogue (Bartericin A from *Dorstenia angusticornis*) is known to be very active against some bacteria and yeasts associated with human pathologies [85]. Both chalcones are known to also have potential antiprotozoal activities [86], e.g., against *Plasmodium falciparum* [87]. Vitexin, on the other hand, is known for its antioxidative and [88] spasmolytic effects [89]. The compound is known to be abundant in plants of the genus *Vitex* (Verbenaceae), which is known to exert insect antifeeding activities, among others [90]. These compounds could now be tested in biological assays for potential PRK1 inhibition.

Acknowledgements

A.N. is currently a doctoral candidate financed by the German Academic Exchange Services (DAAD), Germany. F.N.K. acknowledges a Georg Forster fellowship from the Alexander von Humboldt Foundation, Germany.

Competing interests

The authors declare that they have no competing interests.

List of abbreviations

AfroCancer	African Anticancer Natural Products Database
BFE	Binding free energy
EC_{50}	Half maximal effective concentration, i.e., the concentration of a drug, antibody or toxicant which induces a response halfway between the baseline and maximum after a specified exposure time
ED_{50}	The median effective dose, a dose that produces the desired effect in 50% of a population
GI_{50}	The growth inhibition of 50%, drug concentration resulting in a 50% reduction in the net protein increase
IC_{50}	The drug concentration causing 50% inhibition of the desired activity
NANPDB	Northern African Natural Products Database
NP	Natural product
NPACT	Naturally Occurring Plant-based Anti-cancer Compound Activity-Target Database
p-ANAPL	Pan-African natural products library
PDB	Protein databank
PLS	Partial least squares
PRK1	protein kinase C–related kinase
QSAR	Quantitative structure-activity relationship
RMSD	Root mean square deviation
RMSE	Root mean square error
SM	Secondary metabolite
VS	Virtual screening

Author details

Abdulkarim Najjar[1], Fidele Ntie-Kang[1,2]* and Wolfgang Sippl[1]

*Address all correspondence to: ntiekfidele@gmail.com

1 Department of Pharmaceutical Chemistry, Martin-Luther University of Halle-Wittenberg, Halle (Saale), Germany

2 Department of Chemistry, University of Buea, Buea, Cameroon and Department of Pharmaceutical Chemistry, Martin-Luther University of Halle-Wittenberg, Halle, Germany

References

[1] Hanahan D. Rethinking the war on cancer. Lancet. 2014;**383**:558-563. DOI: 10.1016/S0140-6736(13)62226-6

[2] Cragg GM, Grothaus PG, Newman DJ. Impact of natural products on developing new anti-cancer agents. Chemical Reviews. 2009;**109**:3012-3043. DOI: 10.1021/cr900019j

[3] Newman DJ, Cragg GM. Natural products as sources of new drugs from 1981 to 2014. Journal of Natural Products. 2016;**79**:629-661. DOI: 10.1021/acs.jnatprod.5b01055

[4] Harvey AL, Edrada-Ebel R, Quinn RJ. The re-emergence of natural products for drug discovery in the genomics era. Natural Reviews Drug Discovery. 2015;**14**:111-129. DOI: 10.1038/nrd4510

[5] Ntie-Kang F, Lifongo LL, Judson PN, Sippl W, Efange SMN. How "drug-like" are naturally occurring anti-cancer compounds?. Journal of Molecular Modeling. 2014;**20**:2069. DOI: 10.1007/s00894-014-2069-z

[6] Rodrigues T, Reker D, Schneider P, Schneider G. Counting on natural products for drug design. Natural Chemistry. 2016;**8**:531-541. DOI: 10.1038/nchem.2479

[7] Mangal M, Sagar P, Singh H, Raghava GP, Agarwal SM. NPACT: Naturally occurring plant-based anti-cancer compound-activity-target database. Nucleic Acids Research. 2013;**41**:D1124-D1129. DOI: 10.1093/nar/gks1047

[8] American Cancer Society, 2013. Cancer Facts & Figures. 2013. https://www.cancer.org/content/dam/cancer-org/research/cancer-facts-and-statistics/annual-cancer-facts-and-figures/2013/cancer-facts-and-figures-2013.pdf (Accessed 27-01-2017)

[9] Jilg CA, Ketscher A, Metzger E, Hummel B, Willmann D, et al. PRK1/PKN1 controls migration and metastasis of androgen-independent prostate cancer cells. Oncotarget. 2014;**5**:12646-12664. DOI: 10.18632/oncotarget.2653

[10] Heinlein CA, Chang C. Androgen receptor in prostate cancer. Endocrine Reviews. 2004;**25**:276-308. DOI: 10.1210/er.2002-0032

[11] Lonergan PE, Tindall DJ. Androgen receptor signaling in prostate cancer development and progression. Journal of Carcinogensis. 2011;**10**:20. DOI: 10.4103/1477-3163.83937

[12] Metzger E, Yin N, Wissmann M, Kunowska N, Fischer K, et al. Phosphorylation of histone H3 at threonine 11 establishes a novel chromatin mark for transcriptional regulation. Nature Cell Biology. 2008;**10**:53-60. DOI: 10.1038/ncb1668

[13] Wissmann M, Yin N, Müller JM, Greschik H, Fodor BD, et al. Cooperative demethylation by JMJD2C and LSD1 promotes androgen receptor-dependent gene expression. Nature Cell Biology. 2007;**9**:347-353. DOI: 10.1038/ncb1546

[14] Di Croce L, Shiekhattar R. Thrilling transcription through threonine phosphorylation. Natural Cell Biology. 2008;**10**:5-6. DOI: 10.1038/ncb0108-5

[15] Lachmann S, Jevons A, De Rycker M, Casamassima A, Radtke S, et al. Regulatory domain selectivity in the cell-type specific PKN-dependence of cell migration. PLoS One. 2011;**6**:e21732. DOI: 10.1371/journal.pone.0021732

[16] Turner EC, Kavanagh DJ, Mulvaney EP, McLean C, Wikström K, et al. Identification of an interaction between the TPα and TPβ isoforms of the human thromboxane A2 receptor with protein kinase C-related kinase (PRK) 1: implications for prostate cancer. Journal of Biological Chemistry. 2011;**286**:15440-15457. DOI: 10.1074/jbc.M110.181180

[17] Köhler J, Erlenkamp G, Eberlin A, Rumpf T, Slynko I, et al. Lestaurtinib inhibits histone phosphorylation and androgen-dependent gene expression in prostate cancer cells. PLoS One. 2012;**7**:e34973. DOI: 10.1371/journal.pone.0034973

[18] Slynko I, Schmidtkunz K, Rumpf T, Klaeger S, Heinzlmeir S, et al. Identification of highly potent protein kinase C-related kinase 1 inhibitors by virtual screening, binding free energy rescoring, and *in vitro* testing. ChemMedChem. 2016;**11**:2084-2094. DOI: 10.1002/cmdc.201600284

[19] Slynko I, Scharfe M, Rumpf T, Eib J, Metzger E, et al. Virtual screening of PRK1 inhibitors: Ensemble docking, rescoring using binding free energy calculation and QSAR model development. Journal of Chemical Information and Modeling. 2014;**54**:138-150. DOI: 10.1021/ci400628q

[20] Mukai H, Ono Y. A novel protein kinase with leucine zipper-like sequences: Its catalytic domain is highly homologous to that of protein kinase C. Biochemical and Biophysical Research Communications. 1994;**199**:897-904. DOI: 10.1006/bbrc.1994.1313

[21] Mukai H. The structure and function of PKN, a protein kinase having a catalytic domain homologous to that of PKC. Journal of Biochemistry. 2003;**133**:17-27. PMID: 12761194

[22] Lim WG, Tan BJ, Zhu Y, Zhou S, Armstrong JS, et al. The very C-terminus of PRK1/PKN is essential for its activation by RhoA and downstream signaling. Cell Signal. 2006 Sep;**18**(9):1473-1481. DOI: 10.1016/j.cellsig.2005.11.009

[23] Kannan N, Haste N, Taylor SS, Neuwald AF. The hallmark of AGC kinase functional divergence is its C-terminal tail, a *cis*-acting regulatory module. Proceedings of National Academy Science USA. 2007;**104**:1272-1277. DOI: 10.1073/pnas.0610251104

[24] Chamberlain P, Delker S, Pagarigan B, Mahmoudi A, Jackson P, et al. Crystal structures of PRK1 in complex with the clinical compounds lestaurtinib and tofacitinib reveal ligand induced conformational changes. PLoS One. 2014;**9**:e103638. DOI: 10.1371/journal.pone.0103638

[25] Metzger E, Müller JM, Ferrari S, Buettner R, Schüle R. A novel inducible transactivation domain in the androgen receptor: implications for PRK in prostate cancer. EMBO Journal. 2003;**22**:270-280. DOI: 10.1093/emboj/cdg023

[26] Rester U. From virtuality to reality - Virtual screening in lead discovery and lead optimization: a medicinal chemistry perspective. Current Opinion in Drug Discovery and Developments. 2008;**11**:559-568. PMID: 18600572

[27] Rollinger JM, Stuppner H, Langer T. Virtual screening for the discovery of bioactive natural products. Progress in Drug Research. 2008;**65**:211,213-249. PMID: 18084917

[28] Lavecchia A, Di Giovanni C. Virtual screening strategies in drug discovery: A critical review. Current Medicinal Chemistry. 2013;**20**:2839-2860. DOI: 10.2174/09298673113209990001

[29] Heikamp K, Bajorath J. The future of virtual compound screening. Chemical Biology and Drug Design. 2013;**81**:33-40. DOI: 10.1111/cbdd.12054

[30] Schneider G. Virtual screening: An endless staircase?. Natural Reviws Drug Discovery. 2010;**9**:273-276. DOI: 10.1038/nrd3139

[31] McInnes C. Virtual screening strategies in drug discovery. Current Opinion in Chemical Biology. 2007;**11**:494-502. DOI: 10.1016/j.cbpa.2007.08.033

[32] Cheng T, Li Q, Zhou Z, Wang Y, Bryant SH. Structure-based virtual screening for drug discovery: A problem-centric review. AAPS Journal. 2012;**14**:133-141. DOI: 10.1208/s12248-012-9322-0

[33] Sun H. Pharmacophore-based virtual screening. Current Medicinal Chemistry. 2008;**15**:1018-1024. DOI: 10.2174/092986708784049630

[34] Ripphausen P, Nisius B, Bajorath J. State-of-the-art in ligand-based virtual screening. Drug Discovery Today. 2011;**16**:372-376. DOI: 10.1016/j.drudis.2011.02.011

[35] Anighoro A, Bajorath J. Three-dimensional similarity in molecular docking: prioritizing ligand poses on the basis of experimental binding modes. Journal of Chemical Information and Modeling. 2016;**56**:580-587. DOI: 10.1021/acs.jcim.5b00745

[36] Ballester PJ, Westwood I, Laurieri N, Sim E, Richards WG. Prospective virtual screening with ultrafast shape recognition: The identification of novel inhibitors of arylamine N-acetyltransferases. Journal of Royal Society Interface. 2010;**7**:335-342. DOI: 10.1098/rsif.2009.0170

[37] Li GB, Yang LL, Yuan Y, Zou J, Cao Y, et al. Virtual screening in small molecule discovery for epigenetic targets. Methods. 2015;**71**:158-166. DOI: 10.1016/j.ymeth.2014.11.010

[38] Verma J, Khedkar VM, Coutinho EC. 3D-QSAR in drug design - A review. Current Topics in Medicinal Chemistry. 2010;**10**:95-115. DOI: 10.2174/156802610790232260

[39] Winkler DA. The role of quantitative structure - activity relationships (QSAR) in biomolecular discovery. Briefings in Bioinformatics. 2002;**3**:73-86. PMID: 12002226

[40] Ntie-Kang F, Nwodo JN, Ibezim A, Simoben CV, Karaman B, et al. Molecular modeling of potential anticancer agents from African medicinal plants. Journal of Chemical Information and Modeling. 2014;**54**:2433-2450. DOI: 10.1021/ci5003697

[41] Kumar R, Chaudhary K, Gupta S, Singh H, Kumar S, et al. CancerDR: Cancer drug resistance database. Scientific Reports. 2013;**3**:1445. DOI: 10.1038/srep01445

[42] Tao W, Li B, Gao S, Bai Y, Shar PA, et al. CancerHSP: Anticancer herbs database of systems pharmacology. Scientific Reports. 2015;**5**:11481. DOI: 10.1038/srep11481

[43] Hastings J, Owen G, Dekker A, Ennis M, Kale N, et al. ChEBI in 2016: Improved services and an expanding collection of metabolites. Nucleic Acids Research. 2016;**44**:D1214-D1219. DOI: 10.1093/nar/gkv1031

[44] Gaulton A, Hersey A, Nowotka M, Bento AP, Chambers J, et al. The ChEMBL database in 2017. Nucleic Acids Research. 2017;**45**:D945-D954. DOI: 10.1093/nar/gkw1074

[45] Fang X, Shao L, Zhang H, Wang S. CHMIS-C: A comprehensive herbal medicine information system for cancer. Journal of Medicinal Chemistry. 2005;**48**:1481-1488. DOI: 10.1021/jm049838d

[46] Wishart DS, Knox C, Guo AC, Shrivastava S, Hassanali M, Stothard P, Chang Z, Woolsey J. DrugBank: A comprehensive resource for *in silico* drug discovery and exploration. Nucleic Acids Research. 2006;**34**:D668-D672. DOI: 10.1093/nar/gkj067

[47] Mysinger MM, Carchia M, Irwin JJ, Shoichet BK. Directory of useful decoys, enhanced (DUD-E): Better ligands and decoys for better benchmarking. Journal Medicinal Chemistry. 2012;**55**:6582-6594. DOI: 10.1021/jm300687e

[48] Loharch S, Bhutani I, Jain K, Gupta P, Sahoo DK, Parkesh R. EpiDBase: A manually curated database for small molecule modulators of epigenetic landscape. Database (Oxford). 2015;**2015**.pii: bav013. DOI: 10.1093/database/bav013

[49] Vetrivel U, Subramanian N, Pilla K. InPACdb - Indian plant anticancer compounds database. Bioinformation. 2009;**4**:71-74. PMID: 20198172

[50] Ashfaq UA, Mumtaz A, Qamar TU, Fatima T. MAPS database: Medicinal plant activities. Phytochemical and structural database. Bioinformation. 2013;**9**:993-995. DOI: 10.6026/97320630009993

[51] Ntie-Kang F, Telukunta KK, Döring K, Simoben CV, Moumbock, et al. The Northern African Natural Products Database (NANPDB); 2017. www.african-compounds.org/nanpdb/

[52] Milne GW, Nicklaus MC, Driscoll JS, Wang S, Zaharevitz D. National cancer institute drug information system 3D database. Journal of Chemical Information and Computer Science. 1994;**34**:1219-1224. DOI: 10.1021/ci00021a032

[53] Ko Y, Tan SL, Chan A, Wong YP, Yong WP, et al. Prevalence of the coprescription of clinically important interacting drug combinations involving oral anticancer agents in Singapore: A retrospective database study. Clinical Therapy. 2012;**34**:1696-1704. DOI: 10.1016/j.clinthera.2012.06.025

[54] Hatherley R, Brown DK, Musyoka TM, Penkler DL, Faya N, et al. SANCDB: A South African natural compound database. Journal of Cheminformatics. 2015;**7**:29. DOI: 10.1186/s13321-015-0080-8

[55] Goede A, Dunkel M, Mester N, Frommel C, Preissner R. SuperDrug: A conformational drug database. Bioinformatics. 2005;**21**:1751-1753. DOI: 10.1093/bioinformatics/bti295

[56] Rammensee H, Bachmann J, Emmerich NP, Bachor OA, Stevanović S. SYFPEITHI: Database for MHC ligands and peptide motifs. Immunogenetics. 1999;**50**:213-219. DOI: 10.1007/s002510050595

[57] Lin YC, Wang CC, Chen IS, Jheng JL, Li JH, et al. TIPdb: A database of anticancer, antiplatelet, and antituberculosis phytochemicals from indigenous plants in Taiwan. Scientific World Journal. 2013;**2013**:736386. DOI: 10.1155/2013/736386

[58] Ntie-Kang F, Amoa Onguéné P, Fotso GW, Andrae-Marobela K, Bezabih M, et al. Virtualizing the p-ANAPL library: A step towards drug discovery from African medicinal plants. PLoS One. 2014;**9**:e90655. DOI: 10.1371/journal.pone.0090655

[59] Kim S, Thiessen PA, Bolton EE, Chen J, Fu G, et al. PubChem substance and compound databases. Nucleic Acids Research. 2016;**44**:D1202-D1213. DOI: 10.1093/nar/gkv951

[60] Sterling T, Irwin JJ. ZINC 15 - ligand discovery for everyone. Journal of Chemical Information and Modeling. 2015;**55**(11):2324-2327. DOI: 10.1021/acs.jcim.5b00559

[61] Ha H, Debnath B, Odde S, Bensman T, Ho H, et al. Discovery of novel CXCR2 inhibitors using ligand-based pharmacophore models. Journal of Chemical Information and Modeling. 2015;**55**:1720-1738. DOI: 10.1021/acs.jcim.5b00181

[62] Zhu YM, Webster SJ, Flower D, Woll PJ. Interleukin-8/CXCL8 is a growth factor for human lung cancer cells. British Journal of Cancer. 2004;**91**:1970-1976. DOI: 10.1038/sj.bjc.6602227

[63] Rubie C, Kollmar O, Frick VO, Wagner M, Brittner B, et al. Differential CXC receptor expression in colorectal carcinomas. Scandinavian Journal of Immunology. 2008;**68**:635-644. DOI: 10.1111/j.1365-3083.2008.02163.x

[64] Murphy C, McGurk M, Pettigrew J, Santinelli A, Mazzucchelli R, et al. Nonapical and cytoplasmic expression of interleukin-8, CXCR1, and CXCR2 correlates with cell proliferation and microvessel density in prostate cancer. Clinical Cancer Research. 2005 ;**11**:4117-4127. DOI: 10.1158/1078-0432.CCR-04-1518

[65] Yang G, Rosen DG, Liu G, Yang F, Guo X, et al. CXCR2 promotes ovarian cancer growth through dysregulated cell cycle, diminished apoptosis, and enhanced angiogenesis. Clinical Cancer Research. 2010;**16**:3875-3886. DOI: 10.1158/1078-0432.CCR-10-0483

[66] Kumar AV, Mohan K, Riyaz S. Structure guided inhibitor designing of CDK2 and discovery of potential leads against cancer. Journal of Molecular Modeling. 2013;**19**:3581-3589. DOI: 10.1007/s00894-013-1887-8

[67] Al-Sha'er MA, Khanfar MA, Taha MO. Discovery of novel urokinase plasminogen activator (uPA) inhibitors using ligand-based modeling and virtual screening followed by *in vitro* analysis. Journal of Molecular Modeling. 2014;**20**:2080. DOI: 10.1007/s00894-014-2080-4

[68] Ren JX, Li LL, Zheng RL, Xie HZ, Cao ZX, et al. Discovery of novel Pim-1 kinase inhibitors by a hierarchical multistage virtual screening approach based on SVM model, pharmacophore, and molecular docking. Journal of Chemical Information and Modeling. 2011;**51**:1364-1375. DOI: 10.1021/ci100464b

[69] Li L, Khanna M, Jo I, Wang F, Ashpole NM, et al. Target-specific support vector machine scoring in structure-based virtual screening: Computational validation, in vitro testing in kinases, and effects on lung cancer cell proliferation. Journal of Chemical Information and Modeling. 2011;**51**:755-759. DOI: 10.1021/ci100490w

[70] Khanfar MA, Taha MO. Elaborate ligand-based modeling coupled with multiple linear regression and k nearest neighbor QSAR analyses unveiled new nanomolar mTOR

inhibitors. Journal of Chemical Information and Modeling. 2013;**53**:2587-2612. DOI: 10.1021/ci4003798

[71] B-Rao C, Subramanian J, Sharma SD. Managing protein flexibility in docking and its applications. Drug Discovery Today. 2009;**14**:394-400. DOI: 10.1016/j.drudis.2009.01.003

[72] Bjerrum EJ. Machine learning optimization of cross docking accuracy. Computational Biology and Chemistry. 2016;**62**:133-144. DOI: 10.1016/j.compbiolchem.2016.04.005

[73] Tan C, Yang L, Luo R. How well does Poisson-Boltzmann implicit solvent agree with explicit solvent? A quantitative analysis. Journal of Physical Chemistry B. 2006;**110**:18680-18687. DOI: 10.1021/jp063479b.

[74] Wang J, Tan C, Chanco E, Luo R. Quantitative analysis of Poisson-Boltzmann implicit solvent in molecular dynamics. Physical Chemistry Chemical Physics. 2010;**12**:1194-1202. DOI: 10.1039/b917775b

[75] Mateos-Aparicio G. Partial least squares (PLS) methods: Origins, evolution, and application to social sciences. Communications in Statistics - Theory and Methods. 2011;**40**:2305-2317. DOI: 10.1080/03610921003778225

[76] Gasteiger J, Marsili M. Iterative partial equalization of orbital electronegativity-A rapid access to atomic charges. Tetrahedron. 1980;**36**:3219-3228. DOI: 10.1016/0040-4020(80)80168-2

[77] Kiralj R, Ferreira MMC. 2009. Basic validation procedures for regression models in QSAR and QSPR studies: Theory and application. Journal of Brazilian Chemical Society. 2009;**20**:770-787. DOI: 10.1590/S0103-50532009000400021

[78] Veerasamy R, Rajak H, Jain A, Sivadasan S, Varghese CP, et al. Validation of QSAR models - Strategies and importance. International Journal of Drug Design Discovery. 2011;**2**:511-519

[79] Golbraikh A, Tropsha A. Predictive QSAR modeling based on diversity sampling of experimental datasets for the training and test set selection. Molecular Diversity. 2002;**5**:231-243. PMID: 12549674

[80] Golbraikh A, Tropsha A. Beware of q^2! Journal of Molecular Graphics and Modeling. 2002;**20**: 269-276. DOI: 10.1016/S1093-3263(01)00123-1

[81] Nahum OE, Yosipof A, Senderowitz H. A multi-objective genetic algorithm for outlier removal. Journal of Chemical Information Modeling. 2015;**55**:2507-2518. DOI: 10.1021/acs.jcim.5b00515

[82] Pratim Roy P, Paul S, Mitra I, Roy K. On two novel parameters for validation of predictive QSAR models. Molecules. 2009;**14**:1660-1701. DOI: 10.3390/molecules14051660

[83] Omisore NOA, Adewunmi CO, Iwalewa EO, Ngadjui BT, Adenowo TK, et al. Antitrichomonal and antioxidant activities of *Dorstenia barteri* and *Dorstenia convexa*. Brazilian Journal of Medical and Biological Research. 2005;**38**:1087-1094. DOI: 10.1590/S0100-879X2005000700012

[84] Bouaziz M, Simmonds MS, Grayer RJ, Kite GC, Damak M. Flavonoids from *Hyparrhenia hirta* Stapf (Poaceae) growing in Tunisia. Biochemical Systematics and Ecology. 2001;**29**:849-851. DOI: 10.1016/S0305-1978(01)00028-X

[85] Kuete V, Konga Simo I, Ngameni B, Bigoga DJ, Watchueng J, et al. Antimicrobial activity of the methanolic extract, fractions and four flavonoids from the twigs of *Dorstenia angusticornis* Engl. (Moraceae). Journal of Ethnopharmacology. 2007;**112**:271-277. DOI:10.1016/j.jep.2007.12.017

[86] Fotie J. The antiprotozoan potential of flavonoids. Pharmacognosy Reviews. 2008;**2**:6-19

[87] Ngameni B, Watchueng J, Boyom FF, Keumedjio F, Ngadjui BT, et al. Antimalarial prenylated chalcones from the twigs of *Dorstenia barteri* var. *subtriangularis*. Arkivoc. 2007;**13**:116-123

[88] Kim JH, Lee BC, Kim JH, Sim GS, Lee DH, et al. The isolation and antioxidative effects of vitexin from *Acer palmatum*. Archives of Pharmacal Research. 2005 ;28:195. DOI:10.1007/BF02977715

[89] Ragone MI, Sella M, Conforti P, Volonté MG, Consolini AE. The spasmolytic effect of *Aloysia citriodora*, Palau (South American cedrón) is partially due to its vitexin but not isovitexin on rat duodenums. Journal of Ethnopharmacology. 2007;**113**:258-266. DOI: 10.1016/j.jep.2007.06.003

[90] Hernández MM, Heraso C, Villarreal ML, Vargas-Arispuro I, Aranda E. Biological activities of crude plant extracts from *Vitex trifolia* L. (Verbenaceae). Journal of Ethnopharmacology. 1999;**67**:37-44. DOI: 10.1016/S0378-8741(99)00041-0

Phytocompounds Targeting Cancer Angiogenesis using the Chorioallantoic Membrane Assay

Stefana Avram, Roxana Ghiulai, Ioana Zinuca Pavel,
Marius Mioc, Roxana Babuta, Mirela Voicu,
Dorina Coricovac, Corina Danciu,
Cristina Dehelean and Codruta Soica

Abstract

Cancer is the second cause of mortality worldwide. Angiogenesis is an important process involved in the growth of primary tumors and metastasis. New approaches for controlling the cancer progression and invasiveness can be addressed by limiting the angiogenesis process. An increasingly large number of natural compounds are evaluated as angiogenesis inhibitors. The chorioallantoic membrane (CAM) assay represents an *in vivo* attractive experimental model for cancer and angiogenesis studies as prescreening to the murine models. Since the discovery of tumor angiogenesis, the CAM has been intensively used in cancer research. The advantages of this *in vivo* technique are in terms of low time-consuming, costs, and a lower number of sacrificed animals. Currently, a great number of natural compounds are being investigated for their effectiveness in controlling tumor angiogenesis. Potential reducing of angiogenesis has been investigated by our group for pentacyclic triterpenes, in various formulations, and differences in their mechanism were registered. This chapter aims to give an overview on a number of phytocompounds investigated using *in vitro*, murine models and the chorioallantoic membrane assay as well as to emphasize the use of CAM assay in the study of natural compounds with potential effects in malignancies.

Keywords: phytocompounds, tumor angiogenesis, chorioallantoic membrane assay

1. Introduction

Angiogenesis represents the process by which new vessels are formed from preexisting vessels [1] and has important implications associated with tumor growth and metastasis [2]. Studies have shown that neovascularization is essential for tumor survival and growth, whereas in angiogenic absent conditions, tumor may display necrosis or even apoptosis [3, 4]. The angiogenic switch represents the process in which endothelial cells are led to a rapid growth state induced by stimuli secreted by the tumor microenvironment, comprising tumor and stromal cells, extracellular matrix components, immunologic cells, fibroblasts, adipocytes, muscle cells, and pericytes [5]. The switch may also involve downregulation of endogenous inhibitors of angiogenesis such as endostatin, angiostatin, or thrombospondin.

The undergoing of tumor angiogenesis represents a four-step process [6]: (i) tissue basement membrane injury; (ii) migration of endothelial cells, activated by angiogenic factors; (iii) endothelial cell proliferation and stabilization; (iv) continuous angiogenesis induced by angiogenic factors. Therefore, key elements in the angiogenesis process are the endogenous angiogenic factors. The most relevant angiogenic activators, signal mediators, and signaling effects are represented in **Figure 1**.

A class of proteins that is widely responsible for tumor angiogenesis is represented by growth factors, such as the vascular endothelial growth factor (VEGF), fibroblast growth factor (FGF), platelet-derived endothelial growth factor (PDGF), tumor necrosis factor-α (TNF-α), epidermal growth factor (EGF), placental growth factor (PGF), transforming growth factor (TGF), granulocyte colony stimulating factor (GCSF), hepatocyte growth factor (HGF), angiostatin, and angiogenin [7]. However, VEGF is thought to be the main proangiogenic growth factor, because it induces all four phases of angiogenesis by augmenting vascular permeability, endothelial cell proliferation, endothelial cell migration, and capillary like tube formation [8]. Angiogenic cytokines or other growth factors such as VEGF are expressed under hypoxia conditions or by various oncogenes (e.g., mutant ras, erbB-2/HER2) [9].

As shown in **Figure 1**, after binding the tyrosine kinase specific domain of the receptors, multiple ways of signaling are possible for the angiogenic factors. Important molecular mechanisms involve activation of RAS/RAF1/kinase through the extracellular signal (ERK-1 şi-2), inducing proliferation and differentiation; RAS/p38 mitogen-activated kinase (MAPK) and JUN/kinase 1-3 N-terminal, modulating inflammation, apoptosis, and differentiation; phosfatidyl-3-inositol kinase-1 (PI3K) and AKT dependent, regulating cell survival, mammalian receptor for rapamycin (mTOR), highly involved in proliferation and cell growth. Other inductor factors of the signaling pathways of angiogenesis are found in the cytoplasm (e.g., GAB1, SHC, SRC, PI3K, and phosfolipase γ C) [10].

VEGF and its receptors, the VEGFR family, remain intensively researched for targeting angiogenesis in different tumors. At the same time, other angiogenesis suppressing-related targets are being studied for the development of anticancer therapies for tumors resistant to anti-VEGF therapy. A number of therapeutic agents are currently in use for several malignancies: monoclonal antibodies against angiogenic growth factors (e.g., antibody against VEGF, Bevacizumab), inhibitors of angiogenic factors synthesis (e.g., mTOR inhibitor Rapamycin), and inhibitors of angiogenic factor receptors (tyrosine-kinase inhibitors, e.g., imatinib and sorafenib) [11]. Unfortunately, clinical response to the new molecular advances in cancer therapy by targeting angiogenesis is unsatisfactory. Resistance and low survival rates are signaled. New therapeutic approaches with minimal side effects are desired to act by targeting the multiple factors that are activated during tumor progression.

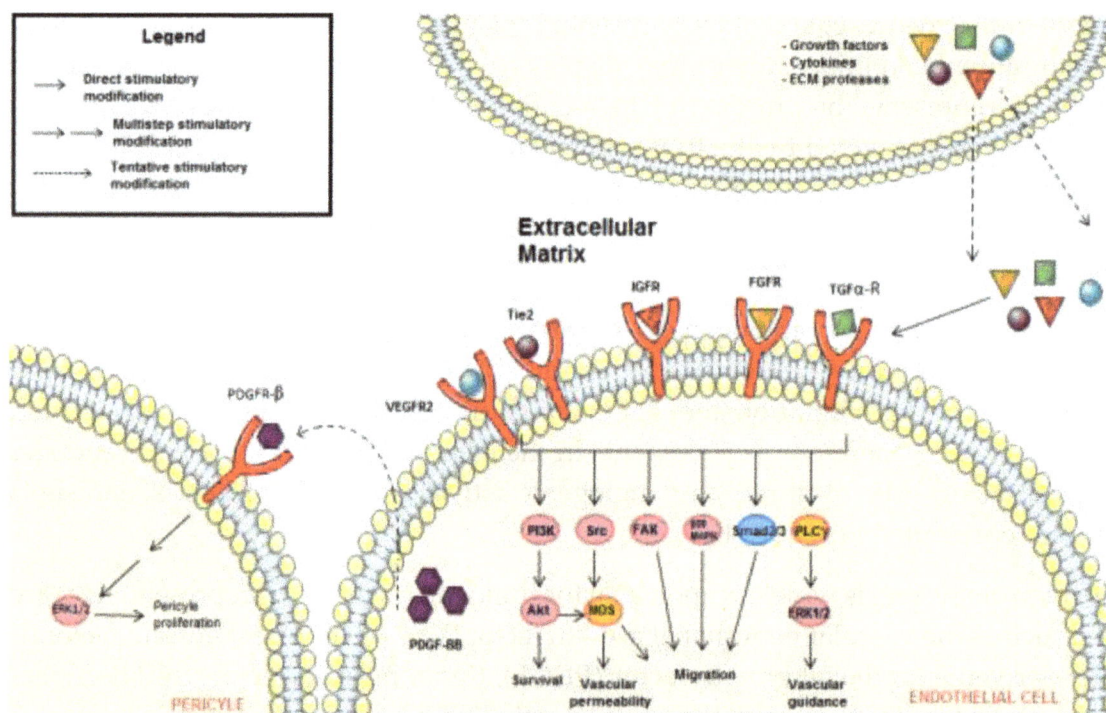

Figure 1. Angiogenic factors and signaling pathways involved in angiogenesis mediation. Abbreviations: Akt, RAC-alpha serine/threonine-protein kinase, ERK1/2, mitogen-activated protein kinase 1/2, FAK, focal adhesion kinase; FGFR, fibroblast growth factor receptor; IGFR, insulin growth factor receptor; MAPK, mitogen-activated protein kinases; NOS, nitric oxide synthase; p38, mitogen-activated protein kinase 11; PDGFR, olated-delivered endothelial growth factor receptor; PI3K, phosphatidylinositol 4,5-bisphosphate 3-kinase; PLCγ, phospholipase C gamma; Smad, Smad protein; Src, proto-oncogene tyrosine-protein kinase; TGFα-R, transforming growth factor α receptor; Tie, angiopoietin receptor; VEGFR, vascular endothelial growth factor receptor.

Based on the preventive effect that healthy diets have on the epidemiology of cancer, medicinal plants, spices, fruits, and vegetables represent an interesting source of phytochemicals. Natural compounds or even plant extracts are now considered important and accessible therapeutic or chemopreventive agents in cancer. In the search of the suitable phytocompounds to test for specific effects, virtual screening methods can be successfully applied in the selection of selective compounds for specific targets [12]. To avoid lack of selectivity, computational filtering schemes can be used [ ]. Extensive studies demonstrate the high potential of plant-derived chemicals in controlling tumor angiogenesis with minimal secondary effects and drug resistance, by targeting multiple key pathways in a synergistic manner.

2. Experimental models for tumor angiogenesis: focus on the CAM assay

An important issue in angiogenesis studies is the appropriate choice of the assays. To evaluate the efficacy of potential phytocompounds and to identify potential targets within the angiogenic process, several methods both *in vitro* and *in vivo* can be applied. Each of them having one or more drawbacks, ideally more techniques are to be applied. *In vitro* techniques are used by co-culturing endothelial cell and other tumor microenvironment factors with tumor cells in 2D or even 3D models which facilitate the identification of the involved molecular mechanisms. Despite the advances made in the direction of designing *in vitro* assays, the *in vivo* environment can be difficultly reproduced with such protocols [14]. To better assess the key aspects of tumor angiogenesis and therapeutic approaches, *in vivo* assays can be applied, such as the chick chorioallantoic membrane (CAM), the zebrafish, the sponge implantation, the corneal, or dorsal air sac and tumor angiogenesis models in rodents or rabbits [15]. Several drawbacks can still be cited, especially for the murine models, including high costs, complex technical and surgical abilities, and important quantities of test compounds.

2.1. Chorioallantoic membrane assay

The chorioallantoic membrane (CAM) assay represents an attractive *in vivo* experimental model for angiogenesis and cancer studies. The advantages of this *in vivo* technique in terms of costs, time, simplicity, reproducibility, and ease of the approval by the ethic committee make it a good prescreening assay to murine models in the research of biological systems and new therapeutic targets. Especially tumor angiogenesis and metastasis protocols benefit for a much shorter time for the tumor to grow and metastasize than the classical animal models.

The limitations of the model include a restricted number of reagents to work with due to low compatibility, nonspecific inflammatory reactions, keratinization of the membrane, and a vascular reaction that interferes with the visualization of vascular modifications. Technical skills may be significant to counteract these limitations [16, 17].

The chorioallantoic membrane is the vascularized respiratory extraembryonic tissue of avian species. First, this biologic system has been used for embryologic, immunological, and tumor grafting studies [18], and more recently, since the discovery of tumor angiogenesis [19], it is intensively applied in cancer research [20]. During the stages of embryo development, the immunologic, nervous, and nociceptive systems are not fully developed [21]. Several types of CAM assay protocols have been developed.

2.2. Uses in biological studies

The method can be applied for bioengineering development, morphology, biochemistry, transplant biology, cancer research, and drug development, but also in immunology, wound healing, tissue repair, or drug toxicity [22, 23]. The possibilities of imaging and evaluation have attracted many research studies. Nutritional therapeutics is an example of products approved by the U.S. Food and Drug Administration (FDA) that were preclinically evaluated in the CAM model [16].

Phytocompounds can be tested in order to evaluate their potential bioavailability, tolerability, and lack of irritation effects. For this purpose, the variations of the HET-CAM protocol can be applied, according the Interagency Coordinating Committee on the Validation of Alternative Methods (ICCVAM) recommendations published in November 2006 in Appendix G of reference [24]. Our previous evaluations proved its applicability in testing different sets of compounds, i.e., surfactants and aflatoxins [25].

In the attempt of finding new means for cancer chemoprevention, the chorioallantoic membrane assay can be used to test natural compounds that could reduce or inhibit several pathways involved in malignancies, especially pro-inflammatory cytokine activation and excessive angiogenesis. Tumor microenvironment, including inflammation and angiogenesis next to the development of new therapeutic targets for these pathological conditions, is intensively researched on murine models [26]. Previously, we have evaluated mast cell involvement in the angiogenesis process implementing a mastocytoma model on the CAM assay [27], which can be further developed for the evaluation of natural compounds on mast cells as key participants in the tumor microenvironment.

2.3. General *in ovo* method

Ex ovo or *in ovo* techniques are applicable. The *ex ovo* protocol involves the transfer of the egg content on day 3 of incubation into a Petri dish. It facilitates the visualization of the experiment, but the unnatural milieu of development of the embryo is detrimental to the survival rate of the specimens. Therefore, we prefer the *in ovo* protocol and is the type of method described here.

Fertilized eggs are horizontally incubated 7 days prior to use, at 37°C, in a controlled wet atmosphere. On the third day of incubation, in order to detach the chorioallantoic membrane, a volume of 2–3 ml of albumen is aspired through a perforation at the more pointed end of the eggs. The hole is resealed and returned to the incubator. The next day, a window is cut and resealed on the superior side of the shell. The eggs are returned to incubation until the day of the experiment [28]. Generally, 5–10 eggs are used for each test sample. Samples are applied inside a sterile plastic ring on the surface of the membrane. Samples are applied in triplicate. *In ovo* investigation by means of a stereomicroscope is performed throughout the experiment. Photographs are recorded for further analysis (**Figure 2**).

Starting with day 11 of incubation, samples can be considered active on excessive angiogenesis. The rapid growth of the vessels occurs during days 7–11; therefore, applying substances during this interval can be evaluated in terms of antiangiogenic effects. Morphometric evaluation of the angiogenic reaction can be conducted using a 0–5 arbitrary scale, the mean values expressing the vascular density around the site of application [20]. Finally, specimens are sacrificed and membranes are submitted to histological and immunohistological evaluation. On slides with immunohistochemical marked vessels, the mean microvascular density can be determined using the hotspot method, and counting the blood vessels, to calculate an antiangiogenic index, with the aid of the formula: $AAI = 1 - No_{BVtest}/No_{BVcontrol,}$ AAI = antiangiogenic index, BV = blood vessels [29].

2.4. Tumor angiogenesis model on CAM

Tumor cells are used on the CAM in order to obtain tumors, to study their microenvironment and the effects that phytochemicals might have. Tumor grafts can be used as well. Usually, cultured cancer cells are inoculated on the surface of the CAM, on day 10 of incubation, after being trypsinized and resuspended in culture medium to final concentrations in the range of 10^5–10^6 ml^{-1}. Cells can be applied directly on the CAM using a plastic ring for localizing the cells or using Matrigel impregnated with cells. Further, test compound solutions diluted with minimal DMSO (dimethyl sulfoxide) concentration in phosphate buffer can be applied on the

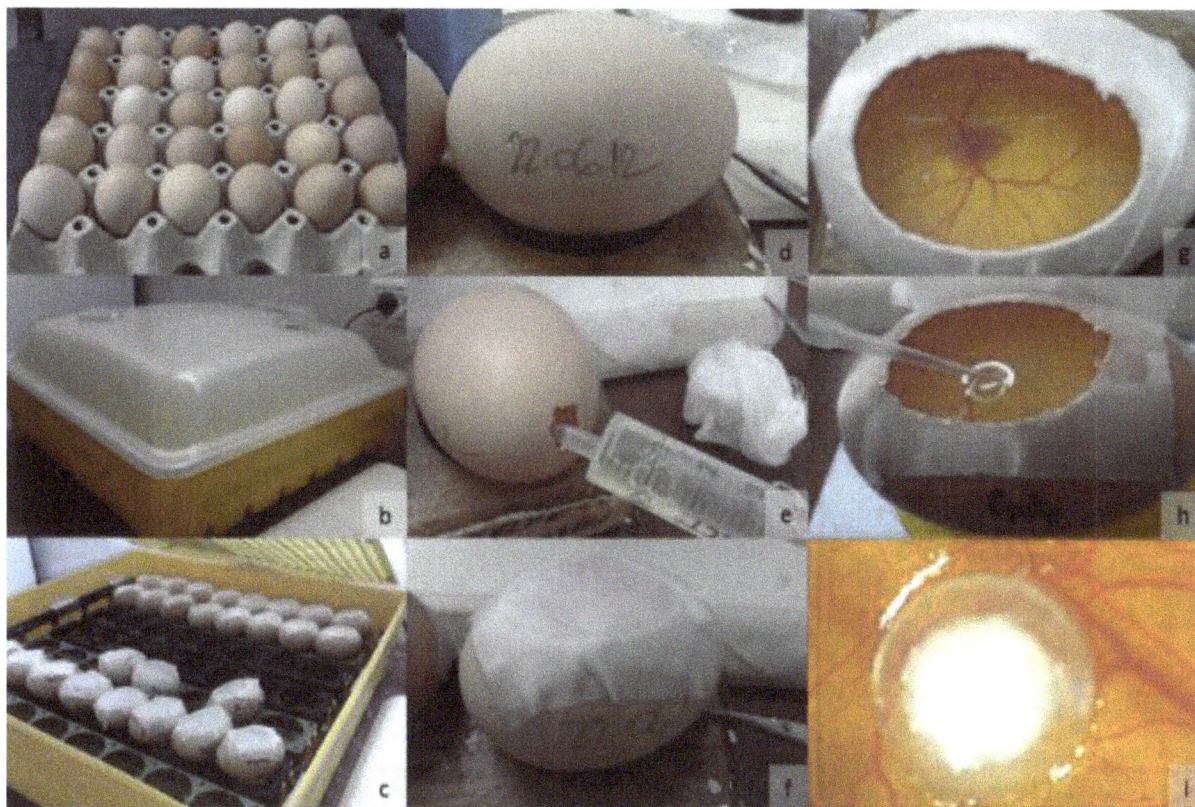

Figure 2. Chorioallantoic membrane assay—*in ovo* practical approach: incubation of the eggs (a–c); albumen removal, shell opening, and resealing (d–f); visualization of the CAM, sample application, and sample application inside a plastic ring (g–i) [30].

same spot as the cancer cell samples. *In ovo* stereomicroscopic follow-up is performed daily to register the changes in the vascular response around the tumor developing area that will be used for the morphometric analysis. On the final day of the experiment, after sacrificing the embryos, tumor masses are measured; the chorioallantoic membrane, the formed tumors, and some organs suspected to have metastasis are harvested and histologically processed.

In order to observe morphologic changes in the chorioallantoic membrane, hematoxylin eosin staining is analyzed. Different panels of immunohistochemical markers can be further applied: tumor cell markers and specific antibodies for different key proteins involved in the tumor microenvironment (e.g., endothelial cell marker-factor VIII, smooth muscle actin (SMA) marker, vascular endothelial growth factors, and its receptors, mast cells marker— Tryptase, the proliferation marker—Ki67). Results can reveal molecular modifications and serve to vascular density quantification.

Our experience is related to testing phytocompounds and plant extracts for the effect on angio-genesis. Using the angiogenesis method in the rapid stage of CAM development, we found that pentacyclic triterpenes, betulinic (BA) acid, and betulin (Bet) in various formulations with cyclodextrin and in nanoemulsion are potential antiangiogenic compounds, acting differently, both through direct and indirect mechanisms [31, 32]. Immunohistochemical staining for smooth muscle actin (SMA) on the specimens treated with betulin in nanoemulsion, next to blank and control samples, are shown in **Figure 3**. The low expression of the marker in the betulin-treated specimen indicates a minimal implication of pericytes in the angiogenesis process [32]. On the contrary, we found that betulinic acid determined rapid maturation of the vessels and high levels of SMA [31]. We also evaluated triterpenes and other types of natural compounds in melanoma models on CAM, which confirms the inhibitory effect on tumor angiogenesis (data not published).

Most studies that use the CAM assay are evaluated through stereomicroscopy that allows a series of quantitative measurements, and by histologic an immunohistological interpretation. Advances in the evaluation techniques include fluorescence microscopy, confocal micros-copy, microCT scanning, and imaging, *in situ* hybridization (ISH), quantitative PCR (qPCR) determination of specific targets [16, 33].

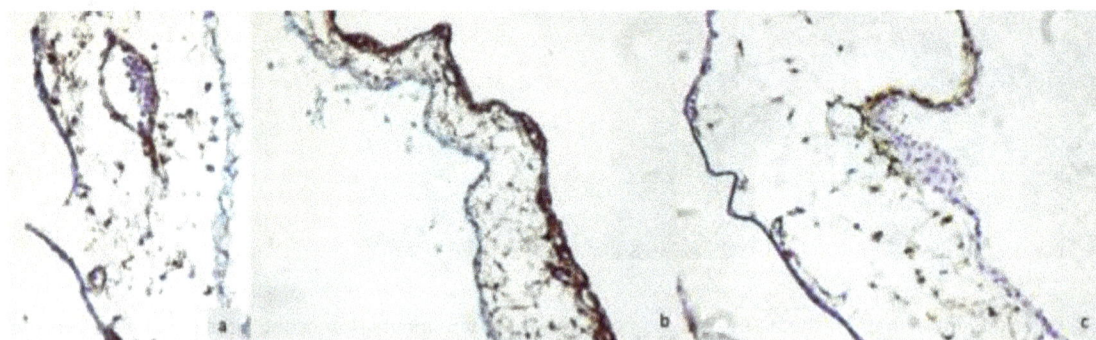

Figure 3. Light microscopic evaluation of CAM sections from ID 11 smooth muscle actin marker: (a) blank specimen, ×40, (b) control specimen treated with nanoemulsion, ×40, (c) specimen treated with betulin in nanoemulsion, ×40 [32].

3. Phytocompounds targeting cancer angiogenesis: *in vitro*, on the chorioallantoic membrane assay, in animal model

Chemicals derived from plant sources as well as various types of extracts have been already investigated for their effects on angiogenesis and on cancer. Currently, based on the failure of the approved therapeutics and also by crediting the traditional medicine philosophy that pathologies are imbalances that have to be rebalanced, the idea of multiple targeting through synergetic phytocompounds mixtures is gaining more attention. Extensive research is being dedicated to the understanding of their mechanism and their efficacy using *in vitro* and *in vivo* methods. The most in depth evidence comes from the results on cell cultures. *In vivo* methods also offer other accurate data on their effects. The chorioallantoic membrane assay is being used by more and more researchers for the evaluation of plant-derived chemicals or extracts. Correlations can be made using the results obtained for *in vitro*, animal and CAM assays, which will improve the knowledge and the future analysis to perform for the active compounds. We reviewed here some of the most investigated phytocompounds concerning the results obtained on all the three experimental models (**Table 1**).

Phytochemical class	Compound	Chemical structure	Plant source	In vitro effects	Effects on CAM	In vivo effects
Polyphenols	Curcumin		Curcuma longa L.	MiaPaCa-2; BxPC-3; Panc-1; MPanc-96 prostate cancer cell lines Reduced expression of NF-κB [34]	Angiogenesis inhibitor on small capillaries [35]	Athymic nude mice xenograft with prostate cancer cells Reduced expression of NFκB-p65, STAT3 and SRC; Reduced expression of ANXA2 and VEGFR2 [36]
	Epigallocatechin-gallate		Camellia sinensis L.	Hepatocellular carcinoma Inhibition of the VEGF-VEGFR axis [37]	Inhibition of fibroblast growth factor (FGF) and inhibition of mean branch formation and tumor weight of neuroblastoma-induced angiogenesis [38]	BGC-823 human gastric cancer xenograft mice model Reduction of VEGF [39]
Phloroglucinol derivative	Hyperforin		Hypericum perforatum L.	BAE – bovine aortic endothelial cell MDA-MB231 human breast cancer and NIH-3T3 mouse fibroblast cell Inhibition of capillary tube formation; Inhibition of urokinase and MMP2 [40]	Multiple target angiogenesis inhibitor [40]	Wistar rats inoculated with MT-450 at mammary tumor cells Suppression tumor-induced lymphangiogenesis [41]
Stilbene phytoalexin derivative	Resveratrol		Vitis vinifera L., Polygonum cuspidatum L.	YUZAZ6, M14, A375 melanoma cell lines Downregulation of VEGF and upregulation of TSP1 [42]	Significant reduction in angiogenesis in higher doses [43]	C57BL/6 Mice inoculated with Lewis lung carcinoma cells Inhibition of neovascularization [44]

Phytochemical class	Compound	Chemical structure	Plant source	In vitro effects	Effects on CAM	In vivo effects
Phenols	Carnosic acid		Rosmarinus officinalis L	HT-1080 Human fibrosarcoma cells, HL60 Human promyelocytic leukemia cells, HUVECs cells Inhibition of capillary tube formation; Decrease in the endothelial cells MMP-2 activity [45]	Antiangiogenic effect; emphasized activity for carnosic acid [45]	DMBA-induced hamster buccal Pouch carcinogenesis Suppressed expression of Cyclin D1 and NFκB; modulation of VEGF [46]
	Carnosol		Rosmarinus officinalis L	HT-1080 Human fibrosarcoma cells, HL60 Human promyelocytic leukemia cells, HUVECs cells capillary tube formation; Decrease in the endothelial cells MMP-2 activity [45]	Antiangiogenic effect; emphasized activity for carnosic acid [45]	n/a
	Capsaicin		Capsicum sp.	Hy-A549CoCl2-stimulated A549 lung cancer cells Inhibition of VEGF by downmodulation of HIF-1α; Increased p53 level [47]	Potent inhibitor of tumor-induced angiogenesis [48]	C57BL/6 mice Inhibition of VEGF and hemoglobin [48]
Isoflavones	Daidzein		Trifolium pratense L., Glycine maxima L.	LNCaP, PC-3, and DU-145 PCa cells - Down-regulation of ECGF1, FGF1, IGF1, FGFR3, IL-1β, IL-6, IL-8, PECAM1[49]	Antiangiogenic effect, anti-inflammatory effect with no membrane-irritating and toxic side effects[50]	n/a
	Genistein		Trifolium pratense L., Glycine maxima L.	BME cloned bovine microvascular endothelial cells Inhibition of bFGF [51]	Antiangiogenic effect, anti-inflammatory effect with no membrane-irritating and toxic side effects[50]	BALB/C nu/nu mice inoculated with Bel 7402 hepatocellular carcinoma Significant decrease of positive unit (PU) of the microvessels[52]

Phytochemical class	Compound	Chemical structure	Plant source	In vitro effects	Effects on CAM	In vivo effects
Flavonoids	Quercetin		*Camelia sinensis* L., *Angelica keiskei*, *Momordica cochinchinensis,*	PC-3 prostate cells Inhibition of VEGF [53]	Potent angiogenesis inhibitor [53]	DMBA-induced experimental mammary carcinoma in rats Inhibition of H-ras protein; inhibition of VEGF and bFGF [54]
	Naringenin		*Citrus* sp.	Aspc-1 and panc-1 prostate cancer cells Inhibition of TGF-β1-induced migration; Decreased expression of MMP2 and MMP9 proteins [55]	Potent angiogenesis inhibitor [56]	n/a
	Apigenin		*Entada africana*, *Matricaria chamomilla* L	PC-3 and DU145 prostate cancer cells Inhibition of HIF-1α and VEGF LNCaP prostate cancer cells, HCT-8 colon cancer cells, and MCF-7breast cancer cells Inhibition of hypoxia-induced HIF-1α and VEGF[57]	Promising antiangiogenic effect [58]	BALB/cA-nu nude mice injected with PC-3 prostate cancer cells and OVCAR-3 ovarian cancer cells Inhibition of blood vessels formation; Inhibition of hemoglobin levels [57]
	Isoliquiritigenin		*Glycyrrhiza glabra* L	ACC-M, ACC-2 adenoid cystic carcinoma cells and EAhy926 endothelial hybridoma cell line Prevention of tube formation; Downregulation of VEGF [59]	Angiogenesis suppressor [60]	BALB/c nude mice injected with ACC-M cells Reduction in S6 phosphorylation; Decreased VEGF; Inhibition of the mTOR signaling pathway[59]
	Silibinin		*Silybum marianum* L	SW480, HT-29 and LoVo colorectal cancer cells Inhibition of NF-κB; Reduction of MMP9, COX-2 and VEGF[61]	dose-dependent suppressive on angiogenesis [62]	A/J mice with Urethane-induced lung tumors Inhibition of new microvessels formation; Decreased levels of IL-1α,-6, -9, -13, -16, IFN-γ and TNF-α[63]

Phytochemical class	Compound	Chemical structure	Plant source	In vitro effects	Effects on CAM	In vivo effects
Alkaloids	Vinblastine		*Vinca* sp.	Human neuroblastoma cell lines Downmodulation of VEGF and VEGF-R2 [64]	Angiostatic activity [64]	Athymic (Nude-nu) mice injected with GI-LI-N cells Decrease of CD31-positive blood vessels; Downmodulation of VEGF and VEGF-R2 [64]
	Vincristine		*Vinca* sp.	Glioblastoma cells — decreased expression of VEGF mRNA and the level of HIF-1α protein [65]	Antiangiogenic effects in neuroblastoma tumors in high doses [66]	Swiss nu/nu mice injected with Caki-1 and Caki-2 renal carcinoma cells Inhibition of angiogenesis [67]
Pentacyclic triterpenes	Betulin		*Betula pendula, Prunus dulcis*	Apoptotic induction in MCF-7, A431 [68]	Strong direct antiangiogenic effects [32]	Balb/C mice DMBA/TPA skin carcinoma model Decreased expression of VEGF [32]
	Betulinic acid		*Betula pendula, Prunus dulcis*	SK-MEL2 melanoma and LNCaP prostate cancer cells - Decreased expression of Sp1, Sp3, Sp4, and VEGF [69]	Strong antiangiogenic effects [31]	Athymic nude mice with LNCaP cells as xenografts Tumor tissue less vascular; Decreased expression of Sp1, Sp3, Sp4, AR, and VEGF [69]
Tetracyclic Triterpenoid saponins	Ginsenoside Rg3		*Panax ginseng*	Eca-109 – human esophageal carcinoma cell line and 786-0 renal cell carcinoma cell line Downregulation of VEGF expression via COX-2 pathway; Reduction of STAT3 phosphorylation; Decreased HIF-1α protein expression in Eca-109 cells [70]	Strong, multi-target inhibition of neovascularization, without affecting endothelial cell proliferation; lack of cytotoxicity [71]	C57BL/6 mice injected with LLC Lewis lung carcinoma cells Decreased tube formation of circulating progenitor cells; Suppression of VEGF dependent p38 and ERK signal pathways [72]

Phytochemical class	Compound	Chemical structure	Plant source	In vitro effects	Effects on CAM	In vivo effects
Flavones	Baicalein		Scutellaria baicalensis Georgi	H-460 cells assessed using BrdU assay Significant antiproliferative and pro apoptotic; inhibit bFGF-induced HUVEC tube formation in Matrigel stronger than baicalin [74, 75]	Dose-dependent antiangiogenic activity [74]	H-460 athymic nude mice, tumor growth and survival low expression of 12-LOX, VEGF and FGFR-2 gene [73]
	Baicalin		Scutellaria baicalensis Georgi	Growth and survival, MMP-2 expression, inhibit bFGF-induced HUVEC tube formation in Matrigel [74]; increases VEGF expression by activating the ERRα/PGC-1α pathway [75]	Dose-dependent antiangiogenic activity [74]	Inhibit growth of S180 solid tumor in mice [76]
Steroids	Withaferin A		Withania somnifera Dunal	Antiangiogenic activity in primary endothelial cells HUVEC [77]	Significant antiangiogenic activity [78]	Inhibits FGF-2 Induced angiogenesis in C57BL/6J mice [77]

Table 1. Common phytocompounds with *in vitro* and *in vivo* antiangiogenic activity.

4. Clinical trials correlation

Implementation of clinical trials is vital for the validation and future use of the active phyto-compounds as additional therapies to the oncologic protocols or as chemopreventive strategies. These types of experiments are difficult to implement and therefore not many trials are finalized for the evaluation of antiangiogenic effect in cancer. Two of the above-listed phyto-chemicals (**Table 1**) benefit from large investigations among which some are clinical trials, but the modulation of the angiogenic process does not appear as a distinct evaluation, cancer effects being the first ones to be described.

Most of the controlled clinical trials of curcumin supplementation in cancer patients aimed to determine its feasibility, tolerability, safety, and to provide early evidence of efficacy [79]. For patients with advanced colorectal cancer, oral doses up to 3.6 g/day for 4 months were well tolerated, although the systemic bioavailability of oral curcumin was low [80]. For this dose, trace levels of curcumin metabolites were measured in liver tissue, but curcumin itself was not detected [81]. These findings suggested that oral curcumin is effective as a therapeutic agent in cancers of the gastrointestinal tract. Other trials found that combining curcumin with anticancer drugs like gemcitabine in pancreatic cancer [82], docetaxel in breast cancer [83], and imatinib in chronic myeloid leukemia may confer additional benefits to conventional drugs against different types of cancer.

Green tea made from *Camellia sinensis* L. leaves, originated in China, is one of the most extensively consumed beverages and achieved significant attention due to health benefits against cancer. Representative compounds are polyphenols and catechins with therapeutic potential against cancer [84]. Recent clinical trials proved that green tea extract and epigallocatechin gallate (EGCG) can be active in several forms of cancer. There is an increasing trend to employ green tea extract and EGCG as conservative management for patients diagnosed with less advanced prostate cancer. Combinations of chemopreventive agents should be carefully investigated because mechanisms of action may be additive or synergistic [85]. Several clinical examinations reported different molecular mechanisms regarding green tea beneficial effects against oral cancer chemoprevention [86–88]. Lung cancer induction may also be inhibited by tea polyphenols. Some studies suggest that individuals who never drank green tea have an elevated lung cancer risk compared to those who drank green tea at least one cup per day, and the effect is more pronounced in smokers [88]. Hepatocellular carcinoma (HCC) usually develops in a cirrhotic liver due to hepatitis virus infection. Green tea catechins (GTCs) may possess potent anticancer and chemopreventive properties for a number of different malignancies, including liver cancer. Antioxidant and anti-inflammatory activities are key mechanisms through which GTCs prevent the development of neoplasms, and they also exert cancer chemopreventive effects by modulating several signaling transduction and metabolic pathways where angiogenesis is exacerbated. Several interventional trials in humans have shown that GTCs may ameliorate metabolic abnormalities and prevent the development of precancerous lesions [89].

5. Conclusion

Currently, a great number of natural compounds are being investigated for their potential effectiveness in controlling tumor angiogenesis and therefore the reduction of tumor growth and metastasis. Observing the high number of molecular pathways that are deregulated in tumor angiogenesis and that many phytocompounds are active on several key factors, it is recommendable that more *in vivo* studies should investigate mixture of compounds for broader targeting, having eventually lower secondary effects and resistance. The optimal experimental technique is an important factor in order to get a useful output. More types of assays are always a good choice, including *in vivo* assays. The chorioallantoic membrane protocol is a good candidate for one type of "golden standardized method" in tumor angiogenesis, being a versatile, rapid, easy, and cheap method to apply in the research of phytocompounds. A great number of plant-derived chemicals, alone or in combination, are studied using this method, but standardization, next to applying new analysis techniques will outcome useful data that will be easier translated to clinical trials.

Acknowledgements

This work was supported by a grant of the Romanian National Authority for Scientific Research and Innovation, CNCS—UEFISCDI, project number PN-II-RU-TE-2014-4-2842 to S.A., R.G., I.Z.P. and D.C. Special thanks to the Histology and Angiogenesis Department, University of Medicine and Pharmacy Victor Babes Timisoara, for the technical support and help in setting up the CAM assay.

Author details

Stefana Avram[1], Roxana Ghiulai[2]*, Ioana Zinuca Pavel[1], Marius Mioc[2], Roxana Babuta[2], Mirela Voicu[3], Dorina Coricovac[4], Corina Danciu[1], Cristina Dehelean[4] and Codruta Soica[2]

*Address all correspondence to: roxana.ghiulai@umft.ro

1 Department of Phamacognosy, Faculty of Pharmacy, Victor Babeș University of Medicine and Pharmacy, Timisoara, Romania

2 Department of Pharmaceutical Chemistry, Faculty of Pharmacy, Victor Babeș University of Medicine and Pharmacy, Timisoara, Romania

3 Department of Phamacology, Faculty of Pharmacy, Victor Babeș University of Medicine and Pharmacy, Timisoara, Romania

4 Department of Toxicology, Faculty of Pharmacy, Victor Babeș University of Medicine and Pharmacy, Timisoara, Romania

References

[1]   Ribatti D, Djonov V. Intussusceptive microvascular growth in tumors. Cancer Letters. 2012;**316**(2):126-131

[2]   Folkman J. Tumor angiogenesis: Therapeutic implications. The New England Journal of Medicine. 1971;**285**(21):1182-1186

[3]   Holmgren L, O'Reilly MS, Folkman J. Dormancy of micrometastases: Balanced proliferation and apoptosis in the presence of angiogenesis suppression. Nature Medicine. 1995;**1**:149-153

[4]   Parangi S, O'Reilly M, Christofori G, Holmgren L, Grosfeld J, Folkman J, Hanahan D. Antiangiogenic therapy of transgenic mice impairs de novo tumor growth. Proceedings of the National Academy of Sciences of the United States of America. 1996;**93**(5):2002-2007

[5]   Ziyad S, Iruela-Arispe ML. Molecular mechanisms of tumor angiogenesis. Genes Cancer. 2011;**2**(12):1085-1096

[6]   Denekamp J. Angiogenesis, neovascular proliferation and vascular pathophysiology as targets for cancer therapy. The British Journal of Radiology. 1993;**66**(783):181-196

[7]   Nishida N, Yano H, Nishida T, Kamura T, Kojiro M. Angiogenesis in cancer. Vascular Health and Risk Management. 2006;**2**(3):213-219

[8]   Prager GW, Poettler M, Unseld M, Zielinski CC. Angiogenesis in cancer: Anti-VEGF escape mechanisms. Translational Lung Cancer Research. 2012;**1**(1):14-25

[9]   Ferrara N, Kerbel RS. Angiogenesis as a therapeutic target. Nature. 2005;**438**(7070):967-974

[10] Oklu R, Walker TG, Wicky S, Hesketh R. Angiogenesis and current antiangiogenic strategies for the treatment of cancer. Journal of Vascular Interventional Radiology. 2010;**21**(12):1791-805; quiz 1806

[11] Wang Z, Dabrosin C, Yin X, Fuster MM, Arreola A, Rathmell WK, Generali D, Nagaraju GP, El-Rayes B, Ribatti D, Chen YC, Honoki K, Fujii H, Georgakilas AG, Nowsheen S, Amedei A, Niccolai E, Amin A, Ashraf SS, Helferich B, Yang X, Guha G, Bhakta D, Ciriolo MR, Aquilano K, Chen S, Halicka D, Mohammed SI, Azmi AS, Bilsland A, Keith WN, Jensen LD. Broad targeting of angiogenesis for cancer prevention and therapy. Seminars in Cancer Biology. 2015;**35**:S224–S243

[12] Bora A, Avram S, Ciucanu I, Raica M, Avram S. Predictive models for fast and effective profiling of kinase inhibitors. Journal of Chemical Information and Modeling. 2016;**56**(5):895-905

[13] Avram SI, Pacureanu LM, Bora A, Crisan L, Avram S, Kurunczi L. ColBioS-FlavRC: A collection of bioselective flavonoids and related compounds filtered from high-throughput screening outcomes. Journal of Chemical Information and Modeling. 2014;**54**(8):2360-2370

[14] Roudsari LC, West JL. Studying the influence of angiogenesis in in vitro cancer model systems. Advanced Drug Delivery Reviews. 2016;**97**:250-259

[15] Staton CA, Reed MWR, Brown NJ. A critical analysis of current in vitro and in vivo angiogenesis assays. International Journal of Experimental Pathology. 2009;**90**(3):195-221

[16] Dupertuis YM, Delie F, Cohen M, Pichard C. In ovo method for evaluating the effect of nutritional therapies on tumor development, growth and vascularization. Clinical Nutrition Experimental. 2015;**2**:9-17

[17] Nowak-Sliwinska P, Segura T, Iruela-Arispe ML. The chicken chorioallantoic membrane model in biology, medicine and bioengineering. Angiogenesis. 2016;**17**(4):779-804

[18] Harris RJ. Multiplication of Rous No. 1 sarcoma agent in the chorioallantoic membrane of the embryonated egg. British Journal of Cancer. 1954;**8**(4):731-736

[19] Folkman J, Cotran R. Relation of vascular proliferation to tumor growth. International Review of Experimental Pathology. 1976;**16**:207-248

[20] Ribatti D. The Chick Embryo Chorioallantoic Membrane in the Study of Angiogenesis and Metastasis. Springer Netherlands; 2010

[21] Friend JV, Crevel RW, Williams TC, Parish WE. Immaturity of the inflammatory response of the chick chorioallantoic membrane. Toxicology In Vitro. 1990;**4**(4-5):324-326

[22] Rashidi H, Sottile V. The chick embryo: Hatching a model for contemporary biomedical research. Bioessays. 2009;**31**(4):459-465

[23] Vargas A, Zeisser-Labouèbe M, Lange N, Gurny R, Delie F. The chick embryo and its chorioallantoic membrane (CAM) for the in vivo evaluation of drug delivery systems. Advanced Drug Delivery Reviews. 2007;**59**(11):1162-1176

[24] Scheel J, Kleber M, Kreutz J, Lehringer E, Mehling A, Reisinger K, Steiling W. Eye irritation potential: Usefulness of the HET-CAM under the globally harmonized system of classification and labeling of chemicals (GHS). Regulatory Toxicology and Pharmacology. 2011;**59**(3):471-492

[25] Ardelean S, Feflea S, Ionescu D, Năstase V, Dehelean CA. Toxicologic screening of some surfactants using modern in vivo bioassays. Revista Medico-Chirurgicala a Societatii De Medici Si Naturalisti Din Iasi Nat. din Iaşi. 2011;**115**(1):251-258

[26] Lokman NA, Elder ASF, Ricciardelli C, Oehler MK. Chick chorioallantoic membrane (CAM) assay as an in vivo model to study the effect of newly identified molecules on ovarian cancer invasion and metastasis. International Journal of Molecular Sciences. 2012;**13**(8):9959-9970

[27] (Feflea) Avram S, Cimpean AM, Raica M. Behavior of the P1.HTR mastocytoma cell line implanted in the chorioallantoic membrane of chick embryos. Brazilian Journal of Medical and Biological Research. 2013;**46**(1):52-57.

[28] Ribatti D. The chick embryo chorioallantoic membrane in the study of tumor angiogenesis. Romanian Journal of Morphology and Embryology. 2008;**49**(2):131-135

[29] Demir R, Peros G, Hohenberger W. Definition of the 'Drug-Angiogenic-Activity-Index' that allows the quantification of the positive and negative angiogenic active drugs: A study based on the chorioallantoic membrane model. Pathology and Oncology Research. 2011;**17**(2):309-313

[30] Feflea S. Stimulators and Inhibitors Of Angiogenesis in Experimental Model. (Doctoral Dissertation). University of Medicine and Pharmacy Victor Babes Timisoara; Timisoara;2013

[31] Dehelean CA, Feflea S, Ganta S, Amiji M. Anti-angiogenic effects of betulinic acid administered in nanoemulsion formulation using chorioallantoic membrane assay. Journal of Biomedical Nanotechnology. 2011;**7**(2):317-324

[32] Dehelean CA, Feflea S, Gheorgheosu D, Ganta S, Cimpean AM, Muntean D, Amiji MM. Anti-angiogenic and anti-cancer evaluation of betulin nanoemulsion in chicken chorioallantoic membrane and skin carcinoma in Balb/c mice. Journal of Biomedical Nanotechnology. 2013;**9**(4):577-589

[33] Xue X, Xiaoying Z, Huixin M, Zhang J, Huang G, Zhang Z, Li P. Chick chorioallantoic membrane assay: A 3D animal model for study of human nasopharyngeal carcinoma. PLoS One. 2015;**10**(6):e0130935

[34] Kunnumakkara AB, Guha S, Krishnan S, Diagaradjane P, Gelovani J, Aggarwal BB. Curcumin potentiates antitumor activity of gemcitabine in an orthotopic model of pancreatic cancer through suppression of proliferation, angiogenesis, and inhibition of nuclear factor-kappa B-regulated gene products. Cancer Research. 2007;**67**(8):3853-3861

[35] Gururaj AE, Belakavadi M, Venkatesh DA, Marmé D, Salimath BP. Molecular mechanisms of anti-angiogenic effect of curcumin. Biochemical and Biophysical Research Communications. 2002;**297**(4):934-942

[36] Ranjan AP, Mukerjee A, Helson L, Gupta R, Vishwanatha JK. Efficacy of liposomal curcumin in a human pancreatic tumor xenograft model: Inhibition of tumor growth and angiogenesis. Anticancer Research. 2013;**33**(9):3603-3609.

[37] Shirakami Y, Shimizu M, Adachi S, Sakai H, Nakagawa T, Yasuda Y, Tsurumi H, Hara Y, Moriwaki H. (-)-Epigallocatechin gallate suppresses the growth of human hepatocellular carcinoma cells by inhibiting activation of the vascular endothelial growth factor-vascular endothelial growth factor receptor axis. Cancer Science. 2009;**100**(10):1957-1962

[38] Siddiqui IA, Adhami VM, Bharali DJ, Hafeez BB, Asim M, Khwaja SI, Ahmad N, Cui H, Mousa SA, Mukhtar H. Introducing nanochemoprevention as a novel approach for cancer control: Proof of principle with green tea polyphenol epigallocatechin-3-gallate. Cancer Research. 2009;**69**(5):1712-1716

[39] Wu H, Xin Y, Xu C, Xiao Y. Capecitabine combined with (-)-epigallocatechin-3-gallate inhibits angiogenesis and tumor growth in nude mice with gastric cancer xenografts. Experimental and Therapeutic Medicine. 2012;**3**(4):650-654

[40] Martínez-Poveda B, Quesada AR, Medina MÁ. Hyperforin, a bio-active compound of St. John's Wort, is a new inhibitor of angiogenesis targeting several key steps of the process. International Journal of Cancer. 2005;**117**(5):775-780

[41] Rothley M, Schmid A, Thiele W, Schacht V, Plaumann D, Gartner M, Yektaoglu A, Bruyère F, Noël A, Giannis A, Sleeman JP. Hyperforin and aristoforin inhibit lymphatic endothelial cell proliferation in vitro and suppress tumor-induced lymphangiogenesis in vivo. International Journal of Cancer. 2009;**125**(1):34-42

[42] Trapp V, Basmina P, Papazian V, Lyndsay W, Fruehauf JP. Anti-angiogenic effects of resveratrol mediated by decreased VEGF and increased TSP1 expression in melanoma-endothelial cell co-culture. Angiogenesis. 2010;**13**:305-315

[43] Wang H, Zhou H, Zou Y, Liu Q, Guo C, Gao G, Shao C, Gong Y. Resveratrol modulates angiogenesis through the GSK3β/β-catenin/TCF-dependent pathway in human endothelial cells. Biochemical Pharmacology. 2010;**80**(9):1386-1395

[44] Kimura Y, Okuda H. Resveratrol isolated from Polygonum cuspidatum root prevents tumor growth and metastasis to lung and tumor-induced neovascularization in Lewis lung carcinoma-bearing mice. The Journal of Nutrition. 2001;**131**(6):1844-1849

[45] López-Jiménez A, García-Caballero M, Medina MÁ, Quesada AR. Anti-angiogenic properties of carnosol and carnosic acid, two major dietary compounds from rosemary. European Journal of Nutrition. 2013;**52**(1):85-95

[46] Rajasekaran D, Manoharan S, Silvan S, Vasudevan K, Baskaran N, Palanimuthu D. Proapoptotic, anti-cell proliferative, anti-inflammatory and anti-angiogenic potential of carnosic acid during 7,12 dimethylbenz[a]anthracene-induced hamster buccal pouch carcinogenesis. African Journal of Traditional, Complementary and Alternative Medicine. 2012;**10**(1):102-112

[47] Chakraborty S, Adhikary A, Mazumdar M, Mukherjee S, Bhattacharjee P, Guha D, Choudhuri T, Chattopadhyay S, Sa G, Sen A, Das T. Capsaicin-induced activation of p53-SMAR1 auto-regulatory loop down-regulates VEGF in non-small cell lung cancer to restrain angiogenesis. PLoS One. 2014;**9**(6):e99743

[48] Min J-K. Capsaicin inhibits in vitro and in vivo angiogenesis. Cancer Research. 2004;**64**(2):644-651

[49] Mahmoud AM, Yang W, Bosland MC. Soy isoflavones and prostate cancer: A review of molecular mechanisms. The Journal of Steroid Biochemistry and Molecular Biology. 2014;**140**:116-132

[50] Krenn L, Paper DH. Inhibition of angiogenesis and inflammation by an extract of red clover (Trifolium pratense L.). Phytomedicine. 2009;**16**(12):1083-1088

[51] Fotsis T, Pepper M, Adlercreutz H, Fleischmann G, Hase T, Montesano R, Schweigerer L. Genistein, a dietary-derived inhibitor of in vitro angiogenesis. Proceedings of the National Academy of Sciences of the United States of America. 1993;**90**(7):2690-2694

[52] Gu Y, Zhu C-F, Iwamoto H, Chen J-S. Genistein inhibits invasive potential of human hepatocellular carcinoma by altering cell cycle, apoptosis, and angiogenesis. World Journal of Gastroenterology. 2005;**11**(41):6512-6517

[53] Pratheeshkumar P, Budhraja A, Son Y-O, Wang X, Zhang Z, Ding S, Wang L, Hitron A, Lee J-C, Xu M, Chen G, Luo J, Shi X. Quercetin inhibits angiogenesis mediated human prostate tumor growth by targeting VEGFR-2 regulated AKT/mTOR/P70S6K signaling pathways. PLoS One. 2012;**7**(10): e47516. https://DOI.org/10.1371/journal.pone.0047516

[54] Kong L, Wu K, Lin H. Inhibitory effects of quercetin on angiogenesis of experimental mammary carcinoma. Chinese Journal of Clinical Oncology. 2005;**2**(3):631-636

[55] Lou C, Zhang F, Yang M, Zhao J, Zeng W, Fang X, Zhang Y, Zhang C, Liang W. Naringenin decreases invasiveness and metastasis by inhibiting TGF-β-induced epithelial to mesenchymal transition in pancreatic cancer cells. PLoS One. 2012;**7**(12):e50956

[56] Anand K, Sarkar A, Kumar A, Ambasta RK, Kumar P. Combinatorial antitumor effect of naringenin and curcumin elicit angioinhibitory activities in vivo. Nutrition and Cancer. 2012;**64**(5):714-724

[57] Fang J, Zhou Q, Liu LZ, Xia C, Hu X, Shi X, Jiang BH. Apigenin inhibits tumor angiogenesis through decreasing HIF-1α and VEGF expression. Carcinogenesis. 2007;**28**(4): 858-864

[58] Germanò MP, Certo G, D'Angelo V, Sanogo R, Malafronte N, De Tommasi N, Rapisarda A. Anti-angiogenic activity of Entada africana root. Natural Product Research. 2015;**29**(16):1551-1556

[59] Sun Z-J, Chen G, Zhang W, Hu X, Huang C-F, Wang Y-F, Jia J, Zhao Y-F. Mammalian target of rapamycin pathway promotes tumor-induced angiogenesis in adenoid cystic carcinoma: Its suppression by isoliquiritigenin through dual activation of c-Jun NH2-terminal kinase and inhibition of extracellular signal-regulated kinase. Journal of Pharmacology and Experimental Therapeutics. 2010;**334**(2):500-512

[60] Jhanji V, Liu H, Law K, Lee VY-W, Huang S-F, Pang C-P, Yam GH-F. Isoliquiritigenin from licorice root suppressed neovascularisation in experimental ocular angiogenesis models. British Journal of Ophthalmology. 2011;**95**(9):1309-1315

[61] Raina K, Agarwal C, Agarwal R. Effect of silibinin in human colorectal cancer cells: Targeting the activation of NF-κB signaling. Molecular Carcinogenesis. 2013;**52**(3):195-206

[62] Yang S-H, Lin J-K, Huang C-J, Chen W-S, Li S-Y, Chiu J-H. Silibinin inhibits angiogenesis via Flt-1, but not KDR, receptor up-regulation. Journal of Surgical Research. 2005;**128**(1):140-146

[63] Tyagi A, Singh RP, Ramasamy K, Raina K, Redente EF, Dwyer-Nield LD, Radcliffe RA, Malkinson AM, Agarwal R. Growth inhibition and regression of lung tumors by silibinin: Modulation of angiogenesis by Macrophage-Associated cytokines and nuclear

Factor- B and signal transducers and activators of transcription 3. Cancer Prevention Research. 2009;**2**(1):74-83

[64] Marimpietri D, Brignole C, Nico B, Pastorino F, Pezzolo A, Piccardi F, Cilli M, Di Paolo D, Pagnan G, Longo L, Perri P, Ribatti D, Ponzoni M. Combined therapeutic effects of vinblastine and rapamycin on human neuroblastoma growth, apoptosis, and angiogenesis. Clinical Cancer Research. 2007;**13**(13):3977-3988

[65] Park K-J, Yu MO, Park D-H, Park J-Y, Chung Y-G, Kang S-H. Role of vincristine in the inhibition of angiogenesis in glioblastoma. Neurology Research. 2016; 38(10):871-9. doi: 10.1080/01616412.2016.1211231

[66] Michaelis M, Hinsch N, Michaelis UR, Rothweiler F, Simon T, ilhelm Doerr HW, Cinatl J, Cinatl J. Chemotherapy-associated angiogenesis in neuroblastoma tumors. The American Journal of Pathology. 2012;**180**(4):1370-1377

[67] Schirner M, Hoffmann J, Menrad A, Schneider MR. Antiangiogenic chemotherapeutic agents: Characterization in comparison to their tumor growth inhibition in human renal cell carcinoma models. Clinical Cancer Research. 1998;**4**(5):1331-1336.

[68] Dehelean CA, Feflea S, Molnár J, Zupko I, Soica C. Betulin as an antitumor agent tested in vitro on A431, hela and MCF7, and as an angiogenic inhibitor in vivo in the CAM assay. Natural Product Communications. 2012;**7**(8):981-985

[69] Chintharlapalli S, Papineni S, Ramaiah SK, Safe S. Betulinic acid inhibits prostate cancer growth through inhibition of specificity protein transcription factors. Cancer Research. 2007;**67**(6):2816-2823

[70] Chen Q-J, Zhang M-Z, Wang L-X. Gensenoside Rg3 inhibits hypoxia-induced VEGF expression in human cancer cells. Cellular Physiology and Biochemistry. 2010;**26**(6):849-858

[71] Xiu Yu JL, Xu H, Hu M, Luan X, Wang K, Fu Y, Zhang D. Ginsenoside Rg3 bile Salt-Phosphatidylcholine-Based mixed micelles: Design, characterization, and evaluation. Chemical and Pharmaceutical Bulletin. 2015;**63**(5):361-368

[72] Kim J-W, Jung S-Y, Kwon Y-H, Lee J-H, Lee YM, Lee B-Y, Kwon S-M. Ginsenoside Rg3 attenuates tumor angiogenesis via inhibiting bioactivities of endothelial progenitor cells. Cancer Biology & Therapy. 2012;**13**(7):504-515

[73] Cathcart M-C, Useckaite Z, Drakeford C, Semik V, Lysaght J, Gately K, O'Byrne KJ, Pidgeon GP. Anti-cancer effects of baicalein in non-small cell lung cancer in-vitro and in-vivo. BMC Cancer. 2016;**16**(1):707

[74] Liu J-J, Huang T-S, Cheng W-F, Lu F-J. Baicalein and baicalin are potent inhibitors of angiogenesis: Inhibition of endothelial cell proliferation, migration and differentiation. International Journal of Cancer. 2003;**106**(4):559-565

[75] Zhang K, Lu J, Mori T, Smith-Powell L, Synold TW, Chen S, Wen W. Baicalin increases VEGF expression and angiogenesis by activating the ERR /PGC-1 pathway. Cardiovascular Research. 2011;**89**(2):426-435

[76] Xin W, Tian S, Song J, He G, Mu X, Qin X. Research progress on pharmacological actions and mechanism of baicalein and baicalin. Current Opinion In Complementary and Alternative Medicine. 2014;**1**(2):e00010

[77] Vanden Berghe W, Sabbe L, Kaileh M, Haegeman G, Heyninck K. Molecular insight in the multifunctional activities of Withaferin A. Biochemical Pharmacology. 2012;**84**(10):1282-1291

[78] Mathur R, Gupta SK, Singh N, Mathur S, Kochupillai V, Velpandian T. Evaluation of the effect of Withania somnifera root extracts on cell cycle and angiogenesis. Journal of Ethnopharmacology. 2006;**105**(3):336-341

[79] Fanaei H, Khayat S, Kasaeian A, Javadimehr M. Effect of curcumin on serum brain-derived neurotrophic factor levels in women with premenstrual syndrome: A randomized, double-blind, placebo-controlled trial. Neuropeptides. 2016;**56**:25-31

[80] Mall M, Kunzelmann K. Correction of the CF defect by curcumin: Hypes and disappointments. BioEssays. 2005;**27**(1):9-13

[81] Garcea G, Jones DJL, Singh R, Dennison AR, Farmer PB, Sharma RA, Steward WP, Gescher AJ, Berry DP. Detection of curcumin and its metabolites in hepatic tissue and portal blood of patients following oral administration. British Journal of Cancer. 2004;**90**(5):1011-1015

[82] Epelbaum R, Schaffer M, Vizel B, Badmaev V, Bar-Sela G. Curcumin and gemcitabine in patients with advanced pancreatic cancer. Nutrition and Cancer. 2010;**62**(8):1137-1141

[83] Bayet-Robert M, Kwiatkowski F, Leheurteur M, Gachon F, Planchat E, Abrial C, Mouret-Reynier M-A, Durando X, Barthomeuf C, Chollet P. Phase I dose escalation trial of docetaxel plus curcumin in patients with advanced and metastatic breast cancer. Cancer Biology & Therapy. 2010;**9**(1):8-14

[84] Chen L, Zhang HY. Cancer preventive mechanisms of the green tea polyphenol (-)-epigallocatechin-3-gallate. Molecules. 2007;**12**(5):946-957

[85] Davalli P, Rizzi F, Caporali A, Pellacani D, Davoli S, Bettuzzi S, Brausi M, D'Arca D. Anticancer activity of green tea polyphenols in prostate gland. Oxidative Medicine and Cellular Longevity. 2012; 2012. DOI:10.1155/2012/984219

[86] Soulieres D, Senzer NN, Vokes EE, Hidalgo M, Agarwala SS, Siu LL. Multicenter phase II study of erlotinib, an oral epidermal growth factor receptor tyrosine kinase inhibitor, in patients with recurrent or metastatic squamous cell cancer of the head and neck. Journal of Clinical Oncology. 2004;**22**

[87] Lee U-L, Choi S-W. The chemopreventive properties and therapeutic modulation of green tea polyphenols in oral squamous cell carcinoma. ISRN Oncology. 2011;**2011**:1-7

[88] Yang X, Thomas DP, Zhang X, Culver BW, Alexander BM, Murdoch WJ, Rao MN, Tulis DA, Ren J, Sreejayan N. Curcumin inhibits platelet-derived growth factor-stimulated vascular smooth muscle cell function and injury-induced neointima formation. Arteriosclerosis Thrombosis and Vascular Biology. 2006;**26**

[89] Shimizu M, Shirakami Y, Sakai H, Kubota M, Kochi T, Ideta T, Miyazaki T, Moriwaki H. Chemopreventive potential of green tea catechins in hepatocellular carcinoma. International Journal of Molecular Sciences. 2015;**16**(3):6124-6139

Immunotherapy in Pediatric Acute Leukemia: A Novel Magic Bullet or an Illusory Hope?

Monika Barełkowska and Katarzyna Derwich

Abstract

The last decade became the renaissance for investigating and exploring the potential role of immunotherapy in pediatric acute leukemia (AL). It is beyond question that there is an interaction between innate immune system and hematological malignancy. Leukemia cells inhibit the host immune response according to multiple mechanisms, but exploiting the innate immune system mechanisms can overcome the resistance to the conventional treatment. What is the role of immunotherapy in pediatric AL treatment? Does it have the potential to substitute or combine the standard chemotherapy? What is the best possible timing to take advantage of immune interventions? This review is considered to follow through the possible treatment options including their foundation, strong and weak points, but also information about possible implementation into the clinical practice.

Keywords: immunotherapy, acute lymphoblastic leukemia, acute myeloblastic leukemia, children

1. Introduction

Acute leukemia (lymphoblastic and myeloblastic) is the most common malignancy diagnosed in children with an incidence of about 4.2 and 4.9 per 100,000 in the age groups of 0–19 and 0–14, respectively. In the population of children aged 0–19, acute lymphoblastic leukemia (ALL) accounts for approximately 75% while acute myeloblastic leukemia (AML) accounts for 20% of pediatric leukemia cases. Contemporary therapy allows achieving complete remission in approximately 90% of patients with ALL and 70% with AML [1, 2]. It is worth mentioning that 50 years ago acute leukemia was almost universally incurable [3]. The breakthrough has been achieved through standardized and optimized multi-agent therapeutic regimens and through therapy individualization according to the risk stratification. However, even though great progress in therapy is reported, refractory or relapsed leukemia remains one of the major causes of cancer-related mortality. Failure to respond to chemotherapy is almost universally connected with poor prognosis. Survival rates for patients with relapsed or refractory AML receiving a second treatment attempt was estimated between 25 and 30% [4]. In 15% of ALL patients who experience relapse of the disease, long-term survival rates vary from 40 to 50%, even though the remission is achieved in over 70% of patients [5, 6]. What is more, current chemotherapy regimens are consisted of very intensive blocks of treatment that are responsible for multiple acute and long-term sequelae, especially in the pediatric population. According to multiple research, 60% of children after an anticancer treatment present at least one organ late effect [7]. New approaches that redirect treatment toxicity accurately to the neoplastic cells, sparing the normal cells and hematopoietic counterparts, will significantly reduce the possible complications and improve the survivor's quality of life.

1.1. Contemporary treatment strategy for acute leukemia in children

The therapy for ALL and AML in children is based on standardized protocols and is composed of four major phases: remission induction, followed by consolidation, reinduction (intensification), and maintenance. In order to provide the most effective and harmless treatment for every patient, children are classified into three groups based on the risk of treatment failure (standard, intermediate, or high). This way, less toxic regimens can be administered to patients with more favorable prognosis, whereas those children with features showing higher risk of relapse are receiving more aggressive blocks of chemotherapy. Protocols that are currently used in treatment of acute leukemia in Polish children are ALL IC-BFM 2009 and AML-BFM 2012 [8, 9]. Allogeneic hematopoietic stem cell transplantation (allo-HSCT), which is a form of immunotherapy, is generally not recommended in the first remission of pediatric AML patients except for those at high risk. Comparably, only the children with high-risk ALL and additional particular unfavorable prognostic factors, like T-cell ALL, high initial leukocytosis, hypodiploidy, and genetic impairments, like t(9;22) or t(4;11), benefit from allo-HSCT in the first complete remission [10, 11]. Radiotherapy is considered as a treatment option in case of extramedullary organ (central nervous system, testicular) involvement, but also as a prevention of central nervous system relapse in every patient with AML and, in strictly defined circumstances, children with the high-risk ALL. This approach is reserved only for selected group of patients according to an increased risk and severity of ionization-related late sequelae in the pediatric population [12].

Chemotherapy regimens used in acute leukemia in children are distinguished as extremely intensive, especially the treatment in patients with AML. This causes a long period of bone marrow aplasia that causes vulnerability to numerous infectious complications. Notably, 5% of treatment failures using previous versions of chemotherapy regimens were the result of treatment-related deaths in the first complete remission. According to the significant improvement in supportive care and therapy individualization, the treatment-related mortality has decreased gradually over the last decade [13]. However, there are still patients with drug-resistant or recurrent leukemia who require further efforts to identify effective treatment strategies based on the advances in our knowledge, understanding of leukemic cell biology, and interactions between them and the innate immune system. Without searching for new approaches and confining ourselves only to chemotherapy regimens, their prognosis remains unfavorable.

1.2. Rationale for immunotherapy in acute leukemia

The evidence supporting the idea of interactions between immune system and malignant cells is based on multiple observations of leukemia course depending on immune system function. For example, shift reconstitution of the immune system after induction regimens correlates with improved survival, and absolute leukocyte count is an independent prognostic factor for survival in patients with acute leukemia [14]. What is more, it is proven that malignant cells use multiple pathways to interfere the host immune system promoting the number and function of regulatory T cells (T regs) and subsequently reducing the ability of cytotoxic T cells to target leukemia [17].

The most popular and the only undisputed and thoroughly investigated form of immunotherapy, which has been applied in clinical practice for a few decades, is **allogeneic HSCT**. This form of treatment is considered in a subgroup of high-risk patients in the first remission or in refractory and relapsed hematological malignancies. The **graft-versus-leukemia effect (GvL)**, which occurred to be an additional immunological benefit to this approach, is mediated by donor T cells and natural killer (NK) cells against residual leukemia blasts. This phenomenon was discovered according to the observations of a decreased risk of relapse in allogeneic graft recipients compared to patients after syngeneic HSCT or those who received T-depleted grafts to reduce the risk of graft-versus-host-disease (GvHD) [15].

Understanding the impact on immune response against malignant cells was a trigger to further investigations that enabled a better understanding of mechanisms of how leukemia cells manage to evade immune surveillance. This study has laid the foundation for novel approaches using immune interventions. Immunotherapy approaches are mostly investigated in the context of HSCT. However, possible strategies are feasible also in settings which are not related to transplantation. The next chapter indicates the immunotherapeutic approaches that can be potentially implemented into the treatment regimens of acute leukemia in children (**Table 1**).

To boost the immunity	
Inhibiting excessive function of regulatory T cells	CTLA-4 inhibition: Iipilimumab
	PD-1 inhibition: Nivolumab
To enhance the cytotoxic effect	
Using T cells, NK cells, and dendritic cells	Allogeneic HSCT
	Donor lymphocyte infusion (DLI)
	CAR-T cell therapy
	Transfer of allogeneic NK cells
	CAR-engineered NK cell therapy
	Dendritic cell (DC) vaccines

To bridge the tumor cell to the killer	
Monoclonal antibodies	Anti-CD20: Rituximab, Ofatumumab
	Anti-CD22: Epratuzumab
	anti-CD52: Alemtuzumab
	anti-CD33: Lintuzumab
Monoclonal antibodies conjugated to cytotoxic compounds	Anti-CD22 linked to calicheamicin: Inotuzumab ozogamicin
	Anti-CD33 linked to calicheamicin: Gemtuzumab ozogamicin
Bispecific T-cell engagers (BiTEs)	Blinatumomab, anti-CD3, and -CD19

Table 1. Immunotherapeutic strategies in acute leukemia.

1.3. To boost the immunity: potential therapies inhibiting excessive function of regulatory T cells

Regulatory T cells' (T reg, CD4+, CD25+) major role is to control immune tolerance. They are crucial to maintain unresponsiveness against self-antigens, but also to prevent autoimmune diseases and allogeneic graft rejection. In terms of their role in hematological malignancies, they may suppress the anticancer effect mediated by activated T cells. As a consequence of tumor activity, their immunosuppressive effect on T cells may be aggravated compared to healthy individuals (**Figure 1**). Studies show that high plasma and tissue T regs level at the moment of diagnosis correlate with a worse response to chemotherapy and prognosis [16].

One of the mechanisms that leukemia cells tend to interfere T regs function is **overexpression of the FOXP3 gene** and high levels of Foxp3 mRNA, which is considered to be essential for their inhibitory effect. This phenomenon was described in particular subtypes of AML [17], but there are a few reports of Foxp3 overexpression and T regs activity in ALL. However, it

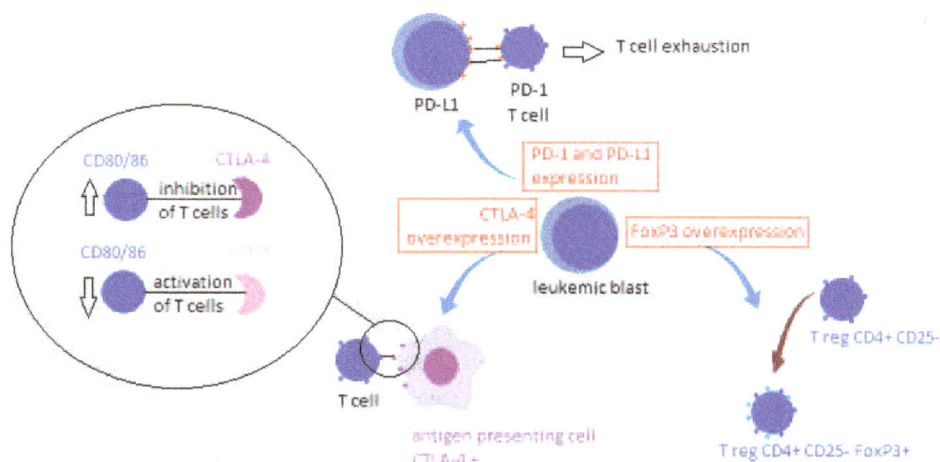

Figure 1. Immune surveillance evasion of leukemic blasts by promoting T regs–inhibitory function.

has been described that B-ALL patients' T regs presented higher immunosuppression than T reg cells from normal healthy individuals. What is more, chemotherapy corresponded to the reduction of Foxp3 and interleukin-10 expression which is also a mediator of cytotoxic T cells suppression [18, 19].

Another way to support inhibitory T regs function mediated by leukemic blasts is the expression of **cytotoxic T-lymphocyte–associated antigen 4 (CTLA-4)** on T cells and the surface of leukemia cells. CTLA-4 binds the ligands which are essential for early T cell activation (CD80 and CD86) and as a result it inhibits T cell activation and increases inhibitory cytokine production by T regs. It has been proved that the higher levels of soluble CTLA-4 and CD86 in B-ALL patients worsen the prognosis and should be considered as potential high-risk factors [20, 21]. Inhibition of CTLA-4 by specific antibody ipilimumab was not yet investigated in acute leukemia in children, but there are ongoing clinical trials assessing its potential in small groups of adults with acute myeloid leukemia, relapsed after allo-HSCT showing promising regression of malignancy, but also immune-related adverse events connected with drug infusion [22–24].

Programmed cell death protein 1 (PD-1) high expression on activated immune system cells and **Programmed cell death ligand 1 (PD-L1)** on blasts due to the tumor influence are mechanisms for leukemia evasion from an immune attack. This molecule induces T cell tolerance by direct inhibition of activated T cells and enhancement of T regs–inhibitory function in myeloid malignancies. Exhausted T cells are no longer capable to produce the cytokines: interleukin 2 (IL-2), tumor necrosis factor-α (TNF-α), and interferon-γ (IFN-γ), which impair their cytotoxic effect. This is also the signal to induce the apoptosis of activated T cells. Overexpression of PD-1 is associated with leukemia relapse after hematopoietic stem cell transplantation [25]. Using PD-1 is being investigated as its inhibition (nivolumab) may have the potential to break immune tolerance to AML cells. It may also enhance the cytotoxic effect of donor-derived cytotoxic T cells [26–28].

1.4. To enhance the cytotoxic effect: potential therapies are promoting innate or using adoptive T cells, NK cells, and dendritic cells

Donor lymphocyte infusion is the basic method of the relapse treatment and prevention after allogeneic HSCT mediated through the GvL effect. Its major complication was the high risk of graft-versus-host-disease, which is associated with a donor lymphocyte reaction against host antigens [29]. Its efficacy is nonetheless assessed as disappointing. A major obstacle is tumor-mediated evasion from the immune surveillance by downregulating surface antigens and costimulatory molecules (CD80 and CD86). As a result, T cells are not appropriately activated in vivo to induce an antitumor response. To improve the efficacy of DLI, multiple methods have been used: costimulation with CD3/CD28 and activation ex vivo [30], enrichment of donor T cells with leukemia-specific antigens (WT1) [31] or tumor-specific and host-restricted minor histocompatibility complex antigens [29, 32].

The DLI and GvL effect were the foundation to search for modified approaches to avoid side effects and use the potential T cells against leukemia. The next step was using **genetically modified and activated autologous T cells** to target tumor-specific antigens. The major advantage of this approach is eliminating the risk of GvHD.

At first, genetic modifying was based on **transferring α/β heterodimer of T-cell receptors (TCRs)** to the autologous T cells, but the limitation was the fact that the TCR receptor was only able to recognize antigens presented by human leukocyte antigen (HLA) molecules, which can be downregulated on the tumor cells avoiding immune surveillance. The next idea was to **transfer chimeric antigen receptors (CARs)** instead that are composed of a single-chain-variable fragment (scFv) antibody, which is specific for tumor antigens. CARs have an ability to recognize and fight the cells presenting any specific antigen without HLA molecules. The engineered cells express antigen receptors against tumor-associated surface antigens, thus redirecting the effector cells and enhancing tumor-specific immunosurveillance [33].

CAR-T cell therapy is now being actively investigated in refractory or relapsed ALL in adults and children. At the moment, majority of patients benefit from this approach having achieved remission when the disease appears to be incurable in terms of using standard chemotherapy. Side effects are mostly immune-related and reversible. The studies were carried out on small groups of patients, and the results are now to be confirmed in the larger multicenter trials [34, 35].

The potential limitation that make a CAR-T therapy ineffective in some groups of patients is the lack of the antigens that would be specific only for leukemia cells and their ability to downregulate the antigens by the neoplastic cells, but also unsatisfactory persistence of CAR-T cells after an adoptive transfer and predominance of an immunosuppressive microenvironment, which is a result of leukemia and the host immune system interactions [36].

One of the major challenges in terms of defining the ideal CAR-T target antigen is identifying a leukemia-specific molecule, expressed primarily, if not exclusively on the neoplastic cells, absent on their normal hematopoietic counterpart. This is an important field of research in terms of immunotherapy efficacy improvement [37]. The antigen that is commonly used as a target against B-linear blasts is CD19; however, this molecule is not a specific one. Another target that is being currently evaluated in a context of CAR-T therapy in ALL is **CD22**. Targeting CD22 turned out to be effective in vitro and is currently investigated in vivo, but its expression is still not limited to leukemia cells as this antigen is naturally presented by HLA class I on dendritic cells (DCs) and macrophages [38, 39]. In AML, **CD33** is one of the most popular among various antigens that are being investigated. However, it is highly expressed on both leukemic cells and their normal hematopoietic counterpart which explains the severe toxicity of immunotherapy targeting CD33 established in the clinical trials [40]. **CD123** molecule has emerged as more specific for AML blasts as it is expressed at low levels by normal progenitor cells, which makes it more applicable [41]. There is no defined target that could be addressed in the treatment of T-linear ALL, which has a worse prognosis in the pediatric population compared to the B-linear analog.

Further investigations led to multiple improvements of the method, like producing NK CAR cells as an alternative to T cells [42, 43], enhancing cytotoxicity of CAR-T cells by the addition of costimulatory molecules (second and third generation) or by adding chemokine receptors to enable the effective infiltration to the tumor site. For example, the expression of CD40 ligand by genetically modified T cells leads to increased proliferation and secretion of proinflammatory TH1 cytokines, but also enhances the immunogenicity of tumor cells by upregulation of costimulatory molecules (CD80 and CD86), adhesion molecules (CD54, CD58, and CD70), and human leukocyte antigen molecules on their surface. Improved survival was confirmed on a model with mice [44]. In terms of managing cytokine release syndrome, the researchers work on the antibody-based switches to mediate the interaction between the CAR-T cell and target cells to improve the safety of therapy [45].

In terms of using NK cells in the treatment of leukemia, a possible strategy is using **adoptive transfer of allogeneic NK cells** or **genetically modified autologous NK cells** (CAR-engineered NK cells). Supremacy of NK cells over T cells is connected with its lower potential to cause GvHD while being donor-derived [46, 47]. The limitation in using autologous NK cells is the overexpression of killer immunoglobulin-like receptors (KIRs) on target cells which counteract the activation of the NK cells and tumor lysis. To overcome this problem, it is more accurate to use allogeneic NK cells, but it is also important to examine the donor and recipient in terms of incompatibility of the KIR ligand (which is presented with HLA-Bw4 and HLA-C) [48]. Only mismatched donor's NK cells would be effective in the treatment of residual disease. The efficacy of using adoptive immunotherapy with NK cells is being examined in AML patients who are not eligible for stem cell transplantation. The results indicate that this approach can help to sustain the remission in patients with AML, but its efficacy is limited in active disease and it was only examined in a small group of elderly patients [46]. There are no reports in applying the therapy in patients with ALL.

Eliciting the T cells immunity can also be performed by using **dendritic cell vaccines**, which are modified to present antigens that are characteristic for leukemia blasts. This way, cytotoxic T cells are activated to kill tumor cells overcoming the mechanisms of evading immune surveillance, like downregulating of surface antigens and then T regs function enhancement are present. DCs can be autologous or allogeneic, but the HLA restriction is essential for the second option. The specific antigen that has been used so far is **Wilms' Tumor-1 (WT1)**, which is a characteristic for myeloblasts, especially in relapse, but it is also detectable in some patients with ALL and different solid tumors. This approach was assessed as effective in several patients with posttransplant-relapsed AML or ALL. The GvHD was assessed as mild and no serious adverse events were reported [49–51]. Ongoing clinical trials are developed to assess WT1 dendritic cell vaccines in larger groups of patients.

1.5. To bridge the tumor cell to the killer

Antigens expressed on leukemic blasts can also be utilized as a target for specific antibodies. Hematological malignancies express surface molecules that are accessible in the circulation. Epitopes presented exclusively on leukemic cells would be preferential for the antibody therapy. However, identifying unique ones, characteristic only for the neoplastic cells and not for their normal hematopoietic counterparts, is challenging. There are several mechanisms that can be used to eliminate blasts including internalization of toxins or drugs that are conjugated to the antibodies, antibody-dependent cellular toxicity (ADCC), complement-dependent cytotoxicity (CDC), induction of apoptosis, and direct-engaging endogenous T cells at the leukemic cells surroundings. Antigens that are candidates for antibody therapy in ALL are mostly characteristic for B-linear differentiation, like CD19, CD20, and CD22, but it is necessary to look for the targets not only presented on B-linear blasts, like CD52. Epitope that is targeted in AML is CD33 [52].

Monoclonal antibodies (MoAbs) are capable of eliminating blasts not only by promoting cytotoxic or complement-dependent cell lysis but also by blocking the effects that are advantageous for neoplastic cells, mediated by growth signals and various agonists. They are selective to the targeted molecules so that the treatment-related toxicity can be reduced. Also, the treatment response can be improved by using monoclonal antibodies as they sensitize leukemic blasts to the conventional chemotherapy. Their efficacy is generally limited when employed as a single agent, but in combination with the standard regimens they improve the overall survival even in chemoresistant or posttransplantation-relapsed patients [53, 54].

CD20 was the first epitope that was successfully applied in the therapy of hematological malignancies. **Rituximab** is a chimeric monoclonal antibody, approved in 1997 by the Food and Drug Administration (FDA) in the treatment of non-Hodgkin's lymphoma and chronic lymphocytic leukemia, but its efficacy is also being assessed in combination with chemotherapy in adults with B-cell acute lymphoblastic leukemia. In several studies, targeting CD20 was related to obtaining a prominent improvement of chemotherapy results in the Philadelphia chromosome-negative BCP-ALL [55–57]. **Ofatumumab** is also developed to target CD20; however, its binding site is closer to the cell membrane and with greater avidity than rituximab. This **second-generation anti-CD20** monoclonal antibody is considered to be more effective, even in patients who did not benefit from rituximab. Unconjugated monoclonal antibody that targets **CD22** is called **epratuzumab**. Treatment with epratuzumab was assessed in combination with conventional chemotherapy showing its feasibility in children with relapsed CD22-positive ALL. In several clinical trials, majority of patients achieved early responses [58, 59].

Alemtuzumab is a humanized monoclonal antibody against **CD52**. CD52 is expressed in about 50% of leukemia blasts, including B- and notably in T-ALL and AML. It was assessed in small groups of patients in combination with granulocyte-colony-stimulating factor (G-CSF) to boost antibody-dependent cell cytotoxicity mediated by neutrophils showing transient good responses [60]. One of the promising monoclonal antibodies that can be potentially used in AML is anti-**CD33, lintuzumab** [61, 62]. Clinical trials revealed high efficacy in the reduction of leukemic blasts, but remissions were only reported after effective cytoreduction, not in patients with high tumor burden [63].

To improve leukemic-targeted toxicity, we can also take one step further. If a target is known to internalize on binding, it is effective to use **monoclonal antibodies conjugated to cytotoxic compounds**, producing an additional mechanism for cytotoxicity. For example, CD22 is proven to be internalized on antibody binding. **Inotuzumab ozogamicin** is the antibody targeting **CD22 linked to calicheamicin** that showed improvement over chemotherapy including complete hematologic remission, longer progression-free, and overall survival [64, 65]. The analog that could have been potentially used in AML is **gemtuzumab ozogamicin**, targeting **CD33**. However, according to its toxicity and increased risk of veno-occlusive disease (VOD), it has been withdrawn in 2010. Another approach using antibody-dependent mechanisms of tumor cell lysis is using **immunotoxins**, which are recombinant anti-CD22 or anti-CD19 conjugated with Pseudomonas or Diphtheria endotoxins. **Radioimmunoconjugates** are monoclonal antibodies linked to radioactive isotopes that can be beneficial as the part of hematopoietic stem cell transplantation regimens, but they are non-preferential to be used in children.

Bispecific T-cell engagers (BiTEs) are designed to redirect and activate cytotoxic T cells precisely at the site of a tumor. The idea is to create antibody-based constructs that temporarily bridge T-cells and cancer cells. The most popular and widely investigated bispecific antibody, **Blinatumomab, targets CD3 and CD19.** Based on multiple clinical studies that have shown an achievement of durable complete remission and acceptable safety profile, the FDA granted accelerated approval for blinatumomab for the treatment of Philadelphia chromosome-negative relapsed or refractory B-cell precursor acute lymphoblastic leukemia in 2014 [66–68]. AML treatment requires using BiTEs that are compatible to antigens on myeloblasts. **AMG 330** is designed to target **CD33 and CD3.** Clinical studies indicate that this approach is efficient in relapsed AML, especially when combined with blockade of the PD-1/PD-L1 [26].

2. Conclusions

In the era of discovering new approaches to improve survival in childhood hematological malignancies, immunotherapy has a strong position. Potential benefits that can be achieved by implementation of highly active targeted therapies in pediatric acute leukemia are numerous. Improved overall survival and event-free survival is the major advantage, but the possibility to reduce treatment-related toxicity is also extremely important for improving the convalescent's quality of life. Treatment strategies are now actively investigated in multiple clinical trials, mostly in adults, but also in the pediatric population and the results are promising. However, they can be evaluated only in situations when there are no longer better treatment strategies present in refractory or relapsed leukemia, which means that their efficacy is being assessed in desperate settings with high blasts burden and more aggressive neoplastic cells mutated according to the previous treatment [69]. It would be important to evaluate the role of immunotherapy combined with frontline regimens, whether this approach optimizes the treatment efficacy. For example, remission induction is the phase of impaired T regs number and function, which indicates that it is potentially beneficial to combine the T regs depletion with cytoreduction. What is more, it has been proven that the combination of different immunotherapeutic strategies has the synergistic effect. T regs depletion with CAR-T or bispecific antibodies straightens the efficacy of T cells cytotoxicity [26, 62].

There are still many challenges and difficulties to overcome to make the treatment of childhood acute leukemia more effective and safe. Apart from numerous studies that provide a better understanding of the biology and genetics of leukemia, the impact of immunological processes that influence the treatment response was underestimated for a couple of years. Significant breakthroughs achieved in immunotherapy that improved survival in patients with the most resistant disease triggered a renewed interest in this field of treatment. Immunotherapeutic strategies are being constantly improved using the advances of engineering techniques and a better understanding of immunological mechanisms that play a role in tumor surveillance. The assortment is impressive at the moment and is getting even wider, but it appears that in everyday clinical practice the opportunities are not adequately utilized.

Author details

Monika Barełkowska* and Katarzyna Derwich

*Address all correspondence to: monika.barelkowska@gmail.com

Department of Pediatric Oncology, Hematology and Transplantology, Poznan University of Medical Sciences, Poznan, Poland

References

[1] National Cancer Institute. SEER Cancer Statistics Review 1975-2010. [Internet]. Updated June 14, 2013. Available from: https://seer.cancer.gov/archive/csr/1975_2010/results_merged/sect_28_childhood_cancer.pdf [Accessed: February 13, 2017]

[2] Creutzig U, van den Heuvel-Eibrink MM, Gibson B, Dworzak MN, Adachi S, de Bont E, et al. Diagnosis and management of acute myeloid leukemia in children and adolescents: Recommendations from an international expert panel. Blood. 2012;**120**(16):3187-3205. DOI: 10.1007/s12254-012-0061-9

[3] Adamson PC. Improving the outcome for children with cancer: Development of targeted new agents. CA Cancer Journal for Clinicians. 2015;**65**(3):212-220. DOI: 10.3322/caac.21273

[4] Gorman MF, Ji L, Ko RH, Barnette P, Bostrom B, Hutchinson R, Raetz E, Seibel NL, Twist CJ, Eckroth E, Sposto R, Gaynon PS, Loh ML. Outcome for children treated for relapsed or refractory acute myelogenous leukemia (rAML): A therapeutic advances in childhood leukemia (TACL) consortium study. Pediatric Blood & Cancer. 2010;**55**(3):421-429. DOI: 10.1002/pbc.22612

[5] Ceppi F, Duval M, Leclerc JM, Laverdiere C, Delva YL, Cellot S, Teira P, Bittencourt H. Improvement of the outcome of relapsed or refractory acute lymphoblastic leukemia in children using a risk-based treatment strategy. PLoS One. 2016;**11**(9): e0160310. DOI: 10.1371/journal.pone.0160310

[6] Ko RH, Ji L, Barnette P, Bostrom B, Hutchinson R, Raetz E, Seibel NL, Twist CJ, Eckroth E, Sposto R, Gaynon PS, Loh ML. Outcome of patients treated for relapsed or refractory acute lymphoblastic leukemia: A therapeutic advances in childhood leukemia consortium study. Journal of Clinical Oncology. 2010;**28**(4):648-654. DOI: 10.1200/JCO.2009.22.2950

[7] Krawczuk-Rybak M, Panasiuk A, Muszyńska-Rosłan K, Stachowicz-Stencel T, Drożyńska E, Balcerska A, Pobudejska A, et al. Health status of Polish children and adolescents after ending of anticancer treatment. (Stan zdrowia polskich dzieci i młodzieży po zakończonym leczeniu przeciwnowotworowym). Polish Oncology (Onkologia Polska). 2012;**15**(3):96-102

[8]   International BFM Study Group. Registry ALL IC-BFM 2009 – final version of the therapy protocol from August 14, 2009

[9]   AML-BFM Study Group. Registry AML-BFM 2012. English version no. 1 from July 1, 2012

[10] Schrauder A, Reiter A, Gadner H, Niethammer D, Klingebiel T, Kremens B, et al. Superiority of allogeneic hematopoietic stem-cell transplantation compared with chemotherapy alone in high-risk childhood T-cell acute lymphoblastic leukemia: Results from ALL-BFM 90 and 95. Journal of Clinical Oncology. 2006;**24**(36):5742-5749. DOI:10.1200/JCO.2006.06.2679

[11] Balduzzi A, Valsecchi MG, Uderzo C, De Lorenzo P, Klingebiel T, Peters C, et al. Chemotherapy versus allogeneic transplantation for very-high-risk childhood acute lymphoblastic leukaemia in first complete remission: Comparison by genetic randomisation in an international prospective study. Lancet. 2005;**366**(9486):635-6342. DOI: 10.1016/S0140-6736(05)66998-X

[12] Taskinen M, Oskarsson T, Levinsen M, Bottai M, Hellebostad M, Jonsson OG, et al. The effect of central nervous system involvement and irradiation in childhood acute lymphoblastic leukemia: Lessons from the NOPHO ALL-92 and ALL-2000 protocols. Pediatric Blood & Cancer. 2017;**64**(2):242-249. DOI: 10.1002/pbc.26191

[13] Prucker C, Attarbaschi A, Peters C, Dworzak MN, Pötschger U, Urban C, et al. Induction death and treatment-related mortality in first remission of children with acute lymphoblastic leukemia: A population-based analysis of the Austrian Berlin-Frankfurt-Münster study group. Leukemia. 2009;**23**(7):1264-1269. DOI: 10.1038/leu.2009.12

[14] Behl D, Porrata LF, Markovic SN, Letendre L, Pruthi RK, Hook CC, et al. Absolute lymphocyte count recovery after induction chemotherapy predicts superior survival in acute myelogenous leukemia. Leukemia. 2006;**20**(1):29-34. DOI: 10.1038/sj.leu.2404032

[15] Weiden PL, Flournoy N, Thomas ED, Prentice R, Fefer A, Buckner CD, et al. Antileukemic effect of graft-versus-host disease in human recipients of allogeneic-marrow grafts. The New England Journal of Medicine. 1979;**300**(19):1068-1073. DOI: 10.1056/NEJM197905103001902

[16] Szczepanski MJ, Szajnik M, Czystowska M, Mandapathil M, Strauss L, Welsh A, et al. Increased frequency and suppression by regulatory T cells in patients with acute myelogenous leukemia. Clinical Cancer Research. 2009;**15**(10):3325-3332. DOI: 10.1158/1078-0432.CCR-08-3010

[17] Assem M, Osman A, Kandeel E, Elshimy R, Nassar H, Ali R. Clinical impact of overexpression of FOXP3 and WT1 on disease outcome in Egyptian acute myeloid leukemia patients. Asian Pacific Journal of Cancer Prevention. 2016;**17**(10):4699-4711. DOI: 10.22034/APJCP.2016.17.10.4699

[18] Bhattacharya K, Chandra S, Mandal C. Critical stoichiometric ratio of CD4(+) CD25(+) FoxP3(+) regulatory T cells and CD4(+) CD25(-) responder T cells influence

immunosuppression in patients with B-cell acute lymphoblastic leukaemia. Immunology. 2014;**142**(1):124-139. DOI: 10.1111/imm.12237

[19] Luo X, Tan H, Zhou Y, Xiao T, Wang C, Li Y. Notch1 signaling is involved in regulating Foxp3 expression in T-ALL. Cancer Cell International. 2013;**13**(1):34. DOI: 10.1186/1475-2867-13-34

[20] Mansour A, Elkhodary T, Darwish A, Mabed M. Increased expression of costimulatory molecules CD86 and sCTLA-4 in patients with acute lymphoblastic leukemia. Leukemia & Lymphoma. 2014;**55**(9):2120-214. DOI: 10.3109/10428194.2013.869328

[21] Hui L, Lei Z, Peng Z, Ruobing S, Fenghua Z. Polymorphism analysis of CTLA-4 in childhood acute lymphoblastic leukemia. Pakistan Journal of Pharmaceutical Science. 2014 Jul;**27**(4 Suppl):1005-1013

[22] Bashey A, Medina B, Corringham S, Pasek M, Carrier E, Vrooman L, et al. CTLA4 blockade with ipilimumab to treat relapse of malignancy after allogeneic hematopoietic cell transplantation. Blood. 2009;**113**(7):1581-1588. DOI: 10.1182/blood-2008-07-168468

[23] Slavin S, Moss RW, Bakacs T. Control of minimal residual cancer by low dose ipilimumab activating autologous anti-tumor immunity. Pharmacological Research. 2014;**79**:9-12. DOI: 10.1016/j.phrs.2013.10.004

[24] Davids MS, Kim HT, Bachireddy P, Costello C, Liguori R, Savell A, et al. Ipilimumab for patients with relapse after allogeneic transplantation. The New England Journal of Medicine. 2016;**375**(2):143-153. DOI: 10.1056/NEJMoa1601202

[25] Kong Y, Zhang J, Claxton DF, Ehmann WC, Rybka WB, Zhu L, et al. PD-1(hi)TIM-3(+) T cells associate with and predict leukemia relapse in AML patients post allogeneic stem cell transplantation. Blood Cancer Journal. 2015;**5**:e330. DOI: 10.1038/bcj.2015.58

[26] Choi DC, Tremblay D, Iancu-Rubin C, Mascarenhas J. Programmed cell death-1 pathway inhibition in myeloid malignancies: Implications for myeloproliferative neoplasms. Annals in Hematology. 2017;**96**(6):919-927. DOI: 10.1007/s00277-016-2915-4

[27] Zou W. Immunosuppressive networks in the tumor environment and their therapeutic relevance. Nature Review Cancer. 2005;**5**(4):263-274. DOI: 10.1038/nrc1586

[28] Krupka C, Kufer P, Kischel R, Zugmaier G, Lichtenegger FS, Köhnke T, et al. Blockade of the PD-1/PD-L1 axis augments lysis of AML cells by the CD33/CD3 BiTE antibody construct AMG 330: Reversing a T-cell-induced immune escape mechanism. Leukemia. 2016;**30**(2):484-491. DOI: 10.1038/leu.2015.214

[29] Stamouli M, Gkirkas K, Tsirigotis P. Strategies for improving the efficacy of donor lymphocyte infusion following stem cell transplantation. Immunotherapy. 2016;**8**(1):57-68. DOI: 10.2217/imt.15.100

[30] Porter DL, Levine BL, Bunin N, Stadtmauer EA, Luger SM, Goldstein S, et al. A phase 1 trial of donor lymphocyte infusions expanded and activated ex vivo via CD3/CD28 costimulation. Blood. 2006;**107**(4):1325-1331. DOI: 10.1182/blood-2005-08-3373

[31] Rezvani K, Yong AS, Savani BN, Mielke S, Keyvanfar K, Gostick E, et al. Graft-versus-leukemia effects associated with detectable Wilms tumor-1 specific T lymphocytes after allogeneic stem-cell transplantation for acute lymphoblastic leukemia. Blood. 2007;**110**(6):1924-1932. DOI: 10.1182/blood-2007-03-076844

[32] Warren EH, Greenberg PD, Riddell SR. Cytotoxic T-lymphocyte-defined human minor histocompatibility antigens with a restricted tissue distribution. Blood. 1998;**91**(6): 2197-2207

[33] Davila ML, Brentjens RJ. CD19-Targeted CAR T cells as novel cancer immunotherapy for relapsed or refractory B-cell acute lymphoblastic leukemia. Clinical Advances in Hematology & Oncology. 2016;**14**(10):802-808

[34] Maude SL, Frey N, Shaw PA, Aplenc R, Barrett DM, Bunin NJ, et al. Chimeric antigen receptor T cells for sustained remissions in leukemia. New England Journal of Medicine. 2014;**371**(16):1507-1517. DOI: 10.1056/NEJMoa1407222

[35] Lee DW, Kochenderfer JN, Stetler-Stevenson M, Cui YK, Delbrook C, Feldman SA, et al. T cells expressing CD19 chimeric antigen receptors for acute lymphoblastic leukaemia in children and young adults: A phase 1 dose-escalation trial. Lancet. 2015;**385**(9967):517-528. DOI: 10.1016/S0140-6736(14)61403-3

[36] Zhang E, Hanmei Xu. A new insight in chimeric antigen receptor-engineered T cells for cancer immunotherapy. Journal of Hematology & Oncology. 2017;**10**:1. DOI: 10.1186/s13045-016-0379-6

[37] Orentas RJ, Nordlund J, He J, Sindiri S, Mackall C, Fry TJ, et al. Bioinformatic description of immunotherapy targets for pediatric T-cell leukemia and the impact of normal gene sets used for comparison. Frontiers in Oncology. 2014;**4**:134. DOI: 10.3389/fonc.2014.00134

[38] American Association for Cancer Research [no authors listed] Anti-CD22 CAR therapy leads to ALL remissions. Cancer Discovery. 2017;**7**(2):120. DOI: 10.1158/2159-8290. CD-NB2017-001

[39] Jahn L, Hagedoorn RS, van der Steen DM, Hombrink P, Kester MG, Schoonakker MP, et al. A CD22-reactive TCR from the T-cell allorepertoire for the treatment of acute lymphoblastic leukemia by TCR gene transfer. Oncotarget. 2016;**7**(44):71536-71547. DOI: 10.18632/oncotarget.12247

[40] Wang QS, Wang Y, Lv HY, Han QW, Fan H, Guo B, et al. Treatment of CD33-directed chimeric antigen receptor-modified T cells in one patient with relapsed and refractory acute myeloid leukemia. Molecular Therapy. 2015;**23**(1):184-191. DOI: 10.1038/mt.2014.164

[41] Tettamanti S, Biondi A, Biagi E, Bonnet D. CD123 AML targeting by chimeric antigen receptors: A novel magic bullet for AML therapeutics? Oncoimmunology. 2014;**3**:e28835. DOI: 10.4161/onci.28835

[42] Romanski A, Uherek C, Bug G, Seifried E, Klingemann H, Wels WS, et al. CD19-CAR engineered NK-92 cells are sufficient to overcome NK cell resistance in B-cell malignancies. Journal of Cell & Molecular Medicine. 2016;20(7):1287-1294. DOI: 10.1111/jcmm.12810

[43] Glienke W, Esser R, Priesner C, Suerth JD, Schambach A, Wels WS, et al. Advantages and applications of CAR-expressing natural killer cells. Frontiers in Pharmacology. 2015;6:21. DOI: 10.3389/fphar.2015.00021

[44] Curran KJ, Seinstra BA, Nikhamin Y, Yeh R, Usachenko Y, van Leeuwen DG, et al. Enhancing antitumor efficacy of chimeric antigen receptor T cells through constitutive CD40L expression. Molecular Therapy. 2015;23(4):769-778. DOI: 10.1038/mt.2015.4

[45] Rodgers DT, Mazagova M, Hampton EN, Cao Y, Ramadoss NS, Hardy IR, et al. Switch-mediated activation and retargeting of CAR-T cells for B-cell malignancies. Proceedings of the National Academy of Science United States of America. 2016;113(4):E459-E468. DOI: 10.1073/pnas.1524155113

[46] Curti A, Ruggeri L, D'Addio A, Bontadini A, Dan E, Motta MR, et al. Successful transfer of alloreactive haploidentical KIR ligand-mismatched natural killer cells after infusion in elderly high risk acute myeloid leukemia patients. Blood. 2011;118(12):3273-3279. DOI: 10.1182/blood-2011-01-329508

[47] Ruggeri L, Capanni M, Urbani E, Perruccio K, Shlomchik WD, Tosti A, et al. Effectiveness of donor natural killer cell alloreactivity in mismatched hematopoietic transplants. Science. 2002;295(5562):2097-2100. DOI: 10.1126/science.1068440

[48] Norell H, Moretta A, Silva-Santos B, Moretta L. At the Bench: Preclinical rationale for exploiting NK cells and γδ T lymphocytes for the treatment of high-risk leukemias. Journal of Leukocyte Biology. 2013;94(6):1123-1139. DOI: 10.1189/jlb.0613312

[49] Saito S, Yanagisawa R, Yoshikawa K, Higuchi Y, Koya T, Yoshizawa K, et al. Safety and tolerability of allogeneic dendritic cell vaccination with induction of Wilms tumor 1-specific T cells in a pediatric donor and pediatric patient with relapsed leukemia: A case report and review of the literature. Cytotherapy. 2015;17(3):330-335. DOI: 10.1016/j.jcyt.2014.10.003

[50] De Haar C, Plantinga M, Blokland NJ, van Til NP, Flinsenberg TW, Van Tendeloo VF, et al. Generation of a cord blood-derived Wilms Tumor 1 dendritic cell vaccine for AML patients treated with allogeneic cord blood transplantation. Oncoimmunology. 2015;4(11):e1023973. DOI: 10.1080/2162402X.2015.1023973

[51] Seledtsov VI, Goncharov AG, Seledtsova GV. Clinically feasible approaches to potentiating cancer cell-based immunotherapies. Human Vaccines & Immunotherapy. 2015;11(4):851-869. DOI: 10.1080/21645515.2015.1009814

[52] Papadantonakis N, Advani AS. Recent advances and novel treatment paradigms in acute lymphocytic leukemia. Therapy Advances in Hematology. 2016;7(5):252-269. DOI: 10.1177/2040620716652289

[53] Maino E, Bonifacio M, Scattolin AM, Bassan R. Immunotherapy approaches to treat adult acute lymphoblastic leukemia. Expert Review in Hematology. 2016;9(6):563-577. DOI: 10.1586/17474086.2016.1170593

[54] Jabbour E, O'Brien S, Ravandi F, Kantarjian H. Monoclonal antibodies in acute lymphoblastic leukemia. Blood. 2015;125(26):4010-4016. DOI: 10.1182/blood-2014-08-596403

[55] Loeff FC, van Egmond HM, Nijmeijer BA, Falkenburg JH, Halkes CJ, Jedema I. Complement-dependent cytotoxicity induced by therapeutic antibodies in B-cell acute lymphoblastic leukemia is dictated by target antigen expression levels and augmented by loss of membrane-bound complement inhibitors. Leukemia & Lymphoma. 2017(1):1-14.

[56] Huguet F, Tavitian S. Emerging biological therapies to treat acute lymphoblastic leukemia. Expert Opinion on Emerging Drugs. 2017;22(1):107-121. DOI: 10.1080/1472 8214.2016.1257606

[57] Maury S, Chevret S, Thomas X, Heim D, Leguay T, Huguet F, et al. Rituximab in B-lineage adult acute lymphoblastic leukemia. The New England Journal of Medicine. 2016;375(11):1044-1053. DOI: 10.1056/NEJMoa1605085

[58] Raetz EA, Cairo MS, Borowitz MJ, Blaney SM, Krailo MD, Leil TA, et al. Chemoimmunotherapy reinduction with epratuzumab in children with acute lymphoblastic leukemia in marrow relapse: A Children's Oncology Group Pilot Study. Journal of Clinical Oncology. 2008;26(22):3756-3762. DOI: 10.1200/JCO.2007.15.3528

[59] Chevallier P, Chantepie S, Huguet F, Raffoux E, Thomas X, Leguay T, et al. Hyper-CVAD + epratuzumab as salvage regimen for younger patients with relapsed/refractory CD22+ precursor B-cell ALL. Haematologica. 2017;102(5):e184-e186. DOI: 10.3324/haematol.2016.159905

[60] Gorin NC, Isnard F, Garderet L, Ikhlef S, Corm S, Quesnel B, Legrand O, Cachanado M, Rousseau A, Laporte JP. Administration of alemtuzumab and G-CSF to adults with relapsed or refractory acute lymphoblastic leukemia: Results of a phase II study. European Journal of Haematology. 2013;91(4):315-321. DOI: 10.1111/ejh.12154

[61] Montalban-Bravo G, Garcia-Manero G. Novel drugs for older patients with acute myeloid leukemia. Leukemia. 2015;29(4):760-769. DOI: 10.1038/leu.2014.244

[62] Jurcic JG, Rosenblat TL. Targeted alpha-particle immunotherapy for acute myeloid leukemia. American Society of Clinical Oncology Educational Book. 2014:e126-e131. DOI: 10.14694/EdBook_AM.2014.34.e126

[63] Borthakur G. Precision 're'arming of CD33 antibodies. Blood. 2013;122(8):1334. DOI: 10.1182/blood-2013-06-509638

[64] Thota S, Advani A. Inotuzumab ozogamicin in relapsed b-cell acute lymphoblastic leukemia. European Journal of Haematology. 2017;98(5):425-434. DOI:10.1111/ejh.12862

[65] Kantarjian HM, DeAngelo DJ, Stelljes M, Martinelli G, Liedtke M, Stock W, et al. Inotuzumab ozogamicin versus standard therapy for acute lymphoblastic leukemia. The New England Journal of Medicine. 2016;**375**(8):740-753. DOI: 10.1056/NEJMoa1509277

[66] Gökbuget N, Zugmaier G, Klinger M, Kufer P, Stelljes M, Viardot A, et al. Long-term relapse-free survival in a phase 2 study of blinatumomab for the treatment of patients with minimal residual disease in B-lineage acute lymphoblastic leukemia. Haematologica. 2017;**102**(4):132-135. DOI: 10.3324/haematol.2016.153957

[67] Duell J, Dittrich M, Bedke T, Mueller T, Eisele F, Rosenwald A, Rasche L, Hartmann E, Dandekar T, Einsele H, Topp MS. Frequency of regulatory T cells determines the outcome of the T cell engaging antibody blinatumomab in patients with B precursor ALL. Leukemia. Advance online publication 24 February 2017. DOI: 10.1038/leu.2017.41

[68] Bumma N, Papadantonakis N, Advani AS. Structure, development, preclinical and clinical efficacy of blinatumomab in acute lymphoblastic leukemia. Future Oncology. 2015;**11**(12):1729-1739. DOI: 10.2217/fon.15.84

[69] Ishii K, Barrett AJ. Novel immunotherapeutic approaches for the treatment of acute leukemia (myeloid and lymphoblastic). Therapeutic Advances in Hematology. 2016;**7**(1):17-39. DOI: 10.1177/2040620715616544

Permissions

All chapters in this book were first published in NPCDD&UAACDD, by InTech Open; hereby published with permission under the Creative Commons Attribution License or equivalent. Every chapter published in this book has been scrutinized by our experts. Their significance has been extensively debated. The topics covered herein carry significant findings which will fuel the growth of the discipline. They may even be implemented as practical applications or may be referred to as a beginning point for another development.

The contributors of this book come from diverse backgrounds, making this book a truly international effort. This book will bring forth new frontiers with its revolutionizing research information and detailed analysis of the nascent developments around the world.

We would like to thank all the contributing authors for lending their expertise to make the book truly unique. They have played a crucial role in the development of this book. Without their invaluable contributions this book wouldn't have been possible. They have made vital efforts to compile up to date information on the varied aspects of this subject to make this book a valuable addition to the collection of many professionals and students.

This book was conceptualized with the vision of imparting up-to-date information and advanced data in this field. To ensure the same, a matchless editorial board was set up. Every individual on the board went through rigorous rounds of assessment to prove their worth. After which they invested a large part of their time researching and compiling the most relevant data for our readers.

The editorial board has been involved in producing this book since its inception. They have spent rigorous hours researching and exploring the diverse topics which have resulted in the successful publishing of this book. They have passed on their knowledge of decades through this book. To expedite this challenging task, the publisher supported the team at every step. A small team of assistant editors was also appointed to further simplify the editing procedure and attain best results for the readers.

Apart from the editorial board, the designing team has also invested a significant amount of their time in understanding the subject and creating the most relevant covers. They scrutinized every image to scout for the most suitable representation of the subject and create an appropriate cover for the book.

The publishing team has been an ardent support to the editorial, designing and production team. Their endless efforts to recruit the best for this project, has resulted in the accomplishment of this book. They are a veteran in the field of academics and their pool of knowledge is as vast as their experience in printing. Their expertise and guidance has proved useful at every step. Their uncompromising quality standards have made this book an exceptional effort. Their encouragement from time to time has been an inspiration for everyone.

The publisher and the editorial board hope that this book will prove to be a valuable piece of knowledge for researchers, students, practitioners and scholars across the globe.

List of Contributors

Christel L. C. Seegers, Rita Setroikromo and Wim J. Quax
Department of Chemical and Pharmaceutical Biology, Groningen Research Institute of Pharmacy, University of Groningen, Groningen, The Netherlands

Wei Guo, Ning Wang and Yibin Feng
School of Chinese Medicine, Li Ka Shing Faculty of Medicine, The University of Hong Kong, China

Aurélien F.A. Moumbock
Department of Chemistry, University of Buea, Buea, Cameroon

Fidele Ntie-Kang
Department of Chemistry, University of Buea, Buea, Cameroon
Department of Pharmaceutical Chemistry, Martin-Luther University of Halle-Wittenberg, Halle, Germany

Conrad V. Simoben and Wolfgang Sippl
Department of Pharmaceutical Chemistry, Martin-Luther University of Halle-Wittenberg, Halle, Germany

Ludger Wessjohann
Leibniz Institute of Plant Biochemistry, Halle, Germany

Stefan Günther
Pharmaceutical Bioinformatics, Albert-Ludwig-University Freiburg, Freiburg, Germany

Filiz Bakar
Department of Biochemistry, Faculty of Pharmacy, Ankara University, Ankara, Turkey

Pongtip Sithisarn
Department of Pharmacognosy, Faculty of Pharmacy, Mahidol University, Bangkok, Thailand

Piyanuch Rojsanga
Department of Pharmaceutical Chemistry, Faculty of Pharmacy, Mahidol University, Bangkok, Thailand

Codruţa Şoica, Diana Antal, Florina Andrica, Roxana Băbuţa, Alina Moacă, Florina Ardelean, Roxana Ghiulai, Stefana Avram, Corina Danciu, Dorina Coricovac and Cristina Dehelean
Faculty of Pharmacy, "Victor Babeş" University of Medicine and Pharmacy, Timişoara, Romania

Virgil Păunescu
Faculty of Medicine, "Victor Babeş" University of Medicine and Pharmacy, Timişoara, Romania

Kazim Sahin, Nurhan Sahin and Cemal Orhan
Veterinary Faculty, Firat University, Elazig, Turkey

Shakir Ali
Department of Biochemistry, School of Chemical and Life Sciences, Jamia Hamdard, New Delhi, India

Omer Kucuk
Winship Cancer Institute, Emory University, Atlanta, Georgia, USA

Abdulkarim Najjar and Wolfgang Sippl
Department of Pharmaceutical Chemistry, Martin-Luther University of Halle-Wittenberg, Halle (Saale), Germany

Fidele Ntie-Kang
Department of Pharmaceutical Chemistry, Martin-Luther University of Halle-Wittenberg, Halle (Saale), Germany

Stefana Avram, Ioana Zinuca Pavel and Corina Danciu
Department of Phamacognosy, Faculty of Pharmacy, Victor Babeş University of Medicine and Pharmacy, Timisoara, Romania

Roxana Ghiulai, Marius Mioc, Roxana Babuta and Codruta Soica
Department of Pharmaceutical Chemistry, Faculty of Pharmacy, Victor Babeş University of Medicine and Pharmacy, Timisoara, Romania

Mirela Voicu
Department of Phamacology, Faculty of Pharmacy, Victor Babeş University of Medicine and Pharmacy, Timisoara, Romania

Dorina Coricovac and Cristina Dehelean
Department of Toxicology, Faculty of Pharmacy, Victor Babeş University of Medicine and Pharmacy, Timisoara, Romania

Monika Barełkowska and Katarzyna Derwich
Department of Pediatric Oncology, Hematology and Transplantology, Poznan University of Medical Sciences, Poznan, Poland

Index

www.ingramcontent.com/pod-product-compliance
Lightning Source LLC
Chambersburg PA
CBHW080250230326
41458CB00097B/4217

9 781632 418777

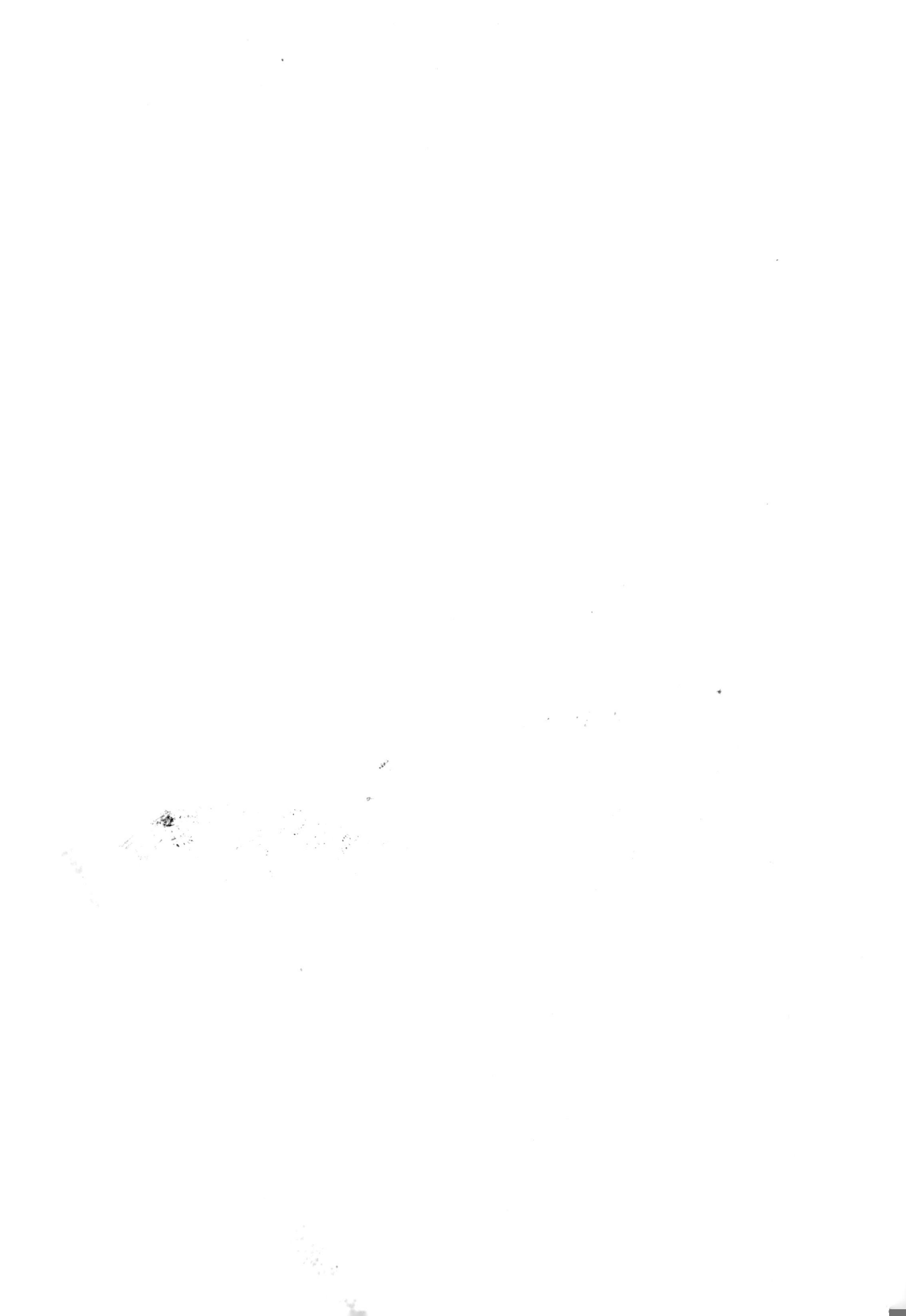